DENTAL ASSISTANT REVIEW

Course Synopses and Review Questions

SECOND EDITION

Stuart M. Hirsch, B.A., D.D.S.
Assistant Dean for Allied Health Programs
and
Chairperson and Associate Professor
Department of Operative Dentistry
New York University College of Dentistry

Michael Ostrofsky, B.S., M.S., M.S., D.D.S.
Director, Dental Auxiliary Utilization and
Dental Team Practice Program
and
Assistant Professor, Department of Operative Dentistry
New York University College of Dentistry

Edited by

Marie E. Gallagher, B.A., M.A., M.P.A.
Administrator, David B. Kriser Institute for
the Rehabilitation of Disabled Dentists
and
Instructor, Dental Assistant Training Program
New York University College of Dentistry

APPLETON & LANGE
Norwalk, Connecticut/San Mateo, California

0-668-05365-8

Copyright © 1978, 1983 by Arco Publishing, Inc.
Published by Appleton & Lange, a division of Prentice Hall.

91 92 93 94 95 / 10 9 8

Prentice Hall International (UK) Limited, *London*
Prentice Hall of Australia Pty. Limited, *Sydney*
Prentice Hall Canada, Inc., *Toronto*
Prentice Hall Hispanoamericana, S.A., *Mexico*
Prentice Hall of India Private Limited, *New Delhi*
Prentice Hall of Japan, Inc., *Tokyo*
Simon & Schuster Asia Pte. Ltd., *Singapore*
Editora Prentice Hall do Brasil Ltda., *Rio de Janeiro*
Prentice Hall, *Englewood Cliffs, New Jersey*

Library of Congress Cataloging-in-Publication Data
Hirsch, Stuart M.
    Dental assistant review.

    (Arco medical review series)
    Rev. ed. of: Dental assistants examination review.
© 1978.
    1. Dental assistants—Examinations, questions, etc.
2. Dentistry—Examinations, questions, etc. I. Ostrofsky,
Michael. II. Gallagher, Marie. III. Title. IV. Series.
RK60.5.H57   1982   617.6'0076   82-8676
ISBN 0-668-05365-8   AACR2

PRINTED IN THE UNITED STATES OF AMERICA

*TO
MARY ANN, LINDA,
DAVID, LISA, KAREN,
AND OUR FRIENDS*

Contributors

All chapters in this text are authored principally by Drs. Stuart M. Hirsch and Michael Ostrofsky and edited by Ms. Marie E. Gallagher. However, the following individuals provided invaluable contributions in their areas of expertise.

Emanuel Barouch, B.S., D.D.S.
Assistant Professor, Department of Operative Dentistry
New York University College of Dentistry
DENTAL MATERIALS

Judith L. Cleary, C.D.A., B.A., M.A.
Director, Dental Assistant Training Program
and Clinical Assistant Professor,
Department of Behavioral Science and Community Health
New York University College of Dentistry
FIRST AID

Sheilah B. Galanti, B.A., C.D.A.
Former Instructor, Dental Assistant Training Program
New York University College of Dentistry
DENTAL MATERIALS

Ilene G. Gold, R.D.H., B.A.
Coordinator, Dental Hygiene Affiliation Program
and Instructor, Dental Assistant Training Program
New York University College of Dentistry
ORAL ANATOMY AND PREVENTIVE DENTISTRY

Wayne Graber, B.A., D.D.S.
Former Instructor, Dental Assistant Training Program
New York University College of Dentistry
BIOMEDICAL SCIENCE

Eugene Hittelman, B.A., M.A., Ed.D.
Acting Chairperson and Associate Professor
Department of Behavioral Science and Community Health
and Instructor, Dental Assistant Training Program
New York University College of Dentistry
BEHAVIORAL SCIENCE

James M. Kaim, B.S., D.D.S.
Associate Professor and Director of Dental Anatomy
and Pre-Clinical Operative Dentistry,
Department of Operative Dentistry,
New York University College of Dentistry
ORAL ANATOMY

Sheryle A. Neuffer, C.D.A., A.A.S., B.S.
Instructor, Dental Assisting Training Program
New York University College of Dentistry
RADIOLOGY

Sharyn West-Samuels, C.D.A.
Former Instructor, Dental Assisting Training Program
New York University College of Dentistry
CHAIRSIDE ASSISTING

Lois Winter, B.A., M.A.
Director of Career Services, Clinical Associate Professor,
Department of Family Practice
and Instructor, Dental Assisting Training Program
New York University College of Dentistry
PRACTICE MANAGEMENT

Acknowledgment

We wish to express our sincere gratitude to Ms. Suzanne Montagne, who illustrated this book and spent countless hours in the preparation of this manuscript. Her talents and diligence are appreciated. Additionally, our appreciation is extended to Mary T. Quinones and Yvonne Martinez, who assisted in the preparation of final copy.

We also wish to thank the faculty and staff of the Dental Assistant Training Program and the Dental Auxiliary Utilization/Dental Team Practice Program at New York University College of Dentistry for their feedback and valuable assistance.

Contents

Preface

This book provides a comprehensive review of various dental subject areas. The principal purpose in preparing a text of this nature was to furnish dental assistant students with a source of information to facilitate studying for examinations, particularly The National Certification Examination. (Students should read each chapter, answer the multiple-choice questions, and then check their answers and note the explanations provided.) This text is not a course in dental assisting; it is a supplement that should be used in conjunction with course texts and study aids. Additional references are also provided in each of the subject areas.

1

Biomedical Sciences

Course Synopsis

Physical Science—Properties of Matter

Matter exists in three different states: solid, liquid, and gas. By altering temperature and pressure, most materials can be changed to any one of the three states. Temperature is a measure of the intensity of heat. The amount of heat evolved or absorbed during a chemical reaction is called the heat of reaction. If heat is evolved, or given off, the reaction is described as exothermic. If heat is absorbed, the reaction is endothermic. The setting of dental stone and acrylic exhibits exothermic reactions; caution must be exercised when using these materials intraorally, to avoid damaging the pulpal tissues and oral mucosa.

Heat is measured in either Fahrenheit or centigrade degrees. However, temperature expressed by one system can easily be converted to the other. To convert degrees Fahrenheit to centigrade (or Celsius), the following formula is used:

$$°C = 5/9 \ (°F - 32)$$

Example: Convert 68°F to degrees centigrade.

$$°C = 5/9 \ (68 - 32) = 5/9 \times 36$$
$$°C = 20°C$$

To convert degrees centigrade to Fahrenheit, the following formula is used:

$$°F = 9/5 \ °C + 32$$

Example: Convert 45°C to degrees Fahrenheit.

$$°F = 45 \times 9/5 + 32 = 81 + 32$$
$$°F = 113$$

Metric System

Most countries use the metric system of measurement, especially in scientific fields. The advantage of the metric system is that it is based on multiples of 10. The standard of length is the meter; of mass, the kilogram; and of volume, the liter.

	Fundamental Unit	Quality	Numerical Value
Length	Meter (m)	Kilometer	1000 m
		Centimeter	0.01 m
		Millimeter	0.001 m
Mass	Gram (g)	Kilogram	1000 g
		Milligram	0.001 g
		Microgram	0.000001 g
Volume	Liter (l)	Milliliter	0.001 l

Dentistry uses the metric system. The depth of cavity preparations is described in millimeters. The length of files, reamers, broaches, and other dental instruments is expressed in millimeters. Increments of grams and milligrams are employed when drugs are prescribed. When taking an alginate impression, the amount of water used is expressed in milliliters.

Cytology and Histology

Cytology is the study of cells, whereas histology is the study of the structure and arrangement of the tissues of an organism. Cytology and histology are the basic sciences that deal with the fundamental building blocks of the oral tissues. The ability to recognize different types of tissues and to differentiate between the normal and abnormal tissues enables the dentist and the assistant to treat and heal diseases of the oral cavity.

The cell is the basic unit of life, and its morphology (structure) is composed of basic units (Fig. 1).

The nucleus is the "brain" of the cell and controls all cellular functions. In short, it is the nucleus that gives out instructions that guide the life process of the cell.

Mitochondria are known as the powerhouses of the cell. They are responsible for energy production and respiration.

Lysosomes are vesicles that store many powerful digestive enzymes. They are called upon to process bulk material that enters the cell and are enclosed within a membrane to prevent the release of these enzymes and to protect the cell from self-destruction.

The endoplasmic reticulum is a system of membranes within the cell that functions to transport various cellular material. There are two types of endoplasmic reticulum: smooth endoplasmic reticulum, which functions in fat synthesis, and rough endoplasmic reticulum characterized by connected ribosomes, which function in the synthesis of protein.

The Golgi apparatus consists of groups of small membranes that function in the storage and modification of secretory products.

Centrioles are paired cylindrical structures lying adjacent to the nucleus that have a role in cell division.

Vacuoles are fluid-filled sacs that contain food products and waste material; they play a part in the fluid balance of the cell.

The cell membrane defines the shape of the cell and permits certain materials to enter and leave the cell.

Cytoplasm is the gel-like substance in which the above organelles are suspended.

Cells have three major functions: respiration, reproduction, and locomotion. The respiratory process is carried out by a series of complex chemical reactions that produce the energy necessary to support cellular function.

Cell division, known as mitosis, involves two distinct processes: division of the nucleus and division of cytoplasm. The result of mitosis is the production of a second cell that contains identical genetic materials (chromosomes) as the original cell.

Cells move by shifting the cytoplasm within the cell or by using special projecting structures known as cilia or flagella.

Genetics

Genetics is the study of heredity and patterns of transmission of a given trait (e.g., blue eyes or brown hair) from parent to offspring.

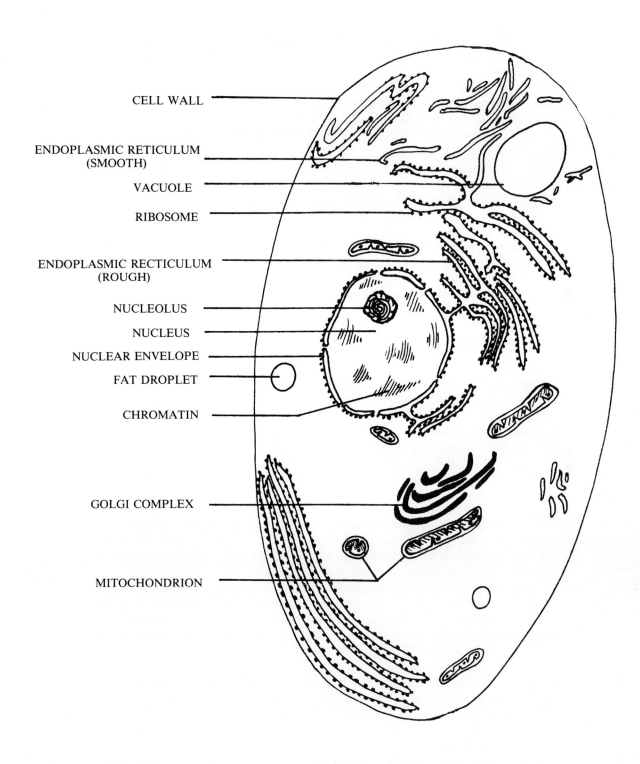

CELL WALL

ENDOPLASMIC RETICULUM
(SMOOTH)

VACUOLE

RIBOSOME

ENDOPLASMIC RECTICULUM
(ROUGH)

NUCLEOLUS

NUCLEUS

NUCLEAR ENVELOPE

FAT DROPLET

CHROMATIN

GOLGI COMPLEX

MITOCHONDRION

Fig. 1. The cell.

Chromosomes are filamentous structures in the cell nucleus along which genes are located. Genes are the basic units of heredity and are capable of self-replication.

Deoxyribonucleic acid (DNA) is the basic carrier of genetic information in the cells; it is included in every cell of the human body. The structure of DNA is described as a double helix, shaped somewhat like a twisted ladder. The structure was delineated by Watson and Crick, who postulated that the DNA molecule is self-replicating. When the two strands that form the "sides" of the ladder break apart, each strand forms a new complementary strand.

Following are several terms commonly used in the study of genetics: a genotype is the genetic constitution or combination of all the genes present in the cells of an organism; a phenotype refers to the physical appearance resulting from the genotype; a mutation is an inheritable change in the genetic material of an organism; a dominant gene is one that exerts its full phenotypic effects; a recessive gene is one whose character is masked by a dominant gene; sex-linked characteristics are genetic characteristics determined by a gene located on the X (female) or Y (male) chromosome.

Examples of genetic manifestations are sex determination, blood type, hemophilia, cleft palate, tooth hardness, saliva flow, and missing teeth. Significant developmental and growth disturbances in the oral cavity have definite genetic implications. Disturbances in the development and growth of teeth, bones, and soft tissues are an important aspect in the study of dentistry.

Reproduction and Fertilization

Humans reproduce sexually. Fertilization is the fusion of the nuclei of the female egg and male sperm. Once a month, an ovum (egg) is emitted from a woman's ovary and enters one of the fallopian tubes. The egg then travels down toward the uterus. If the egg is not fertilized, it degenerates and is discharged from the body. If it is united with the sperm, it becomes what is known as a zygote.

After fertilization, the embryo goes through approximately a 7-day process of complex divisions known as cleavage. It then leaves the fallopian tubes, enters the uterus, and attaches itself to the uterine wall, which has become thick and well vascularized to provide nourishment for the rapidly growing embryo.

An embryo in its later development is known as a fetus. Various physiological developments occur at different time intervals. The face begins to develop between the third and twelfth weeks; teeth begin to develop around the sixth week; and the heart begins to form about the fourth week.

The embryo is nourished through the placenta, a membrane through which oxygen, food, and waste products are exchanged. During the final trimester, the fetus increases greatly in size and weight, and brain cells form rapidly. The fetus also acquires antibodies from the mother, and immunity is transferred. Birth takes place approximately 266 days after conception.

During pregnancy, certain changes occur in the oral cavity of the mother as a result of hormonal fluctuation. The gingiva can become smooth, reddened, and swollen. Increased pocket depth can also occur, causing teeth to become loose. Drugs taken by a pregnant woman can have an effect on the developing fetus. For example, tetracycline taken during the last trimester can cause discoloration of the teeth of the newborn.

It is particularly important to ascertain whether a woman is pregnant before radiographs are taken. The fetus is most vulnerable during the first trimester. If radiographs are necessary, the pregnant woman should be draped accordingly, with a lead-lined apron and exposed to the least amount of radiation possible.

Osteology

Osteology is the study of bone. Bone is a rigid form of connective tissue that contains cells in an intercellular matrix or ground substance. The matrix contains an organic component (fibers) and an inorganic component (salts, such as calcium phosphate and calcium carbonate).

Three types of cells are associated with bone: osteoblasts, osteocytes, and osteoclasts. Osteoblasts are involved with bone formation and are found near those surfaces of bones where the intercellular matrix is deposited. Osteocytes, or matrix bone cells, are osteoblasts that have become trapped within the intercellular matrix. Osteoclasts are giant cells that possess many nuclei and are responsible for the breakdown of bone. Within bone is a substance known as bone marrow. Its function is the production of red blood cells, white blood cells, and platelets, which are the main components of blood.

The Skeleton

The main functions of bone are support and protection. The skeleton, which consists of 206 bones, provides support for the body and enables a human to stand in an erect position. The bones protect many vital organs, provide locations for muscle attachments and store minerals.

The skeleton is divided into two parts: axial and appendicular. The axial skeleton is composed of the skull, vertebrae column, and rib cage. The appendicular skeleton is comprised of bones associated with the body's appendages.

Bones are connected at joints or articulations. There are three types of joints: synarthrotic, amphiarthrotic, and diathrotic.

Synarthrotic joints do not move and join bones in close contact. Examples include the sutures, which are the joints between the bones in the skull.

Amphiarthrotic joints have limited movement and join bones in close proximity, such as those found in the spinal columns.

Diarthrotic joints have the most movement and are the most common joints found in the body. Examples include the elbow, knee, and wrist. The temporomandibular joint, joining the maxilla, and mandible, is a diathrotic joint.

Myology

Myology is the study of muscle. Muscle cells or fibers are grouped into bundles that are responsible for producing movement. Muscle fibers require a rich blood supply in order to work effectively. These blood vessels as well as nerves are carried in connective tissue, which also serves to bind the muscle fibers together.

There are three types of muscle: striated, smooth, and cardiac.

Striated muscles, also known as skeletal or voluntary muscles, are consciously controlled and cause movement of joints and limbs. Striated muscles perform four basic types of movements. When flexed, or contracted, muscles decrease the angle between two bones. Conversely, if extended, the angle is increased. If abducted, muscles move appendages away from the midline of the body and conversely when adducted, toward the midline of the body.

Smooth muscles, also known as involuntary muscles, are not consciously controlled and are located within the wall structures of organ systems such as the digestive and respiratory systems.

Cardiac muscle is specialized muscle found in the heart. It is an involuntary muscle that is responsible for contraction of the heart and circulation of blood.

In simple terms a muscle contraction occurs as a result of muscle filaments sliding over one another. When these filaments slide a contraction takes place and the muscle fiber is shortened. Energy for this process is derived from the breakdown of adenosine triphosphate (ATP) to adenosine diphosphate (ADP) by an enzyme.

Muscle reflexes are actions causing an uncontrollable reaction such as gagging, swallowing and coughing.

When a muscle looses its ability to contract it is known as fatigue. This can happen in situations of strenuous exercise where the amount of ATP needed for energy is depleted.

Neurology

Neurology is the study of the nervous system. Nervous tissue is widely distributed throughout the body. The nervous system consists of those tissues that collect stimuli from the environment, transform the stimuli into impulses, and transmit these impulses to highly organized receptor areas, where they are then interpreted and the appropriate response is made.

The morphology of a nerve cell or neuron consists of a perikaryon or cell body, an axon that arises in the cell body and transmits impulses away from the cell body, and dendrites, which lead impulses toward the cell body.

Nerves respond to stimuli above a particular threshold. As a result of a stimulus, the permeability of the nerve fiber's membrane is altered. Normally, nerve fibers have low concentrations of sodium and high concentrations of potassium. In a response to stimulus, the membrane greatly increases its permeability to sodium ions. Sodium immediately enters the cell and potassium immediately exits, thereby creating a difference in electrical potential. This process continues successively along the nerve fiber allowing propagation of the impulse.

A nerve impulse is transmitted from one nerve to another or from a nerve to a muscle via synapses which are spaces where chemical transmittors mediate propagation of the impulse. These chemicals are released by the ends of axons, cross synapses, and exert their effect on the adjacent nerve or muscle fiber. The chemical mediator is then destroyed by an enzyme. The destruction process is critical to avoid constant stimulation.

There are two major segments of the nervous system: the central nervous system, composed of the brain and the spinal cord, and the peripheral nervous system, composed of all other nerves of the body.

Cranial nerves are 12 paired nerves that control many major functions of the body including sight, smell, and taste.

Cranial Nerves		Function
Number	**Name**	
I	Olfactory	Smell
II	Optic	Sight
III	Oculomotor	Movement of eyes
IV	Trochlear	Movement of eyes
V	Trigeminal	Chewing, conduction of sensation, and movement of the ophthalmic, maxillary, and mandibular nerves to the face
VI	Abducens	Movement of eye
VII	Facial	Secretion of saliva; taste, facial expression

VIII	Auditory (acoustic)	Hearing and balance
IX	Glossopharyngeal	Taste, swallowing, secretion of saliva
X	Vagus	Slowing of heart beat, increase in peristaltic movement, speech
XI	Spinal accessory	Movement of shoulder and head, speech
XII	Hypoglossal	Movement of tongue

Also included in the peripheral nervous system is the autonomic nervous system, composed of neurons that innervate internal organs and that perform such basic life functions as digestion, respiration, and regulation of the heart. The autonomic nervous system is responsible for maintaining bodily homeostasis (equilibrium and physiological stability) and is subdivided into the sympathetic and parasympathetic nervous systems. When stimulated, the sympathetic accelerates the heart beat, produces thick, viscous saliva, and decreases motility and tone of the gastrointestinal tract. Conversely, when the parasympathetic is stimulated, the heart beat is slowed, watery saliva is produced, and motility and tone of the gastrointestinal system are increased. Although these two parts of the autonomic nervous system appear to be antagonistic in nature, it is their dual action that maintains homeostasis.

The nervous system is perhaps one of the most important systems related to dentistry, since stimuli such as pain and anxiety often occur. Nerve fibers are ubiquitous in the oral cavity; therefore, any deviation from the norm usually results in an unpleasant situation. Of primary importance is the use of anesthesia to block the sensation of pain. A local anesthetic prevents a nerve fiber from firing when a stimulus is applied.

Paresthesia, a sensation of anesthesia caused by nerve damage, can result from trauma to a nerve during the administration of anesthesia or from the surgical removal of the tooth. It can be temporary or permanent.

A nerve disturbance involving the oral cavity and face is trigeminal neuralgia. The etiological factors are varied, but the clinical effect is searing or stabbing facial pain. This condition can also be temporary or permanent.

Common diseases associated with the nervous system include Parkinson's disease, epilepsy, and Bell's palsy.

Circulatory System

The circulatory system is comprised of the heart, blood vessels, and the blood. The heart is the specialized organ of the body responsible for initiating the flow of the blood through the body. It is a pump composed of four chambers: left and right atria, and left and right ventricles. Deoxygenated blood enters the right atrium of the heart through the superior and inferior vena cava. It collects in that chamber and, when the auricle is filled, blood flows through valves into the right ventricle. The right ventricle pumps the deoxygenated blood into the pulmonary artery, which leads to the lungs. In the lungs, an exchange of carbon dioxide and oxygen takes place. The oxygenated blood then enters the left atrium, where it collects until the chamber is filled, and then flows into the left ventricle. From the left ventricle, the oxygenated blood is pumped through the aorta and is subsequently distributed throughout the body.

Blood Vessels

After blood leaves the heart, it travels through the arteries, capillaries, and veins. Arteries carry blood away from the heart to all other parts of the body. They are relatively thick elastic vessels that expand and contract as the heart pumps blood. The pulse rate is the number of heart contractions during a given period of time. When the heart contracts, systole occurs; when it is in a relaxed phase, diastole occurs. The measurement of arterial pressure generated during systole and diastole corresponds to the body's blood pressure. For example, the normal pressure is 120/80, measured in millimeters of mercury (mm Hg), which means 120 systole and 80 diastole.

Veins carry blood back to the heart, are thinner than arteries, and possess small valves that prevent blood from flowing backward. Unlike the blood flow in arteries, the blood in veins flows smoothly.

Capillaries are the blood vessels that appear in the greatest number; they are also the smallest blood vessels. It is at the capillary level that the blood and cells exchange nutrients, oxygen, and waste products.

Blood

Each adult has 10 to 12 pints (4.7 to 5.6 liters) of blood. Blood is composed of a liquid component called plasma and of solid components that include red blood cells, white blood cells, and platelets.

Plasma is 90% water; the remaining 10% is divided among plasma proteins (globulin and fibrinogen), inorganic salts, and other products (hormones, antibodies, urea, oxygen, carbon dioxide, and products of digestion.). Globulin functions in the body's defense system, and fibrinogen is an integral component in the clotting of blood.

The solid constituents of blood include the red blood cells, white blood cells, and platelets. Red blood cells, or erythrocytes, are donut-shaped discs that have no nuclei. They are produced in bone marrow and contain hemoglobin, an iron-containing protein responsible for transporting oxygen to the cells.

White blood cells, or leukocytes, are larger than red blood cells and include neutrophils, basophils, and lymphocytes. Some are formed in bone marrow and some in the lymphatic system. Neutrophils are the most common type of white blood cell. They are phagocytes (cell eaters), which function in areas of inflammation by ingesting foreign debris. Basophils are the second most common white blood cells, which function in the production of the anticoagulant heparin. Lymphocytes are an integral part of the body's defense mechanisms.

Platelets, which play a critical role in the clotting process, are actually fragments of larger cells called megakaryocytes, which are formed in bone marrow.

Blood type is inherited and remains unchanged throughout life. There are four basic blood types: A, B, AB, and O. These categories are based on the presence of certain antibodies and the degree to which the red blood cells agglutinate (clump together). In addition, blood types are subdivided by the presence or absence of certain groups of proteins or antigens.

Knowledge of blood type is essential for blood transfusions. If types are not matched properly, or compatible, life-threatening situations can occur. Persons with AB blood are known as universal recipients and can receive any type of blood, but they can donate only to other AB types. Those with type A can receive A or O, but can give to only those with A or AB. Persons with type B can receive B or O, but can donate only to those with B or AB blood. Persons with type O blood are known as universal donors; they can receive only type O blood, but can donate to someone with any type of blood.

An additional factor for blood matching was discovered in 1940. Specifically, the absence or presence of antigens known as the Rh factor were identified. Blood can be further typed as Rh positive or Rh negative. This factor is especially important in Rh-negative women who conceive Rh-positive babies, since Rh-positive babies may require blood transfusions soon after birth.

If a blood vessel is damaged, the flow of blood can be checked or stopped by the clotting process. During this process, platelets liberate a substance that, in conjunction with fibrinogen and calcium, forms a matrix that seals the wounded area.

The dentist and dental assistant must be aware of predisposing factors (e.g., medications and anxiety) that can affect the patient's heart in a dental situation. For example, if a patient is taking certain heart medications without the dentist's knowledge, and the dentist prescribes other medications, dangerous interactions can occur.

Blood pressure should also be carefully monitored. If a patient exhibits high blood pressure, the dentist must decide whether to use a local anesthetic with or without epinephrine. If an anesthetic containing epinephrine is chosen, injection should be slow and aspiration frequent, to determine whether the injection is intravascular, which can cause an increase in heart rate.

In addition, patients who have experienced a myocardial infarction or rheumatic heart disease should be given antibiotics prophylactically in order to prevent dangerous infections that could prove fatal.

Lymphatic System

The lymphatic system works in close association with the circulatory system. Its purpose is to return intercellular fluid and materials to the circulatory system. The fluid and returning materials are called lymph. The lymphatic system also serves to transport absorbed fats from the intestines to the blood and plays an integral part in the body's defense systems.

The organs of the lymphatic system include lymph nodes, tonsils, the thymus, and the spleen. Lymph nodes are encapsulated masses of lymph tissue that filter the lymph fluid and produce lymphocytes and monocytes, which destroy microorganisms in the body. The tonsils and the thymus serve in similar capacities, although their function is still not completely understood. The spleen acts as a storage area for red blood cells and has other important functions.

The lymphatic system is not connected to the arteries, and therefore the fluid in this system is not moved along by the action of the heart. The movement of lymphatic fluid depends on the contraction of the nearby skeletal muscles, which press on lymph vessels. Tissue fluid is absorbed into lymphatic capillaries and flows into connecting lymphatic veins. From there it proceeds into a large vein at the base of the neck.

If large amounts of tissue fluid collect in an area because of a blockage in the lymphatic system or a change in the protein concentration of the surrounding intercellular fluid, a pathology termed edema results. Edema is often symptomatic of other bodily pathologies or of a reaction to a localized inflammatory process, or both.

Lymphadenopathy, or swelling of lymph nodes, should alert the dentist to an infectious process in the patient's body.

Respiratory System

Respiration is the process whereby the oxygen required by each cell for the production of energy is introduced into the bloodstream and carbon dioxide, a waste product of cellular activity, is removed. This transfer of gases occurs in the lungs where thin-walled capillaries are in close proximity to the alveoli, the air sacs of the lungs.

Air is inhaled through the nose and enters the nasal sinuses where it is filtered, warmed, and moistened. The air then travels through the nasopharynx to the pharynx, past the glottis, which is the opening into the larynx and trachea. The epiglottis is a protective flap of tissue that prevents food from entering the lungs. After passing through the glottis, air enters the larynx and subsequently enters the trachea, the major duct leading to the lungs. The trachea branches out into smaller ducts called bronchi, which in turn divide into bronchioles and subsequently alveoli, the smallest components of the respiratory system.

Air is inspired by the expansion of the rib cage and diaphragm, causing a negative air pressure against the lungs. The lungs then expand as air is drawn into them.

After the exchange of gases, air pressure around the lungs increases while the diaphragm and rib case relax. As the air pressure increases, the air is forced out of the lungs.

Digestive System

The digestive system functions to reduce ingested food mechanically and chemically to a state in which it can be used by the body. This process occurs in the alimentary canal, which is composed of five organs: the oral cavity, esophagus, stomach, and small and large intestines. In addition to the alimentary canal there are adjunct organs, including the salivary glands, liver, gallbladder, and pancreas, which assist in the digestive process.

Food enters the oral cavity, where it is acted upon by teeth and saliva. The teeth function to break up food. Incisors are used for biting, canines for tearing, and molars for crushing food. The food bolus is lubricated by saliva, primarily produced in the parotid, submandibular, and sublingual glands.

Saliva is transported to the oral cavity through a system of ducts. In addition to lubricating the food bolus, saliva contains the digestive enzyme ptyalin, which begins the breakdown of starches, in the mouth. The tongue pushes the food bolus downward into the esophagus, which is a long tube that connects the oral cavity to the stomach. Food moves quickly through the esophagus, assisted by waves of muscular contractions in a process called peristalsis. In the stomach, food is churned and acted upon by a variety of gastric enzymes and hydrochloric acid. Some absorption into the bloodstream takes place in the stomach, although this process is conducted mainly in the small intestine. The small intestine is long and is divided into the duodenum, ileum and jejunum. To facilitate absorption, the surface area in the small intestine is greatly increased by numerous folds and ridges and small fingerlike projections called villi. The villi is where absorption occurs. Each villus contains an artery, vein, and lymph vessel. Residual waste products not absorbed into the bloodstream enter the large intestine, or colon, where water is absorbed and the solid waste products are conducted outward from the body.

The liver is involved in the formation of bile, which is important in the intestinal phases of fat digestion. The liver also metabolizes carbohydrates, fats, and proteins for storage or energy utilization. The importance of the liver as a detoxification organ cannot be overemphasized. It detoxifies harmful chemicals that enter the body. Many drugs used in dentistry (e.g., local anesthetics) are broken down in the liver.

The gallbladder stores bile produced by the liver and empties the bile into the small intestine, where it assists in the digestion of fats. The pancreas has a dual function: digestive and hormonal. The pancreas aids in digestion by secreting enzymes into the small intestine.

Nutrition

Nutrition is the process that includes utilization of food in growth, repair and maintenance of body tissues, digestion and absorption of food, and transport of food to the cells.

Basic food elements are essential for proper nutrition. Proteins, made up of amino acids, are either structural, serving as building blocks (e.g., collagen fibers, the major constitutents in skin, bone, and cartilage), or functional, including enzymes and hormones. Primary sources of protein include meat, poultry, fish, eggs, legumes, vegetables, nuts, cheese, and milk.

Carbohydrates provide sources of energy and include sugars (glucose, sucrose, lactose), starches (rice, potatoes, grains), and polysaccharides (cellulose, roughage). Carbohydrates are the principal energy source for most living systems and are the basic materials from which other molecules are built. Excess carbohydrates are stored in the liver.

Fat serves a role both as a structural material and as an energy reserve. It is important to the nervous system in providing insulation for nerves. Fats are found in meats, poultry, fish, oils, and dairy products.

Minerals are important in assisting enzymes in biochemical reactions. Essential minerals include calcium, sulfur, sodium, potassium, magnesium, iron, iodine, chlorine, and copper. Very small amounts of these minerals are needed to maintain adequate nutrition.

Vitamins are organic compounds not synthesized by the body, but necessary for good health. Essential vitamins include A, B, C, D, and K.

Water is essential for all organisms and constitutes 50–70% of total body weight. Without water, we become dehydrated—a minor problem initially, but one that can lead to serious complications, and possibly death.

Metabolism

Metabolism is the process whereby chemical energy is broken down into a form that can be used by the cell to survive and function. It is the sum of all chemical reactions that take place within a cell or organism. Metabolism can take one of two forms: anabolism or catabolism.

Anabolism is the process during which simple products of digestion are built into complex molecules to perform various bodily functions.

Catabolism is the process during which absorbed products of digestion are reduced to simple waste products, such as carbon dioxide, water, and urea.

Carbohydrates are first broken down into glucose, the primary fuel for bodily function. If the glucose is not used, it is changed to glycogen in the liver; similarly, if the glycogen is not used, it is converted to fat. When completely oxidized, the waste products are carbon dioxide and water.

During metabolism, fats are broken down into fatty acids and glycerol, which can be further broken down to glucose and provide direct fuel for the cells. If the body does not need the ingested fat in order to function, it is stored directly as adipose tissue, also known as depot fat. As in carbohydrate metabolism, waste products of fat metabolism are primarily carbon dioxide and water.

Proteins are metabolized and absorbed by the tissues as amino acids. The tissues select and store some of these substances; they are either synthesized into new tissue or used to maintain and repair tissue of each organ.

Heat is produced by every cell during the process of metabolism, especially by the muscles and liver. The heat is conducted by circulating blood and is dissipated through the skin, lungs, urine, and feces.

Excretory System

The excretory system functions to remove waste products from the body, thereby supporting the maintenance of homeostasis. Included in the excretory system are the skin, lungs, intestines, and urinary tract.

The chemical reactions taking place within cells produce certain waste products, such as water, carbon dioxide, urea, as well as heat, which must be eliminated from the body. This elimination process must occur regularly; otherwise, cell functioning will deteriorate, causing eventual death of the cell. The skin, which is the largest organ of the body, functions to eliminate water and various salts through perspiration. As water is eliminated it evaporates, cooling the skin and lowering body temperature.

The lungs function to remove carbon dioxide and water excreted during respiration. The intestines, both small and large, rid the body of solid and liquid waste products. Solid waste products include cellulose, roughage, and nondigestable material. Liquids excreted by the intestines are bile, calcium salts, and water.

The organs of the urinary system include the kidneys, ureters, bladder, and urethra. The two kidneys, located behind the abdominal cavity on each side of the spinal column, function in the balance of osmotic pressure of extracellular fluids. In addition, the kidneys control electrolyte balance and excretion of metabolic wastes, as well as regulating the pH level of body fluids. The functional units of the kidneys are called nephrons. The nephron filters toxic products from the blood to form urine. Urine is about 95% water; the remaining portion is composed of organic and inorganic waste products.

The ureters are tubes that convey the urine from the kidneys to the urinary bladder. The urinary bladder is a hollow muscular organ the function of which is to store urine until it is ready to be excreted. Finally, the bladder passes the urine through the urethra to the external environment.

Endocrine System

The endocrine system is responsible for secreting hormones, which regulate metabolic functions of the body. Hormones are chemicals that are specific in action, continuously secreted, and generally slow acting. Organs of the endocrine system include the pituitary, thyroid, parathyroid, pineal, and adrenal glands, the pancreas, and gonads. The pituitary, located in the cranial cavity, secretes several hormones. Adrenocorticotropic hormone (ACTH) travels to the adrenal gland via the bloodstream and stimulates the secretion of hormones of the adrenal gland. Other hormones secreted by the pituitary are growth hormone (GH), which has a specific effect on the growth of tissues, especially bone and muscle; thyroid stimulating hormone (TSH), which influences secretory activity of the thyroid; follicle stimulating hormone (FSH), which influences ripening of follicle and production of estrogen by the ovaries; luteinizing hormone (LH), which influences secreting cells of the ovaries and testes; and antidiuretic hormone (ADH), which regulates the water and electrolyte balance of body fluids.

The thyroid gland, located in the neck, is acted upon by TSH to release the hormones thyroxine and tri-iodothyronine. The main function of the thyroid hormones is to regulate metabolism.

The parathyroids secrete parathyroid hormone (PTH), which plays an important role in maintaining the normal calcium and phosphorus levels of the blood.

The pineal gland is located in the cranial cavity; its general function is unknown.

The adrenal glands are two small bodies lying on top of each kidney that secrete a group of hormones called corticosteroids, which include the mineralocorticoids and glucocorticoids. The adrenal hormones are released through the influence of the pituitary hormone ACTH. The mineralocorticoids stimulate resorption of sodium in the kidneys, which in turn controls fluid balance in the body. The glucocorticoids predominantly act in the regulation of metabolism of carbohydrates, fats, and proteins. The adrenal gland also secretes epinephrine, which affects all structures of the body innervated by the sympathetic nervous system and thereby reinforces its action (cardiac acceleration, vasoconstriction, and rise in blood pressure).

The pancreas, located in the abdominal cavity, is the site at which insulin and glucagon are released. A specialized group of cells, the isles of Langerhans, secrete insulin. Insulin promotes the utilization of glucose in cells and thereby decreases blood glucose concentration. Insulin is essential for the maintenance of normal levels of blood glucose. A marked increase in the level of blood glucose is known as diabetes mellitus, caused by an inadequate supply of insulin in the body. The pancreatic hormone glucagon increases the blood glucose level. Insulin and glucagon work together to maintain a normal blood glucose level.

The gonads include the female ovary and the male testes. The ovary, under the influence of the pituitary, produces estrogen and progesterone. Estrogen is present in the bloodstream of women from puberty to menopause, reaching its highest concentration before monthly ovulation. Sex hormones in the woman stimulate secondary sexual characteristics, such as enlargement of breasts, growth of pubic hair, broadening of the pelvis, and an increase in the size of the uterus and vagina.

The male hormones, or androgens, promote the development of the male sex organs and of masculine characteristics such as facial hair and deep voice. The primary androgen is testosterone. It should be noted that both male and female sex hormones are produced in both sexes.

A variety of hormones have numerous effects on the oral cavity. For instance, the development and eruption rate of teeth can be severely affected if there is an imbalance in the release of thyroid hormones. The abnormal release of epinephrine from the adrenals can have deleterious effects on the oral mucosa and pulp due to vasoconstriction. In addition, the female sex hormones estrogen and progesterone can exert harmful gingival effects, especially during pregnancy.

The Eye and Ear

The organs of the body that function to produce sight include the eyeball, the optic nerve, and the visual center in the brain.

The Eye

The retina receives images of external objects and transfers these impressions to the visual center of the brain. The macula lutea, a yellow spot located on the retina, is the region of greatest visual activity. The optic nerve enters the eyeball at the optic disc, located on the retina, and transmits visual information to the brain. The cornea is the transparent covering of the anterior portion of the eyeball. The iris is a circular disc suspended in the fluid of the eye in front of the lens and behind the cornea. Pigment in the iris gives a characteristic eye color. The iris expands and contracts to regulate the amount of light that enters the eye. The lens, located behind the iris, focuses light on the retina.

The eye has both intrinsic and extrinsic muscles. The extrinsic muscles serve to roll the eyeball in different directions, while the intrinsic muscles permit constriction and dilation of the pupil (opening at the center of the iris). Eyelids provide protection for the eye, and lacrimal glands secrete tears, which lubricate and maintain the health of the eyes.

The processes necessary for focusing are convergence, change in the size of the pupil, accommodation, and refraction. Convergence, or turning the eyes inward, is necessary to place the image on corresponding points of the two retinae. The change in the size of the pupil, which contracts in bright light and dilates in dim light, plays a role in focusing by regulating the appropriate amount of light. Accommodation is the capacity of the eyes and lenses to adjust so that objects at varying distances can be seen clearly. Refraction is the bending of light rays entering the pupil, bringing them into focus on the retina.

Common optical disorders include myopia, hypermetropia, astigmatism, and glaucoma. Myopia or nearsightedness, results from rays of light converging in front of rather than on the retina. Hypermetropia, or farsightedness, results from rays of light converging behind the retina. Astigmatism is a condition in which the curvature of the refracting surfaces is defective. Glaucoma results from increased interocular pressure, which interferes with blood distribution. This pathology can lead to irreversible damage to visual cells and blindness if left untreated.

In the dental office, safety glasses should be worn by all members of the dental team, including the patient, in order to prevent flying particles from entering and possibly damaging the eyes.

The Ear

The organs involved in hearing include the external, middle, and inner ear; the acoustic nerve; and the acoustic center in the brain.

The external ear consists of the exposed portion of the ear (pinna) and the auditory canal. The middle ear is situated in the temporal bone and is separated from the external ear by the tympanic membrane, or eardrum. The middle ear houses the auditory ossicles, or bones, namely, the malleus (hammer), incus (anvil), and stapes (stirrup). These bones are set in motion by the movements of the tympanic membrane. The internal ear, or labyrinth, consists of the cochlea and semicircular canals, which are suspended in a fluid medium.

Hearing is accomplished when air waves enter the auditory canal, causing the vibration of the tympanic membrane. Vibrations are communicated to the ossicles and are transmitted to the fluid in the internal ear which, in turn, stimulates auditory nerve impulses, which are transmitted to the acoustic center of the brain.

Balance or body equilibrium is regulated by the fluid within the semicircular canals. Movement of the canal fluid resulting from body movement causes information about body position and motion to be transmitted to the acoustic center of the brain. Dysfunction in this process can lead to temporary or permanent inability to maintain equilibrium.

Continued exposure to high-speed drills in the dental office can result in loss of hearing. Consequently, all dental personnel should have hearing tests at regular intervals.

Pharmacology

Pharmacology is the scientific body of knowledge concerned with the properties of drugs and the interactions of chemical compounds within living systems.

Drugs can be used as a means of sustaining and maintaining health. Examples of useful drugs are antibiotics which aid in the defense mechanisms of the body by inhibiting or destroying invading bacteria; central nervous system depressants, such as barbiturates; and stimulants, such as amphetamines. Muscle relaxants such as succinylcholine can be used during certain surgical procedures as a skeletal muscle relaxant. Hormones such as estrogen contained in birth control pills affect the endocrine system.

Methods of Administration

Drugs are administered in a variety of ways, including topically (on the surface), orally, sublingually (under the tongue), rectally, by inhalation, and by injection. Injections can be given intravenously (into a vein), intramuscularly (into a muscle), intradermally (just breaking the skin surface), and subcutaneously (somewhat deeper than intradermally, into subcutaneous tissue). Parenteral administration refers to the introduction of medication in locations of the body other than the gastrointestinal system.

Drugs are most commonly administered orally because of the relative ease of administration and inexpensiveness. A major disadvantage of drugs given orally, however, is that their potency can be diminished or eliminated by interaction with stomach enzymes, such as insulin. Sublingual administration produces rapid onset through the rich vascular network located beneath the tongue. Rectal administration of drugs is advantageous for patients with stomach disorders or for those who are unable to take a drug orally. Drugs administered by inhalation have a very quick onset, but can be easily abused, particularly by adolescents and young adults. Parenteral administration has an almost immediate onset, but it can be extremely dangerous if the drug is toxic to a given patient. It is virtually impossible to remove the drug once it has been given, and treatment usually involves administration of additional drugs containing counteractive properties.

Prescription Writing

A prescription is a written order for a specific drug prepared by a licensed health care provider. The order contains a superscription or Rx, the abbreviation for recipe, which literally means "take thou"; an inscription, indicating the ingredients and the amount of each; a subscription, containing the directions for dispensing; and a signature indicating directions to the patient. In addition to the four major parts indicated above, a prescription contains the doctor's name, address, and Drug Enforcement Agency (DEA) number; the patient's name, address, and age; the date of the prescription; and a statement indicating whether a substitution is permissible (see below).

A number of Latin words in abbreviations and phrases are used when writing prescriptions. Examples are p.o., for per os, or by mouth; q.i.d., meaning four times a day; and stat, for immediately. Shown below is a sample prescription.

John Smith, D.D.S.   License #_____
Address   DEA # _____
Telephone

Name: Date:
Address: Age:

Rx
     Tetracycline USP, 250 mg
     Dispense: 30 capsules
     Signature: Take 2 stat and 1 q.i.d. subsequently

                                    John Smith, D.D.S.

Drugs are classified as either proprietary (brand name) or generic (nonbrand version reflective of chemical composition). It is within the purview of the individual dentist to decide whether to permit generic substitution for specific proprietary medications.

Categories of Medication

Major types of drugs used in dentistry include central nervous system depressants, central nervous system stimulants, anesthetics, and antibiotics.

Central nervous system depressants include barbiturates, which are sedative hypnotics principally used to induce sleep, reduce anxiety, and alleviate convulsions. Common barbiturates are phenobarbitol, secobarbitol, and pentobarbitol. Barbiturates should be dispensed with caution, however, since abuse can lead to respiratory depression, resulting in coma or death. Patients should be told that mixing alcohol with barbiturates is particularly dangerous. Antianxiety drugs, such as diazepam (Valium) and chlordiazepoxide (Librium) are similar in action to barbiturates, but are less potent. These drugs are often used to decrease anxiety and to increase the effectiveness of nitrous oxide.

Narcotics are potent analgesics (pain-relieving drugs) derived from natural opiates or synthetic compounds. Common narcotics include codeine, meperidine (Demerol), and morphine. These drugs greatly elevate the pain threshold and are prescribed for moderate to severe pain. Toxic doses of narcotics can cause marked respiratory depression; furthermore, if abused, dependency can occur.

Non-narcotic analgesics including aspirin, acetaminophen (Tylenol), and propoxyphene hydrochloride (Darvon) alleviate mild to moderate pain. Aspirin, in addition to being an analgesic, has antipyretic (fever-reducing) and anti-inflammatory properties.

Central nervous system stimulants include caffeine, epinephrine, and amphetamines. Caffeine contained in coffee, tea, and chocolate affects the cerebral cortex and causes restlessness and alertness. Epinephrine, which dilates bronchial muscles and increases activity of the heart, is contained in many local anesthetics because of its vasoconstrictive properties. Epinephrine is also administered to patients who show evidence of severe allergic reaction approaching or evidencing anaphylactic shock. Amphetamines are psychomotor stimulants and mood elevators, the disadvantages of which include a mild to moderate letdown after the initial stimulation. Central nervous system stimulants are rarely prescribed by dentists.

Anesthetics are either general or local. General anesthetics induce sleep, eliminate noxious reflexes, and relax muscles. Halothane, nitrous oxide, and sodium thiopental are examples of general anesthesia. Halothane and nitrous oxide are gases administered by inhalation, and sodium thiopental is administered intravenously. The combination of nitrous oxide and oxygen administered by inhalation is the most commonly used analgesia in dentistry. Analgesia is the first stage of anesthesia during which a patient remains conscious, has an increased threshold for pain, and might experience some amnesia. Nitrous oxide and oxygen analgesia are easily controlled, short acting, and relatively safe.

Local anesthesia, administered by injection, causes a short-term reversible loss of sensation in a specific area of the body. Common local anesthesias include procaine (Novocain), lidocaine (Xylocaine), and mepivacaine (Carbocaine). Some local anesthetics contain vasoconstrictors, such as epinephrine, which prevent systemic absorption, thereby making the anesthetic longer acting in the specific area.

Antibiotics are bacteriocidal (bacteria killing) or bacteriostatic (bacteria-controlling agents). Penicillin is a bacteriocidal antibiotic that kills a wide range of microorganisms. It is currently the most frequently prescribed antibiotic in dentistry for the use of both local and systemic infections. Penicillin is often used prophylactically to prevent infection after surgery. Erythromycin and tetracycline are bacteriostatic antibiotics often prescribed for patients who are allergic to penicillin.

Microbiology

Microbiology is the study of biological microorganisms seen only with the aid of a microscope. These organisms are either single celled or multicellular, some beneficial and others harmful to humans. The three major classifications of microorganisms are viruses, fungi, and bacteria.

Viruses are the smallest infectious agents, containing a strand molecule of nucleic acid encased in a protein shell. Viruses are parasites, which replicate only in living cells. There are animal viruses, plant viruses, and bacterial viruses, known as bacteriophages. Examples of pathologies caused by viruses include herpes, influenza, and polio. Antibiotic therapy is usually ineffective for the treatment of viral infections.

Fungi include yeasts and molds. They are widely distributed microorganisms that grow as a mass of branching, interlacing filaments containing nuclei and organelles. A common intraoral disease caused by fungi is thrush. Antifungicides such as nystatin effectively fight fungal infection.

Bacteria are microorganisms that appear in three basic shapes: rod-like, spherical, and spiral. Rod-shaped bacteria are called bacilli; spherical bacteria are called cocci; and spiriform are called spirilla. Bacteria have nuclei and are enclosed in cell walls. They have the ability to replicate themselves and some are motile. Common pathologies caused by bacteria are caries, periodontal disease, pneumonia, and rheumatic fever. Antibiotic therapy is generally used to fight systemic bacterial infections.

Normal microorganism constituents of the mouth include fungi such as *Candida albicans* and bacteria such as *Streptococcus* and *Staphylococcus*. These microorganisms are not harmful in normal amounts. It is only when they proliferate and disrupt homeostasis that pathology occurs.

Infection and Immunity

Infection is the process during which a microorganism enters into a relationship with the host, establishes itself, and multiplies within the host. The tissue environment controls susceptibility or resistance to given microorganisms. If the host lacks sufficient resistance, infection occurs.

Immunity is the property of a host to resist specific infections. Immunity can be produced by an injection of antibodies of one person into another or by the formation of antibodies in a person as a result of previous exposure to a microorganism. Smallpox or poliovirus immunizations are examples of injected immunity, in contrast to the resistance to mumps that results from a previous episode of the disease, an immunity resulting in previously formed antibodies.

Sterilization

Asepsis is the term used to describe an area which is free from pathological microorganisms. Conversely, sepsis refers to the existence of disease-producing organisms. Sterilization and disinfection are methods used, respectively, to destroy pathological microorganisms; completely or partially.

Sterilization is the destruction of microbes by heat and pressure, heat, radiation, or ultrasonic waves. Autoclaves use steam under pressure to sterilize stainless steel (nonrusting) dental instruments, glass slabs, and cloth materials.

Dry-heat ovens use heat alone to sterilize carbon steel instruments and very sharp instruments that would be dulled by the steam of an autoclave.

Boiling water is not as effective as an autoclave or dry heat oven, but it kills most microbes.

Molten metal and glass bead sterilizers are rapid methods of sterilization used for endontic instruments. They are advantageous in the dental office because instruments and other materials can be sterilized immediately before insertion into the mouth.

After sterilization, asepsis must be maintained, or instruments and materials will again become contaminated. Instruments should be removed from the sterilizing unit with sterile instruments and should be stored in areas that will maintain sterility.

Disinfection is the process through which most microorganisms are destroyed; however sterility is not guaranteed. Disinfection is usually accomplished by heating or applying antimicrobial chemicals. When materials are placed in heat sterilizers for shorter than the specified amount of time for sterilization, they are disinfected. Chemical disinfectants used in dentistry are glutaraldehyde (Cidex), alcohol, and sodium hypochlorite solution.

Glutaraldehyde (Cidex) effectively destroys bacteria, fungi, and viruses. Those items that can be submerged in solutions should be submerged at least 10 minutes to ensure disinfection. A 60–75% concentration of ethyl or isopropyl alcohol will destroy bacteria. However, it is not effective against spores. Sodium hypochlorite solution (bleach) is also used as a disinfectant, but it is irritating to the skin.

Instruments and equipment that cannot be soaked can be wiped down with either glutaraldehyde solution or alcohol, making them the weakest link in the aseptic chain.

Question Section

Directions: Each of the questions or incomplete statements below is followed by several suggested answers or completions. Select the BEST answer in each case.

1. Histology is the study of
   1. tissue anatomy
   2. artifacts
   3. internal body pressure
   4. the history of the human species

2. Genetics is the study of
   1. the nervous system
   2. heredity
   3. tissue composition
   4. intercellular fluids

3. Embryology is the study of
   1. humans and their environment
   2. the diseases of humankind
   3. muscular control
   4. the human organism in the uterus

4. Solubility refers to
   1. capillary action
   2. different states of matter
   3. the amount of substance that can be dissolved
   4. the heat of reaction

5. States of matter include
   A. solid
   B. liquid
   C. gas
   D. heat
      1. A, B, and C
      2. A and C only
      3. B and D only
      4. all of the above

6. As the state of matter is changed from solid to liquid to gas, molecular movement is
   1. decreased
   2. unchanged
   3. increased
   4. stopped

7. A flow of electrons is called
   1. resistance
   2. electricity
   3. ductility
   4. malleability

8. The measurement unit of 1°F is
   1. larger than 1°C
   2. smaller than 1°C
   3. the same as 1°C
   4. unrelated to 1°C

9. Metabolism is the combined process of
   A. osmosis
   B. anabolism
   C. passive diffusion
   D. catabolism
      1. A, B, and C
      2. A and C only
      3. B and D only
      4. D only
      5. all of the above

10. The cells that produce bone are
    1. osteoblasts
    2. osteocytes
    3. osteoclasts
    4. fibrocytes

11. The cell organelle that produces energy for the cell is the
    1. lysosome
    2. mitochondrion
    3. cell membrane
    4. nucleus

12. Ribosomes are involved in
    A. energy production
    B. fat synthesis
    C. cell division
    D. protein synthesis
       1. A, B, and C
       2. A and C only
       3. B and D only
       4. D only
       5. all of the above

13. Which tissue has the poorest regenerative capability?
    1. epithelial
    2. connective
    3. nerve
    4. muscle

14. The function of bone marrow is to
    1. add resiliency to bones
    2. produce blood cells
    3. decrease the weight of bones
    4. aid in muscular attachments

15. The axial skeleton refers to bones of the
    A. arm
    B. head
    C. leg
    D. neck
    E. ribs
       1. A, B, and D
       2. B, C, and E
       3. B, D, and E
       4. C, D, and E

16. Which of the following bones are types of vertebrae?
    A. cervical
    B. lumbar
    C. thoracic
    D. patella
    E. tibia
       1. A, B, and C
       2. A, C, and E
       3. B, D, and E
       4. C, D, and E

17. Most ribs are attached to the spinal column and the
    1. scapula
    2. sternum
    3. clavicle
    4. sacrum

18. A joint is the
    1. point of intersection of muscle and bone
    2. junction of bones
    3. overlapping of muscles
    4. center of ossification

19. Joints that do not move are called
    1. hinge joints
    2. ball-and-socket joints
    3. gliding joints
    4. sutures

20. The types of muscle tissues are
    A. smooth
    B. elastic
    C. striated
    D. cardiac
    E. extension
       1. A, C, and D
       2. B, C, and D
       3. B, D, and E
       4. C, D, and E

21. Muscle tissue is present in which system?
    1. circulatory
    2. digestive
    3. respiratory
    4. all of the above

22. Tendons attach
    1. muscle to bone
    2. muscle to nerve
    3. nerve to bone
    4. bone to bone

23. The condition that exists when a muscle loses its ability to contract is
    1. exhaustion
    2. reflex
    3. fatigue
    4. hyperextension

24. A reflex is
    1. an action that can always by controlled
    2. always hormonal in nature
    3. an involuntary response to a stimulus
    4. a response that bypasses the central nervous system

25. An example of a reflex is
    1. writing
    2. wiping one's nose
    3. talking
    4. coughing

26. A nerve impulse is transmitted from nerve to nerve via
    1. the myoneural junction
    2. ligaments
    3. the synaptic junction
    4. foramina

27. A neuron is composed of
    A. dendrites
    B. axons
    C. a perikaryon
    D. epithelium
        1. A, B, and C
        2. A and C only
        3. B and D only
        4. D only
        5. all of the above

28. The central nervous system is covered by a membrane called the
    1. hyaline membrane
    2. meninges
    3. Nasmyth membrane
    4. primary cuticle

29. The portions of the brain are
    A. cerebrum
    B. peripheral nerves
    C. medulla oblongata
    D. spinal nerves
    E. cerebellum
        1. A, B, and D
        2. A, C, and E
        3. B, D, and E
        4. C, D, and E

30. Cranial nerves responsible for the movement of the eye include
    A. abducens
    B. trochlear
    C. oculomotor
    D. optic
        1. A, B, and C
        2. A, and C
        3. B, and D
        4. D only
        5. all of the above

31. Neurons conducting impulses away from the central nervous system are called
    1. afferent nerves
    2. sensory nerves
    3. motor nerves
    4. accessory nerves

32. Involuntary nervous control of the body is determined by the
    1. fifth cranial nerve
    2. autonomic nervous system
    3. cerebellum
    4. none of the above

33. The cranial nerve controlling tongue movements is the
    1. olfactory
    2. trigeminal
    3. vagus
    4. hypoglossal

34. The acoustic nerve controls
    1. taste
    2. eye movements
    3. balance
    4. voice

35. A piece of amalgam flying into an assistant's eye would most likely cause a scratch on the
    1. retina
    2. lens
    3. iris
    4. cornea

36. Endocrine glands affect the body by chemical mediators called
    1. impulses
    2. hormones
    3. catalysts
    4. globulins

37. Which of the following are endocrine glands?
    A. kidneys
    B. pituitary
    C. thyroid
    D. spleen
    E. gonads
        1. A, B, and C

2. B, C, and E
3. B, D, and E
4. C, D, and E

38. The hormone released during times of dental stress is
    1. epinephrine
    2. melatonin
    3. parathormone
    4. testosterone

39. The primary female hormones are
    A. progesterone
    B. testosterone
    C. estrogen
    D. thyroxine
       1. A, B, and C
       2. A and C only
       3. B and D only
       4. D only
       5. all of the above

40. Diabetes mellitus is caused by the lack or inactivity of which hormone?
    1. ACTH
    2. thyroxine
    3. parathormone
    4. insulin

41. The trachea divides directly into the
    1. sinuses
    2. bronchioles
    3. alveoli
    4. bronchi

42. Where does gaseous exchange take place in the lungs?
    1. larynx
    2. bronchioles
    3. alveoli
    4. bronchi

43. The function of the epiglottis is to
    1. regulate the CO_2 and O_2 ratio of inspired air
    2. control the tidal volume of air
    3. support the thyroid gland
    4. prevent liquids and solids from entering the respiratory system

44. Inspiration is caused by
    1. a decrease in size of alveoli
    2. expansion of the pleural cavity
    3. relaxation of the diaphragm
    4. contraction of the chest

45. Blood normally transports
    A. fibrin
    B. oxygen
    C. cellulose
    D. nutrients

E. hormones
   1. A, B, and D
   2. B, C, and E
   3. B, D, and E
   4. C, D, and E

46. The blood vessels that contain valves are
    1. arteries
    2. arterioles
    3. capillaries
    4. veins

47. The function of hemoglobin is to
    1. carry nutrients
    2. fight infection
    3. transport oxygen
    4. stimulate endocrine glands

48. Leukocytes are
    1. a defense mechanism of the body
    2. part of the oxygen transport system
    3. formed by bone marrow
    4. part of the excretory system

49. The fluid portion of blood is known as
    1. megakaryocytes
    2. plasma
    3. erythrocytes
    4. lymph

50. Blood platelets are necessary in
    1. CO_2 elimination
    2. antigen–antibody reactions
    3. allergic reactions
    4. blood clotting

51. The number of chambers in the human heart is
    1. one
    2. two
    3. three
    4. four

52. What type of tissues make up the heart?
    A. muscle
    B. epithelial
    C. nervous
    D. connective
       1. A, B, and C
       2. A and C
       3. B and D
       4. D only
       5. all of the above

53. The blood vessel that conducts blood from the heart to the body is
    1. the superior vena cava
    2. the right atrium
    3. the aorta
    4. the pulmonary vein

54. Valves between the chambers of the heart
    1. regulate the electrical potential of the pressure
    2. prevent the backflow of blood
    3. supply blood to the heart muscles
    4. are vestigial organs

55. The diastolic blood pressure is the pressure exerted by blood on the walls of
    1. arteries when the heart is at rest
    2. veins when the heart pumps
    3. arteries when the heart pumps
    4. veins when the heart is at rest

56. The arterial pulse indicates the
    1. blood pressure
    2. number of times the heart is contracting
    3. temperature of the blood
    4. cardiac output

57. Lymph nodes function to
    1. transport nutrients
    2. produce plasma
    3. produce lymphocytes
    4. all of the above

58. What is the fate of lymph?
    1. absorbed by the body
    2. enters the bloodstream
    3. swallowed and digested
    4. secreted as saliva

59. Digestion begins in the
    1. esophagus
    2. stomach
    3. oral cavity
    4. small intestine

60. The rhythmic movement of the esophagus that moves the food bolus onward is known as
    1. digestion
    2. churning
    3. swallowing
    4. peristalsis

61. Absorption of most nutrients occurs in the
    1. stomach
    2. small intestine
    3. large intestine
    4. esophagus

62. The major function of the large intestine is to
    1. aid in protein metabolism
    2. lubricate the food bolus
    3. aid in water absorption
    4. store nutrients

63. Proteins are made up of
    1. adipose tissue

2. amino acids
3. glycogen
4. lactose

64. Water composes what percentage of body weight?
    1. 0 to 20%
    2. 20 to 40%
    3. 50 to 70%
    4. 70 to 90%

65. Chromosomes are made up of
    1. fats
    2. carbohydrates
    3. nucleic acids
    4. glycogen

66. The union of egg and sperm is known as
    A. an embryo
    B. a yolk sac
    C. a fetus
    D. fertilization
       1. A, B, and C
       2. A and C
       3. B and D
       4. D only
       5. all of the above

67. Congenital refers to
    1. a condition at birth
    2. a condition that worsens during aging
    3. only diseases of the genitalia
    4. none of the above

68. Which dental abnormalities are caused primarily by genetic disorders?
    A. cleft palate
    B. caries
    C. anodontia
    D. bruxing
       1. A, B, and C
       2. A and C
       3. B and C
       4. D only
       5. all of the above

69. A hereditary blood disease that can lead to uncontrolled bleeding is
    1. epidermal dysplasia
    2. sickle cell anemia
    3. A and B blood types
    4. hemophilia

70. Organs found in the excretory system are the
    A. oral mucosa
    B. skin
    C. liver
    D. lungs
    E. kidneys
       1. A, B, and D

2. B, C, and E
3. B, D, and E
4. C, D, and E

71. Organs found in the respiratory system include
    A. nasopharynx
    B. esophagus
    C. bronchi
    D. oral cavity
       1. A, B, and C
       2. A and C
       3. B and D
       4. D only
       5. all of the above

72. Components of the urinary system are the
    A. ureters
    B. uterus
    C. bladder
    D. urethra
    E. liver
       1. A, B, and C
       2. A, C, and D
       3. B, C, and D
       4. C, D, and E

73. The lungs are considered a part of which two systems?
    A. circulatory
    B. respiratory
    C. urinary
    D. excretory
       1. A and B
       2. A and C
       3. B and D
       4. A and D
       5. B and C

74. Structures of the eye include
    A. ciliary body
    B. cornea
    C. lens
    D. cochlea
       1. A, B, and C
       2. A and C only
       3. B and D only
       4. D only
       5. all of the above

75. The presence of bacteria in the urine indicates
    1. a possible infection in the urinary tract
    2. a bacteremia
    3. normal functioning
    4. hypotension

76. The liver functions to
    1. metabolize fat
    2. detoxify harmful substances
    3. manufacture bile
    4. all of the above

77. Which are the smallest microbes?
    1. viruses
    2. fungi
    3. bacteria
    4. algae

78. What do all microbes have in common?
    1. nucleic acid
    2. they are parasitic
    3. chloroplasts
    4. they cause disease

79. Some common shapes of bacteria are
    A. square
    B. round
    C. rods
    D. corkscrew
    E. triangular
       1. A, B, and D
       2. B, C, and D
       3. B, D, and E
       4. C, D, and E

80. Normal fungi found in the mouth include
    1. pyogenes
    2. molds
    3. yeasts
    4. all of the above

81. A medium often used to colonize bacteria is
    1. saliva
    2. urine
    3. agar
    4. dextrose

82. Exotoxins refer to
    1. chemicals secreted by viruses to kill bacteria
    2. intercellular materials produced by liver cells
    3. growth requirements of bacteria
    4. toxic chemicals secreted by bacteria

83. Viruses contain
    A. nuclei
    B. ribosomes
    C. mitochondria
    D. DNA
       1. A, B, and C
       2. A and C
       3. B and D
       4. D only

84. Bactericidal refers to
    1. inhibiting bacterial growth
    2. bacteria in the blood stream
    3. killing bacteria
    4. the effect of bacteria on people

85. A protective nongrowing form of a micro-organism is referred to as a(n)
    1. spore
    2. crypt
    3. egg
    4. virus

86. What becomes contaminated in the dental operatory with each operation?
    1. windows
    2. reception area
    3. floor
    4. all surfaces that come in contact with any microbes from the patient's mouth

87. Who can become infected from contaminated instruments?
    1. the dentist
    2. the dental assistant
    3. the patient
    4. any of the above

88. Instruments are washed before being autoclaved
    1. to prevent rusting
    2. to prevent debris from harboring microbes
    3. to kill any spores
    4. none of the above

89. The ultrasonic cleaner is used to
    1. sterilize handpieces
    2. clean instruments
    3. sterilize instruments
    4. pasteurize fluids

90. If carbon steel instruments are autoclaved, the instruments
    1. will melt
    2. may rust
    3. will be contaminated
    4. will turn green

91. The most effective way to kill microbes is
    1. cold sterilization
    2. boiling
    3. autoclaving
    4. ultraviolet light

92. The instrument best cleaned with 70% alcohol swabs is a(n)
    1. amalgam plugger
    2. air and water syringe
    3. rubber dam clamp
    4. suture needle

93. How can you tell whether a package of instruments has been autoclaved?
    1. temperature-sensitive tape will turn color
    2. instruments are a different color after being autoclaved
    3. the autoclave bags are left open
    4. instruments feel warm

94. Sterilization by autoclave requires what temperature?
    1. 175°C
    2. 121°C
    3. 250°C
    4. 163°C

95. Which materials are best sterilized by autoclaving?
    A. gauze pads
    B. stainless steel hand instruments
    C. handpieces
    D. glass slabs
    E. carbon steel instruments
    F. plastic head-rest covers
    1. A, B, and C
    2. A, B, and D
    3. B, D, and E
    4. D, E, and F

96. Carbon steel instruments are best sterilized by
    1. dry heat
    2. autoclaving
    3. disinfectants
    4. flaming

97. At what temperature are instruments dry-heat sterilized?
    1. 120°–130°C
    2. 212°–240°C
    3. 160°–175°C
    4. 100°–120°C

98. A surgical mask can be used during a dental operation to
    1. avoid odors of various dental materials
    2. protect the patient from inhaling the aerosol created by the high-speed handpiece
    3. protect the operator from inhaling the aerosol created by the high-speed handpiece
    4. avoid the use of high-speed evacuation

99. Which of the following pieces of equipment should be disinfected after treatment of each patient?
    A. handpieces
    B. curettes
    C. light handles
    D. scalpels
    E. chair switches
    F. needles

1. A, C, and D
2. A, C, and E
3. A, E, and F
4. C, E, and F

100. Which microbes can be found in the oral cavity?
    1. bacteria
    2. fungi
    3. viruses
    4. all of the above

101. A person who harbors a disease without feeling its effect is called a
    1. retainer
    2. transmitter
    3. carrier
    4. neophyte

102. Which diseases can be caused by contaminated dental instruments?
    A. trumatic bone cysts
    B. syphilis
    C. ANUG
    D. thrush
    E. hepatitis
       1. A, B, and D
       2. A, C, and D
       3. B, D, and E
       4. C, D, and E

103. Which of the following chemicals is/are used to disinfect instruments?
    A. 70% ethyl alcohol
    B. warm water
    C. eugenol
    D. quaternary ammonium salts
    E. chloroform
       1. A and C
       2. A and D
       3. B and D
       4. C and E

104. The effectiveness of a disinfectant solution is altered by the
    1. number of instruments
    2. dilution of water
    3. room temperature
    4. number of bacteria on the instruments

105. How long should instruments be left in disinfectant solutions before they are ready to be used again?
    1. 30 minutes
    2. 1 hour
    3. 2 hours
    4. 1 day

106. Conditions in an autoclave for effective sterilization include

A. a temperature of 121°C
B. 15–25 pounds of pressure
C. a minimum time of 10–20 minutes
D. ultraviolet light
   1. A, B, and C
   2. A and C
   3. B and D
   4. D only
   5. all of the above

107. Rubber gloves and rubber dams are best sterilized by
    1. quaternary ammonium salts
    2. boiling water
    3. autoclaving
    4. flaming

108. Which of the following is/are used for sterilization?
    A. silver nitrate
    B. gas
    C. alcohol
    D. boiling water
    E. hot glass beads
       1. A, B, and D
       2. B, C, and E
       3. B, D, and E
       4. C, D, and E

109. Mouthwashes are used to
    1. sterilize the mouth
    2. remove plaque
    3. freshen the breath
    4. disinfect the mouth

110. The passage of an infectious microbe from one patient to another is called
    1. plague
    2. rehosting
    3. microbe transfer
    4. cross-infection

111. Bad breath is usually caused by
    1. constipation
    2. a diet high in carbohydrates
    3. odiferous materials in the mouth
    4. insufficient fluids

112. The type of administration that allows the drug the fastest onset is
    1. intramuscular
    2. subcutaneous
    3. intravenous
    4. sublingual

113. Before prescribing any drug
    1. an accurate medical history must be taken
    2. a Snyder test should be performed

3. a complete blood count should be performed
4. a urinalysis should be performed

114. Various methods of drug administration are
     A. intradermal
     B. retroperitoneal
     C. intraradicular
     D. intramuscular
     E. sublingual
        1. A, B, and D
        2. A, D, and E
        3. B, C, and D
        4. C, D, and E

115. Some drugs cannot be taken orally because
     1. they are in liquid form
     2. saliva will dilute them
     3. the enamel will corrode
     4. the digestive system will alter the drug

116. Parental administration of drugs include
     A. subcutaneous
     B. intramuscular
     C. intravenous
     D. intradermal
        1. A, B, and C
        2. A and C
        3. B and D
        4. D only
        5. all of the above

117. When determining the dosage of a drug to be prescribed, an important consideration is the patient's
     1. weight
     2. height
     3. head size
     4. appetite

118. When two drugs have a combined effect greater than the sum of the individual drug taken alone, it is known as
     1. additive
     2. synergism
     3. parasitism
     4. combination

119. If two drugs have a combined effect less than the sum of the individual drugs, it is referred to as
     1. cumulation
     2. summation
     3. desensitization
     4. drug antagonism

120. The condition that necessitates increasing the amount of a drug needed to receive the same effect is called
     1. summation

2. tolerance
3. cumulation
4. combination

121. Various sources of drugs are
     A. electricity
     B. animals
     C. plants
     D. sand
     E. synthetic matcrials
        1. A, B, and C
        2. B, C, and D
        3. B, C, and E
        4. C, D, and E

122. The administration of an excess amount of a drug is known as
     1. an overdose
     2. an overkill
     3. hyperactivation
     4. hypokinesis

123. A written direction to a pharmacist to prepare a drug is called
     1. a prescription
     2. an order blank
     3. a slip
     4. a label

124. The abbreviation q4h means
     1. every 4 days
     2. 4 times a day
     3. every 4 hours
     4. for 4 days

125. Which member of the dental team is responsible for writing drug orders?
     1. dentist
     2. hygienist
     3. assistant
     4. receptionist

126. Which federal agency ensures public safety in relation to drugs?
     1. Federal Safety Commission
     2. Food and Drug Administration
     3. National Health Commission
     4. American Medical Association

127. Antihistamines are used to
     1. delay the effects of a narcotic
     2. premedicate and allay fears
     3. enhance the effects of antibiotics
     4. counteract allergic reactions

128. Tranquilizers are
     1. used in dentistry before root canal therapy
     2. used in dentistry after any surgical procedure

3. used in dentistry whenever antibiotics are used
4. almost never used in dentistry

129. Some analgesics used in dentistry are
A. aspirin
B. codeine
C. acetaminophen
D. phenobarbital
   1. A, B, and C
   2. A and C
   3. B and D
   4. D only
   5. all are correct

130. The type of drug most commonly used to premedicate an anxious patient is
   1. a barbiturate
   2. meperidine
   3. an antibiotic
   4. chloral hydrate

131. The condition that exists when a drug becomes necessary and its discontinuance would cause mental or physical changes is termed
   1. summation
   2. addiction
   3. addition
   4. cumulation

132. Barbiturates are classified according to the
   1. number of milligrams
   2. color of the pill
   3. duration of action
   4. speed of onset

133. The same drug can have various uses, depending on
   1. the method of administration
   2. how it is excreted
   3. the dosage
   4. how the drug is absorbed

134. Alcohol is a(n)
   1. hormone
   2. diuretic
   3. central nervous system depressant
   4. enzyme used in respiration

135. Caffeine is a(n)
   1. depressant
   2. tranquilizer
   3. stimulant
   4. irritant

136. Lidocaine is a
A. barbiturate
B. narcotic
C. general anesthetic
D. local anesthetic
   1. A, B, and C
   2. A and C
   3. B and D only
   4. D only
   5. all are correct

137. A drug used to prevent epileptic attacks is
   1. ampicillin
   2. a tranquilizer
   3. Dilantin
   4. monoamine oxidase

138. Addictive analgesic drugs are known as
   1. narcotics
   2. antihistamines
   3. tranquilizers
   4. stimulants

139. A placebo is a(n)
   1. substance given for psychological effect
   2. antihistamine
   3. stimulant
   4. depressant

140. Some common barbiturates used in dentistry are
A. nitrous oxide
B. secobarbital
C. phenobarbital
D. pentobarbital
E. meperidine
   1. A, B, and D
   2. B, C, and D
   3. B, C, and E
   4. C, D, and E

141. Some narcotics used in dentistry are
A. codeine
B. Tylenol
C. meperidine
D. morphine
E. aspirin
   1. A, B, and C
   2. A, C, and D
   3. B, D, and E
   4. C, D, and E

142. The most commonly used analgesic is
   1. codeine
   2. aspirin
   3. meperidine
   4. morphine

143. Some patients cannot take aspirin because of
   1. a previous heart attack
   2. the gastrointestinal irritation
   3. the production of gas pains
   4. the severe headaches it causes

144. The condition in which a patient lacks oxygen is called
    1. hyperventilation
    2. hypoxia
    3. anoxia
    4. none of the above

145. An alternative drug to aspirin is
    1. a tranquilizer
    2. secobarbital
    3. caffeine
    4. acetaminophen

146. The most commonly used local anesthetic is
    1. Novocain
    2. Xylocaine
    3. Carbocaine
    4. cocaine

147. Epinephrine in local anesthesia causes
    1. increased uptake of the anesthetic by blood vessels
    2. hyperventilation
    3. prolonged effects of the anesthetic
    4. none of the above

148. Under which circumstance would local anesthesia most likely be ineffective?
    1. a toothache in the mandibular premolar area
    2. injection in an inflamed area
    3. injection in elderly patients
    4. injection in a diabetic patient

149. An antibiotic is a drug
    1. produced by a microorganism that destroys other microorganisms
    2. that inhibits viruses
    3. used only for pulmonary infections
    4. that increases circulation

150. The antibiotic of choice for oral infections is
    1. penicillin
    2. streptomycin
    3. sulfa
    4. tetracycline

151. The function of a hemostatic agent is to
    1. thicken the blood
    2. thin the blood
    3. stop bleeding
    4. increase the number of blood platelets in the circulating blood

152. Which antibiotic can cause staining of a child's primary teeth if it is taken by a pregnant woman during her last trimester of pregnancy?
    1. tetracycline
    2. penicillin
    3. erythromycin
    4. streptomycin

153. The use of drugs in cancer therapy is called
    1. radiotherapy
    2. electrocautery
    3. chemotherapy
    4. psychotherapy

154. Having a patient bite on a moist tea bag can
    1. alleviate pain
    2. help stop bleeding
    3. cause a dry socket
    4. impede the clot formation

155. Hydrogen peroxide can be used as a(n)
    1. hemostatic agent
    2. anodyne
    3. oxidizing mouthwash
    4. treatment for herpetic lesions

156. Which of the following drugs are applied topically?
    A. fluoride
    B. penicillin
    C. anesthetic agents
    D. iodine
    E. tetracycline
        1. A, B, and E
        2. A, C, and D
        3. B, C, and D
        4. C, D, and E

157. Drugs that reduce fever are
    1. antiemetics
    2. antihistamines
    3. hypertensives
    4. antipyretics

158. A common drug used in the dental office to decrease anxiety is
    1. nitrous oxide–oxygen
    2. caffeine
    3. aspirin
    4. benzocaine

159. Ethyl chloride can be used as a(n)
    1. general anesthetic
    2. inhalant
    3. topical anesthetic
    4. antiemetic

Answers and Explanations

1. **1** Histology is the microscopic study of tissue anatomy.

2. **2** Genetics is the study of heredity.

3. **4** Embryology is the study of the human organism developing in the uterus.

4. **3** Solubility refers to the amount of a substance, the solute, that can be dissolved in a solvent. For example, salt, the solute, may be dissolved in warm water, the solvent.

5. **1** The three states of matter that exist in nature are solid, liquid, and gas.

6. **3** As the state of matter changes from solid to liquid to gas, the molecular movement is increased. An example is the state of hydrocolloid. The solid state (gel), when heated, causes the molecules to move faster, resulting in a liquid state (sol).

7. **2** Some examples of the use of electricity in dentistry are powering the dental unit, pulp testing, electroplating, and electrosurgery.

8. **2** 1°F is a measurement unit lower than 1°C.

9. **3** Metabolism is the combined process catabolism (breakdown of body materials) and anabolism (buildup of body materials). Growth is dependent on the anabolic reactions exceeding the catabolic reactions.

10. **1** Cells involved in the production, maintenance, and resorption of bone are osteoblasts, osteocytes, and osteoclasts, respectively. Osteoblasts produce a prebony matrix that is then calcified. They then become osteocytes, which are responsible for maintaining bone. Osteoclasts cause the resorption of bone by secreting enzymes that dissolve the bony matrix.

11. **2** Mitochondria are responsible for cellular respiration and production of energy.

12. **4** Ribosomes, small cytoplasmic organelles, are involved in protein synthesis.

13. **3** Nerve tissue has the poorest regenerative capability of any tissue. A severed nerve may regenerate only if its nerve body is not injured.

14. **2** Bone marrow functions to form red blood cells, some white blood cells, and platelets and to destroy old red blood cells.

15. **3** The axial skeleton consists of the head, neck, vertebrae, ribs, and sternum.

16. **1** The vertebrae consist of the cervical, thoracic, and lumbar vertebrae, the sacrum, and the coccyx.

17. **2** Most ribs are attached to the spinal column and the sternum, forming the thorax. The function of the thorax is to protect the heart and lungs and to aid in respiration.

18. **2** A joint is the junction of bones. The types of joints are synarthroses, which do not move, such as those found in the skull; amphiarthroses, those with limited movements, such as those between vertebrae; and diarthroses, the most mobile, such as the temporomandibular joint.

19. **4** A suture is a type of joint that does not move.

20. **1** The three types of muscle tissue are striated (or voluntary), smooth or involuntary, and cardiac.

21. **4** Muscle tissue is present in all body systems including the circulatory, in vessel walls and the heart; the digestive, in the oral cavity and in the wall along the entire length of the tract; and the respiratory, in the diaphragm and intercostal muscles.

22. **1** Tendons are made up of fibrous tissue that attaches skeletal muscle to bone. Ligaments are fibrous tissues that attach bone to bone, limiting movement.

23. **3** Fatigue is the condition in which the ability of a muscle to contract is impaired. It is caused by the accumulation of lactic acid, which is removed by respiration.

24. **3** The simplest type of reflex is the stimulation of an afferent neuron, which transmits an impulse to an efferent neuron, which stimulates an effector to respond voluntarily to the initial stimulation. An example of this is the jerking of a hand from a hot object.

25. **4** Coughing is a protective reflex that attempts to remove an irritating substance from the respiratory tract.

26. **3** A nerve impulse is transmitted from the axon of one nerve to the dendrite of the next nerve over a synaptic junction. The transmission is caused by a chemical released from the axon that can excite or inhibit the next neuron.

27. **1** A neuron (nerve cell) is composed of dendrites, which are fibers that lead impulses toward the cell body (perikaryon), and an axon, which

contains fibers that transmit impulses away from the cell body.

28. **2** The central nervous system is protected by tough coverings called the meninges. The meninges are made up of three membranes: the dura mater, the arachnoid, and the pia mater.

29. **2** The brain can be divided into three parts: the hindbrain, including the medulla oblongata, pons, and cerebellum; the midbrain; and the forebrain, including the cerebrum, thalmus, and hypothalamus.

30. **1** Cranial nerves responsible for eye movements are abducens, trochlear, and oculomotor nerves. The optic nerve is a cranial nerve responsible for sight.

31. **1** Neurons can be classified as motor or efferent, which conduct impulses away from the central nervous system; sensory or afferent, which conduct impulses toward the central nervous system; and internuncial, which connect sensory and motor neurons.

32. **2** Involuntary nervous control of the body is mediated through the autonomic nervous system. This system attempts to maintain homeostasis in the body. It is further broken down into the sympathetic and parasympathetic divisions. The sympathetic is most active during times of stress, and the parasympathetic is most active during quieter times.

33. **4** The hypoglossal nerve controls tongue movement.

34. **3** The acoustic nerve controls balance.

35. **4** A foreign object flying into an assistant's eye could scratch the cornea. This type of injury might cause visual impairment and pain. Wearing safety glasses would prevent such injuries.

36. **2** Endocrine glands produce chemical mediators called hormones. Hormones are proteins distributed via the circulatory system.

37. **2** The endocrine glands are the pituitary, thyroid, gonads, parathyroid, adrenals, pancreas, and pineal.

38. **1** Epinephrine is produced by the medullary portion of the adrenal glands during times of stress. It increases the heart rate, constricts most arterioles, and increases the blood pressure. The effects of epinephrine are similar to the effects of the sympathetic division of the autonomic nervous system.

39. **2** The primary female hormones include estrogen and progesterone, which play an important role in the female reproductive system.

40. **4** Diabetes mellitus is caused by the lack, or inactivity, of the hormone insulin. Insulin functions to lower blood sugar by causing its conversion to glycogen and causing its uptake by cells.

41. **4** The passage of the respiratory tract is nose ⟶ pharynx ⟶ larynx ⟶ trachea ⟶ bronchi ⟶ bronchioles ⟶ alveolar duct ⟶ alveolar sac.

42. **3** In the lungs gaseous exchange takes place between the alveoli and the pulmonary capillaries. Gases diffuse from areas of higher concentration to areas of lower concentration; therefore oxygen, which has a higher concentration in the lungs, diffuses into the blood and carbon dioxide, which has a higher concentration in the blood, diffuses into the alveoli. Blood reaching the cells has a higher concentration of oxygen; therefore, the oxygen will diffuse into the cell. The cell has a higher concentration of carbon dioxide, and the carbon dioxide will therefore diffuse into the blood.

43. **4** The epiglottis prevents solids and liquids from entering the respiratory system, by closing the entrance of the larynx.

44. **2** Inspiration is caused by expansion of the pleural cavity. This is accomplished by the constriction of the diaphragm and the intercostal muscles, causing the alveoli to expand and create a vacuum. Expiration is the reverse of inspiration.

45. **3** Blood transports gases, hormones, nutrients, waste products, and infection-fighting components.

46. **4** Large veins contain valves to stop the backflow of blood. Valves are most commonly found in veins of the extremities. If the valves are not able to stop the backflow of blood the veins become dilated and are known as varicose veins.

47. **3** Hemoglobin is a red pigment in red blood cells that transports oxygen to cells and helps remove carbon dioxide from cells.

48. **1** Leukocytes, also known as white blood cells, function as a protection against infection. There are two groups of leukocytes: granular and nongranular. Leukocytes are transported to the area in which they are needed by blood vessels. They then leave the circulatory system and move to the area of infection to begin the reparative process.

49. **2** Plasma is made up of 90% water. The other 10% includes proteins, glucose, fats, wastes, dissolved gases, hormones, enzymes, and many other components.

50. **4** The sequence in blood clotting is:
    a. broken blood vessels ⟶ breakdown of platelets ⟶ platelet factors
    b. platelet factors + antihemophilic factor ⟶ thromboplastin
    c. prothrombin + thromboplastin ⟶ thrombin
    d. fibrinogen + thrombin ⟶ fibrin

51. **4** The heart is composed of four chambers: two atria and two ventricles. The atria have thinner walls and are collecting chambers, receiving blood from the body and the lungs. The ventricles contain more muscle tissue and pump the blood to the lungs and the body.

52. **5** Heart tissue is made up of muscles (cardiac), epithelium (pericardium), nervous, and connective tissue.

53. **3** The aorta conducts the blood from the left ventricle of the heart to the body. The aorta may be divided into the following parts: ascending aorta, aortic arch, thoracic aorta and abdominal aorta.

54. **2** Heart valves are used to regulate the flow of blood through the heart and prevent blood from flowing backward.

55. **1** Diastolic blood pressure is the pressure exerted by blood on the walls of arteries when the heart is at rest. Systolic blood pressure is the pressure exerted on the walls of arteries when the heart contracts. In healthy young adults the average blood pressure is 120/80.

56. **2** The arterial pulse normally indicates the number of times the heart is contracting. Other characteristics of the pulse, such as rhythm and strength, are indications of the cardiac condition.

57. **3** Lymph nodes function to filter lymph and to produce lymphocytes and antibodies.

58. **2** Lymph moves from smaller to larger vessels and eventually enters the venous system. The function of the lymphatic system is to return to the bloodstream water, proteins and products of cellular metabolism not previously picked up by the bloodstream.

59. **3** The enzyme ptyalin, contained in the saliva, begins the digestion of starch.

60. **4** The movement of food in the digestive tract is caused by peristalsis. The amount of peristalsis is controlled by the autonomic nervous system. Parasympathetic control increases the amount of peristalsis and sympathetic control decreases the amount of peristalsis.

61. **2** Absorption of most nutrients occurs in the small intestine. The surface area of the small intestine is greatly enlarged by the number of surface projections called villi.

62. **3** The function of the large intestine is to absorb water.

63. **2** Proteins are made up of amino acids. There are about 20 amino acids that act as building blocks for proteins. Proteins are used by the body as building structures, enzymes, hormones and a source of energy if needed.

64. **3** Water composes 50–70% of human body weight. Some functions of water in the body are to serve as a solvent, allow chemical reactions to occur, ionize chemicals, and regulate body temperature.

65. **3** Chromosomes are made up of genes, which carry the hereditary message. Genes are made of deoxyribonucleic acid (DNA).

66. **4** The union of an egg and sperm is known as fertilization, which occurs in the fallopian tubes. The fertilized egg is known as a zygote.

67. **1** Congenital refers to a condition that exists at or before birth. Some common congenital defects of the oral cavity are missing teeth, alterations in the enamel and dentin, cleft palate, and many facial defects.

68. **2** Cleft palate and anodontia (absence of teeth) are both dental abnormalities caused by genetic disorders.

69. **4** Hemophilia is a hereditary disease in males that results in prolonged bleeding. The body is not able to produce the antihemophilic factor needed in the clotting mechanism.

70. **3** The organs of the excretory system are the skin, which removes water, minerals and nitrogenous wastes; the lungs, which remove water and carbon dioxide; the digestive tract, which removes solid nondigestible material and some water; and the urinary system, which removes water, toxins, nitrogenous wastes, and minerals.

71. **2** Organs included in the respiratory system are nose, nasopharynx, pharynx, larynx, trachea, bronchi, and lungs, which include bronchioles and alveoli.

72. **2** The urinary system consists of two kidneys, which produce urine; two ureters, which transport it from the kidneys to the bladder; the urinary bladder, which stores it; and the urethra, through which urination occurs.

73. **3** The lungs are considered a part of the respiratory system by the exchange of gases and the excretory system by expelling waste products (primarily carbon dioxide and water vapor).

74. **1** Structures of the eye include the ciliary body which is made up of smooth muscle causing contraction of the lens for accomodation. The action of the ciliary body enables a person to focus on either distant objects or very close objects. The cornea is a transparent covering of the exposed portion of the eye.

75. **1** Bacteria in freshly drawn urine could indicate an infection in the urinary tract and should be further investigated. Other abnormal constitutents of the urine that are indications of problems are blood, pus, albumin, and large amounts of glucose.

76. **4** The liver functions to metabolize fats, carbohydrates, and proteins; to produce bile and blood proteins; to detoxify harmful substances; to produce body heat; and to store vitamins.

77. **1** Viruses, the smallest microbes, are composed of DNA or RNA in a protein coat. Viruses are cuboidal, spherical, elongated, or tadpole-like. Some diseases caused by viruses are herpes simplex, infectious and serum hepatitis, rabies, influenza, and poliomyelitis.

78. **1** All living organisms have nucleic acids, either DNA or RNA. Without nucleic acid it would be impossible to reproduce.

79. **2** Some shapes of bacteria are round (cocci), rodlike (bacilli), and corkscrew (spirochetes).

80. **3** *Candida albicans*, a yeast, is a common inhabitant of the oral cavity. It normally exists in a state of balance with other microbes. If this balance is disrupted, *Candida albicans* can cause a condition called thrush.

81. **3** Some culturing media are agar, blood, and other tissues.

82. **4** Exotoxins are poisons excreted by microbes into the surrounding medium. Three diseases caused by exotoxins are tetanus, botulism, and diphtheria.

83. **4** Viruses do not contain nuclei but do contain DNA. Ribosomes are involved in protein synthesis and mitochondria are involved in energy production in more sophisticated forms of life than viruses.

84. **3** Bactericidal refers to killing bacteria. Bacteriostatic refers to inhibiting bacterial growth. Bacteremia is the presence of bacteria in the bloodstream.

85. **1** Spores are a protective bacterial form. Some bacteria assume this form under unfavorable conditions. When conditions are again favorable the bacteria will emerge from its cystic form and begin to grow again.

86. **4** All surfaces in the operatory that come in contact with microbes from the patient's mouth become contaminated—including instruments, equipment, and people.

87. **4** The dentist, dental assistant and/or patient can become infected from contaminated instruments. Every effort should be made to have instruments as microbe free as possible by sterilization and disinfection.

88. **2** Instruments must be thoroughly washed before any sterilization technique is employed. Debris not removed could harbor bacteria and insulate them from the bactericidal effect of the sterilization technique.

89. **2** Ultrasonic cleaners can be used to clean instruments instead of washing by hand. The cleaned instruments are then sterilized.

90. **2** If carbon steel instruments are autoclaved, the steam can cause them to rust.

91. **3** Autoclaving, steam under pressure, is the most effective way to kill microbes. The heat from the steam sterilizes the instruments.

92. **2** Alcohol disinfection is often used when instruments cannot be heat sterilized or conveniently detached, such as the air–water syringe. Most other instruments can be heat sterilized.

93. **1** A thermochromatic indicator, tape, part of the sterilization package, will change color after it has been autoclaved.

94. **2** Autoclaves are most frequently operated at 121°C for 15–20 minutes at 15 pounds of pressure.

95. **2** Materials can be placed in the autoclave if they do not rust, melt, have to remain sharp, or are otherwise not adversely affected by moist heat. Materials commonly autoclaved are stainless steel instruments, materials such as gauze and cotton, rubber dams, rubber gloves, and glass slabs.

96. **1** Carbon steel instruments are best sterilized by dry heat. This procedure will avoid rusting and dulling of sharp edges.

97. **3** Dry heat sterilization takes place at temperatures between 160° to 175°C for approximately 1 hour. Sterilization of large loads will require longer periods.

98. **3** When using a high-speed handpiece, an aerosol is created that consists of water spray, saliva, microbes from the patient's mouth, and debris (e.g., tooth, filling material). The aerosol could cause respiratory infections or traumatic eye injuries to the operator, assistant, or patient. The use of a surgical mask will avoid the inhalation of the aerosol. Protective glasses will prevent eye injuries from flying debris.

99. **2** The following pieces of equipment should be disinfected after treatment of each patient: handpieces, light handles, chair switches, air–water syringe, countertops, and chair head rest.

100. **4** Microbes found in the oral cavity include bacteria, fungi, viruses, and protozoa.

101. **3** A person who harbors a disease without feeling its effect is a carrier. It might be a person who has never had symptoms of the disease or a person recovering from the disease. A carrier can transmit the disease to other people.

102. **3** Some diseases that can be caused by contaminated dental instruments are syphilis, hepatitis, thrush, skin infections, abscesses,

rheumatic fever, subacute bacterial endocarditis, aphthous ulcers, pneumonia, and tuberculosis.

103. **2** The following chemicals can be used as disinfectants: quaternary ammoninum compounds, 70% ethyl alcohol, formaldehyde, and phenolic compounds.

104. **2** The effectiveness of a disinfectant solution is altered by dilution. Wet instruments placed in disinfectant solution will dilute the concentration; the solution will not kill the organisms it is capable of killing in its correct concentration.

105. **1** Instruments should be left in disinfectant solutions for 30 minutes before they are used again. If a 30-minute cycle is disrupted by the addition of another instrument, the cycle is started all over again.

106. **1** For effective sterilization, materials should be autoclaved for 10–20 minutes at a temperature of 121°C under 15–20 pounds of pressure. Ultraviolet light is not involved in autoclaving.

107. **3** Autoclaving is the most effective method of killing microorganisms; therefore any material that would not be adversely affected by steam heat would be best sterilized by autoclaving.

108. **3** Some methods of sterilization are gas, boiling water, hot glass beads, dry heat, and autoclaving.

109. **3** Mouthwashes are used to freshen the breath for a short time. The mechanical action of rinsing initially decreases the number of bacteria, but it quickly returns to its previous levels.

110. **4** The passage of an infectious microbe from one patient to another is called cross-infection. This is an indirect transmission of disease and may take the following route in dentistry: patient's mouth ⟶ hand instruments ⟶ another patient's mouth.

111. **3** Bad breath is a problem the cause of which is usually localized in the mouth. Frequent and thorough cleaning of the oral cavity will alleviate the problem.

112. **3** Intravenous drug administration has the fastest onset. An intravenous injection introduces the drug directly into the bloodstream. This method is also used to infuse a large amount of fluid into the body.

113. **1** Before prescribing any drugs, an accurate medical history must be taken. Some factors in a patient's history that can influence drug administration are a history of drug allergies, other drugs the patient might be taking, and physical and mental states.

114. **2** Various methods of drug administration are oral, sublingual, inhalation, topical, rectal, and parenteral.

115. **4** Some drugs taken orally might not be absorbed or effective and/or could irritate the lining of the stomach.

116. **5** Parenteral administration of drugs refers to administration in areas of the body other than the digestive system and includes subcutaneous, intradermal, intramuscular, and intravenous administration.

117. **1** When determining dosage, important considerations are the patient's weight, other drugs the patient is taking, route of administration, the disease entity, and past experience the patient has had with the drug.

118. **2** Synergism is the condition that exists when two drugs have a combined effect greater than the sum of the individual drug.

119. **4** Drug antagonism is the condition that exists when two drugs have a combined effect less than the sum of the individual drugs.

120. **2** Tolerance, also called drug resistance, is a condition existing in a patient that necessitates an increase in the dosage of a drug to produce the same effect.

121. **3** The sources of drugs are animal (insulin, adrenalin), plant (opium), mineral (zinc oxide), and synthetic (ampicillin).

122. **1** The administration of an excessive amount of a drug is known as an overdose. The result of an overdose can range from mild toxicity to death.

123. **1** A prescription is a written direction to a pharmacist to prepare a drug. A prescription includes the following information: doctor's name, address and telephone number; patient's name, address and age; date; drug name and dosage; quantity of the drug; directions for use; and doctor's signature and DEA (narcotic registration number).

124. **3** Some common Latin abbreviations are q4h (every 4 hours), qid (4 times a day), prn (as needed), and ac (before meals).

125. **1** The dentist is responsible for prescribing drugs.

126. **2** The Food and Drug Administration is responsible for ensuring public safety in relationship to drugs. Manufacturers of a new drug must prove that the drug is safe and effective before it can be used by the public.

127. **4** Antihistamines are used to treat allergic reactions. A common side effect of these drugs is drowsiness.

128. **4** Tranquilizers are rarely used in dentistry. These drugs are used for their long-range sedating effects.

129. **1** Aspirin and acetaminophin are commonly prescribed for mild to moderate pain following dental treatment. Codeine is an analgesic used for more severe pain.

130. **1** The drug most commonly used to premedicate an anxious patient is a barbiturate.

131. **2** Addiction is the condition existing in a patient where a drug, after repeated use, becomes needed by the body and its cessation would cause mental or physical changes. Addiction includes developing tolerance to the drug being used.

132. **3** Barbiturates are classified according to the duration of action: ultrashort acting, short acting (secobarbital, pentobarbital), intermediate acting, and long acting (phenobarbital).

133. **3** The same drug can have various uses, depending on the dosage. Barbiturates can act as a sedative, hypnotic, or anesthetic, depending on the dose.

134. **3** Alcohol is a central nervous system depressant. There is no use in dentistry for alcohol that is imbibed.

135. **3** Caffeine is a central nervous system stimulant. Side effects of caffeine include stimulation of respiration and the myocardium.

136. **4** Lidocaine is the most common local anesthesia used in dentistry.

137. **3** A drug used to prevent epileptic attacks is diphenylhydantoin (Dilantin). A side effect of this drug is fibrous hyperplasia of the gingiva.

138. **1** Addictive analgesic drugs are narcotics. Care must be taken when these drugs are prescribed, since they can become physiologically habit forming.

139. **1** A placebo is a substance usually thought to be an effective drug by the patient, but that actually has no physical effect.

140. **2** Some common barbiturates used in dentistry are secobarbital, pentobarbital, and phenobarbital.

141. **2** The most common narcotics used in dentistry are codeine, meperidine, and morphine.

142. **2** The most commonly used analgesic is aspirin. Aspirin also functions as an antirheumatic, antipyretic, and anti-inflammatory agent.

143. **2** Some patients claim to have adverse gastrointestinal effects after the ingestion of aspirin. Stomach ulcers have been induced in animals with salicylates.

144. **3** Anoxia is the condition in which a patient lacks oxygen. In the past, nitrous oxide alone was used as a general anesthetic. In some cases this resulted in loss of consciousness caused by anoxia. Subsequently, oxygen was used in conjunction with nitrous oxide as a controlling mechanism to provide an adequate amount of oxygen.

145. **4** Some mild analgesics substituted for aspirin are phenacetin, acetaminophen (Tylenol), and propoxyphene hydrochloride (Darvon).

146. **2** The most commonly used local anesthetic is lidocaine (Xylocaine). Local anesthetics can be classified into four groups: para-aminobenzoic acid, meta-aminobenzoic acid, benzoic acid, and amides.

147. **3** Epinephrine in local anesthesia causes prolonged effects of anesthesia. Epinephrine is a vasoconstrictor; it decreases the size of the blood vessels, hence a decrease of the circulation in the area, and the anesthetic remains active for a longer period of time.

148. **2** Local anesthetics are injected as acids and require the basic pH of the body tissues to become effective. An inflamed area has an acidic pH value and thereby would not activate the anesthetic.

149. **1** An antibiotic is a drug produced by a microorganism that destroys bacteria. Commonly used antibiotics are penicillin, erythromycin, tetracycline, streptomycin, bacitracin, and chloramphenicol.

150. **1** The antibiotic of choice in oral infections is penicillin. It is most active against gram-positive bacteria and it is this type of bacteria that causes most oral infections. Penicillin is also administered prophylactically to prevent infection in patients who have a heart problem.

151. **3** Hemostatic agents stop bleeding by aiding the normal clotting mechanism. Examples of hemostatic agents used in dentistry are absorbable gelatin sponges, absorbable oxidized cellulose, and alum.

152. **1** Tetracycline taken at the time of enamel formation may result in staining of the enamel. Enamel formation takes place during the last trimester of pregnancy through early childhood.

153. **3** The use of drugs in cancer therapy is called chemotherapy. Other modes of treatment for cancer are surgery and radiation.

154. **2** A moist tea bag can stop bleeding due to the tannic acid contained in the tea. Other chemicals used to stop bleeding are thrombin, copper sulfate, epinephrine, and hemostatics.

155. **3** Hydrogen peroxide diluted with water can be used as an oxidizing mouthwash. It is also used as an irrigant in root canal therapy.

156. **2** Drugs applied topically in dentistry include fluoride, anesthetic agents, and Orabase. These

drugs are usually applied intraorally. Iodine and bacitracin can be topically applied externally.

157. **4** Drugs that reduce fever are known as antipyretics. The best known and most widely used antipyretic is aspirin.

158. **1** Nitrous oxide–oxygen is often used as a sedative in the dental office. It is applied to a patient through a nose mask. The sedative effects are eliminated at the end of the procedure by giving the patient pure oxygen.

159. **3** Ethyl chloride can be used as a topical anesthetic. It temporarily freezes the area to which it is applied.

Bibliography

Alexander, G. and Alexander, D.G. *Biology,* 9th ed. New York: Harper & Row Publishers Inc., 1970.

Anthony, C.P. and Thibodeau, G.A. *Basic Concepts in Anatomy and Physiology; A Programmed Presentation,* 4th ed. St. Louis: The C. V. Mosby Co., 1979.

Anthony, C.P. and Thibodeau, G.A. *Structure and Function of the Body,* 6th ed. St. Louis: The C. V. Mosby Co., 1980.

Chen, P.S. *Chemistry: Inorganic, Organic and Biological,* 2nd ed. New York: Harper & Row Publishers Inc., 1980.

Goss, C.M. *Gray's Anatomy,* 29th ed. Philadelphia: Lea & Febiger Publishers, 1973.

Goth, A. *Medical Pharmacology,* 10th ed. St. Louis: The C. V. Mosby Co., 1981.

Ham, A.W. *Histology,* 8th ed. Philadelphia: J. B. Lippincott Co., 1979.

Jawetz, E., et al. *Review of Medical Microbiology,* 12th ed. Los Altos, Calif.: Lange Medical Publications, 1976.

Keeton, W.T. *Biological Science,* 3rd ed. New York: W. W. Norton and Co., 1980.

Miller, F. *College Physics,* 5th ed. New York: Harcourt Brace Jovanovich, Inc., 1982.

Ross, G. *Essentials of Human Physiology,* Chicago: Year Book Medical Publishers Inc., 1978.

2

Oral Anatomy and Oral Pathology

Course Synopsis

Introduction

A dental assistant must be aware of the fundamentals of oral anatomy, dental anatomy, and oral pathology. This chapter presents the basic hard and soft tissue landmarks, as well as the oral pathologies commonly seen in the dental office.

Hard Tissue Landmarks of the Skull

The skull is a bony structure composed of 22 bones. It is divided into the cranium, which protects the brain (eight bones), and the skeleton of the face (14 bones). All the bones of the skull, except the mandible, are joined by immovable joints called sutures (see Figs. 2, 3, and 4).

The upper jaw, or maxilla, contains the upper teeth. This irregularly shaped bone helps form the boundaries of the roof of the mouth, the floor and lateral walls of the nose, the floor of the orbit, and the maxillary sinus.

The maxillary sinus is a large cavity located in the maxilla adjacent to the nose. This open space acts as a resonator that contributes to the quality of the voice and communicates with the nasal cavity.

The lower jaw, or mandible, contains the lower teeth. This horseshoe-shaped bone, the largest and strongest bone of the face, consists of a horizontal structure (body) and a pair of vertical structures (rami). Each ramus has two processes (extensions): the condylar process and the coronoid process. Soft tissue attachments (muscles and ligaments) to these processes enable the jaw to be opened and closed (see Figs. 5 and 6).

The range of motion of the mandible is defined by the temporomandibular joint, which is both a hinge joint and a gliding joint. This joint is a complex articulator composed of several ligaments that contribute to its functioning.

Listed below are the names and locations of other facial bones.

Facial Bone	Location
Frontal	Superior anterior and roof of the skull; contains the front sinuses
Parietal	Superior medial sides and roof of the skull
Temporal	Medial sides of the skull; contains middle ear
Occipital	Posterior of skull; posterior wall and posterior floor of cranial cavity
Sphenoid	Anterior base of skull, behind orbits

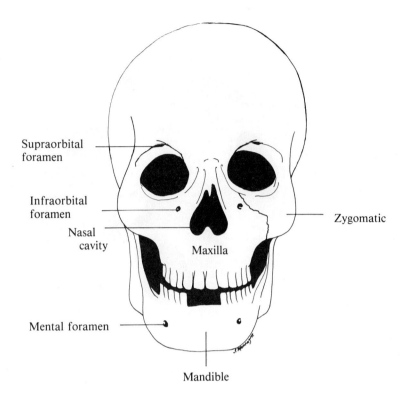

Fig. 2

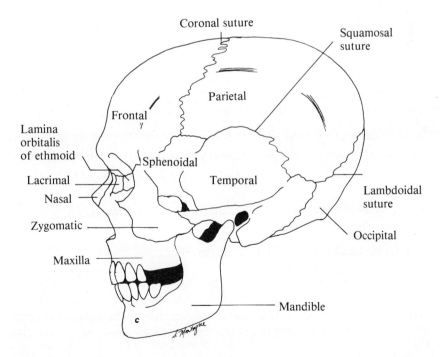

Fig. 3

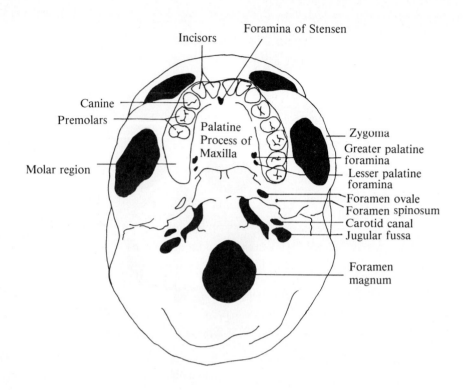

Fig. 4

Facial Bone	Location
Ethmoid	Part of nose, orbits, and floor of cranial cavity
Nasal	Bridge of the nose
Zygomatic	Forms the prominence of the cheeks, lateral wall, and floor of the orbit
Lacrimal	Anterior part of medial wall of the orbit
Palatine	Floor of nasal cavity; floor of the orbit
Vomer	Posterior and inferior portion of nasal septum
Inferior turbinate	Lateral wall of nasal cavity

Soft Tissue Landmarks of the Oral Cavity

The oral cavity is the beginning of the digestive system. It is composed of the vestibule, bounded by the lips and cheeks externally and by the gums internally. The oral cavity proper is bounded by the alveolar arches, teeth, isthmus of fauces, hard and soft palate, and the tongue. It receives secretions from the salivary glands (see Fig. 7).

The oral cavity contains three major glandular systems that produce saliva. Saliva is a liquid medium that distributes basic digestive enzymes, lubricates the oral tissues and ingested food, and functions in the balance of oral bacteria.

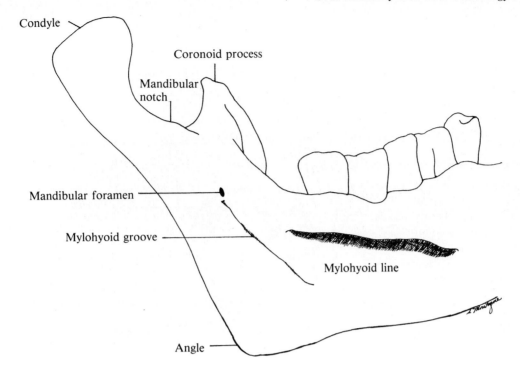

Fig. 5. Medial aspect of mandible.

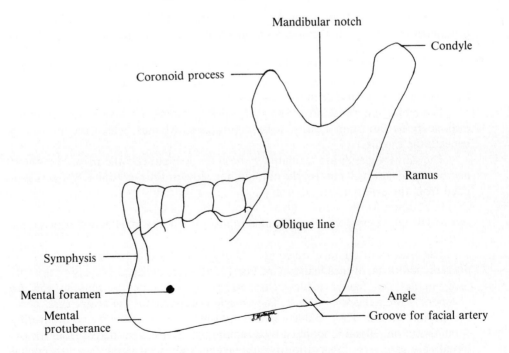

Fig. 6. Lateral aspect of mandible.

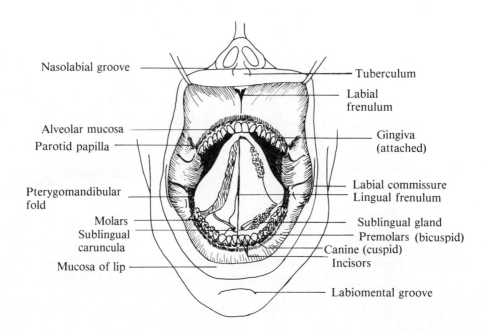

Nasolabial groove

Tuberculum

Labial frenulum

Alveolar mucosa

Parotid papilla

Gingiva (attached)

Pterygomandibular fold

Labial commissure

Lingual frenulum

Molars

Sublingual caruncula

Sublingual gland

Premolars (bicuspid)

Canine (cuspid)

Incisors

Mucosa of lip

Labiomental groove

Fig. 7. Oral cavity.

The parotid glands are located in front of and just below each ear. Their secretions enter the oral cavity through Stenson's ducts located in the cheeks opposite the first or second molars.

The submandibular glands are located on the inner surface of the mandible beneath the tongue. Their secretions enter the oral cavity through Wharton's ducts, located beneath the tongue in the anterior portion of the mouth.

The sublingual glands are the smallest salivary glands. Their secretions enter the oral cavity by Bartholin's ducts or by the ducts of Rivinus, which are all located beneath the tongue.

The salivary glands are regulated by both the sympathetic and parasympathetic nervous systems which control the amount and flow of the secretions. Blood is supplied from the external carotid artery.

In addition to the major salivary glands, the oral cavity contains many minor sets of salivary glands, which are located in the lips, cheeks, palate, and beneath the tongue.

The muscles of the face are composed of two major groups: those of facial expression and those of mastication (see Fig. 8). Muscles of facial expression are surface muscles that have a tendency to merge with other nearby muscles and are grouped by the areas they affect. These basic groups affect the scalp, ears, nose, eyelids, and mouth. They enable expression of personality and influence nonverbal communication. Blood is supplied by a number of arteries that derive from the external carotid artery; innervation is supplied by the facial nerve (seventh cranial nerve).

The muscles of mastication function in the movement of the mandible. Each side of the face has four major muscles: the temporal muscle, the internal pterygoid muscle, the external pterygoid muscle, and the masseter.

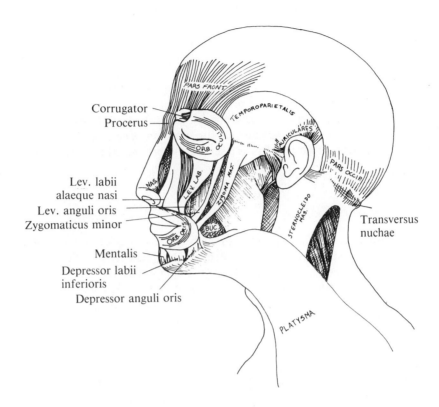

Fig. 8. Muscles of the head and face.

The temporal muscle functions to close and retract the jaw. It originates in the temporal fossa and inserts onto the coronoid process and the anterior border of the ramus.

The internal pterygoid muscle closes the jaw. It originates on the medial surface of the pterygoid plate and inserts onto the lower and posterior borders of the inner surface of the ramus.

The external pterygoid muscle has two functions: to open the jaw and to move it both forward and laterally. It originates on the lateral surface of the sphenoid bone and on the lateral surface of the pterygoid plate and inserts onto the neck of the condoyle and into the articular disc located in the temporomandibular joint.

The masseter muscle closes the jaw. Its origin is in the exterior of the maxilla and zygomatic arch; it inserts onto the lateral surface of the body of the mandible.

The blood for each of the muscles, as with the muscles of facial expression, is supplied by branches of the external carotid artery. All the muscles of mastication are innervated by the trigeminal nerve (the fifth cranial nerve).

Secondary muscles assist the masticatory process as well. These include the buccinator muscle, the myelohyoid muscle, the geniohyoid muscle, and the anterior belly of the digastric muscle. These muscles are innervated and supplied with blood in the same manner as the major muscles of mastication.

The tongue functions in speech, as well as in mastication and deglutition (swallowing) of food. It is also the major organ of taste. The tongue is divided into two identical halves, connected at a medial septum. It contains two sets of muscles: intrinsic and extrinsic. The intrinsic muscles are contained within the tongue entirely and are responsible for altering the shape of the tongue. The extrinsic muscles originate outside the tongue and function to change the positions of the tongue in the oral cavity.

The surface of the tongue contains several types of papillae, which contribute to its texture. Taste buds are located along the surface of the tongue and are found in large numbers in the papillae. Four basic taste senses are experienced: salty, sour, sweet, and bitter (see Fig. 9).

The roof of the mouth is formed by the palate, which is divided into two areas: an anterior area, the hard palate, and a posterior area, the soft palate.

The hard palate separates the oral and nasal cavities and is bound by the alveolar arches and gingiva anteriorly, and by the soft palate posteriorly. The soft palate is mostly muscular in origin and functions in speech and deglutition. Its posterior border hangs free and acts as a separation between the mouth and pharynx (see Fig. 10).

Teeth

Teeth begin their development at approximately the sixth week in utero. The surface tissue of the oral cavity along the future dental arch thickens. This thickening tissue is called the dental lamina. Ten areas along the upper and lower arch possess further growths, causing the appearance of 10 swellings or buds, which are precursors of the future primary and later succedaneous (succeeding) teeth. The proliferating lamina leads to the formation of a shallow invagination of each bud into the oral tissue. From this, three distinct areas for each tooth develop. The first is the enamel organ, which is responsible for the formation of enamel. The second is the dental papillae, which is responsible for the development of dentin and pulp. The third is the dental sac, from which the cementum and periodontal ligament are developed. As growth continues, the teeth undergo a stage during which they all look identical to each other. This process continues until each tooth bud begins to differentiate into its final shape (e.g., incisor, canine, molar). A period of apposition and calcification follows, during which enamel, dentin, and cementum are formed. As each tooth matures, it begins to erupt in its appropriate place in the mouth.

Teeth function primarily in the cutting and grinding of food. They also maintain the integrity of the dental arch, protect the supporting periodontal tissue, function in producing speech sounds, and are a component in each person's facial esthetics. The shape of each tooth is determined by its function.

Each person has two complete sets of teeth during a lifetime. The primary dentition begins to erupt around 6 months of age and is usually completed by the time a child is 2 years of age. This dentition is composed of 20 teeth: a central incisor, a lateral incisor, a canine, and a first and second molar in each quadrant. Primary teeth begin to exfoliate at approximately 6 years of age, when succedaneous teeth begin to erupt. This process continues until the child is approximately 11 years of age, when the exfoliation of the primary dentition is complete. Succedaneous teeth continue to erupt until the child is approximately 13 years of age. With the exception of the third molars, the secondary dentition is complete. Third molars erupt between the ages of 17 and 21 years. Each quadrant in the permanent dentition is composed of a central and lateral incisor, a canine, two premolars, and three molars. In total, there are 32 teeth.

There are several major differences between primary and permanent teeth. Primary teeth are smaller and have less tooth structure protecting the pulp chamber than do their corresponding permanent teeth. Primary teeth also have more pronounced cervical ridges, as well as a more constricted cervical line. Their roots are longer, more slender, and the teeth are lighter in color than succedaneous teeth.

Teeth contained in the permanent dentition are described below.

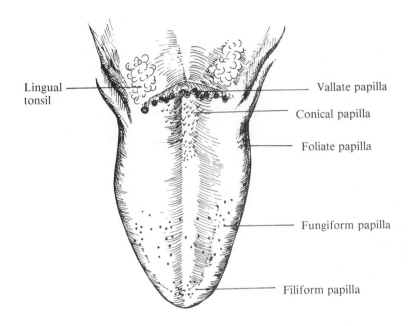

Lingual tonsil

Vallate papilla

Conical papilla

Foliate papilla

Fungiform papilla

Filiform papilla

Fig. 9. The tongue.

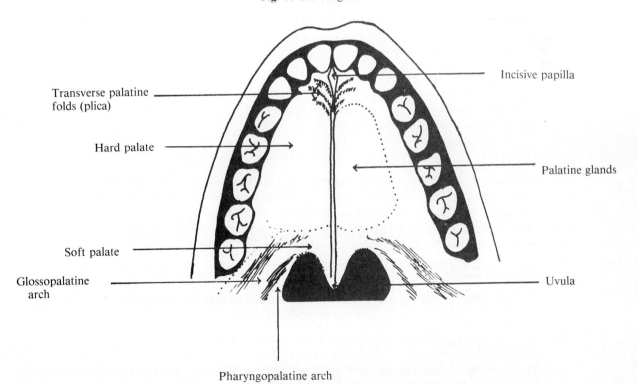

Transverse palatine folds (plica)

Hard palate

Soft palate

Glossopalatine arch

Incisive papilla

Palatine glands

Uvula

Pharyngopalatine arch

Fig. 10. The palate.

Incisors

Incisors act to shear or cut food and affect esthetics and speech. In adult dentition, there are eight incisors: four in the maxilla and four in the mandible.

Maxillary Central Incisors

The permanent central incisors erupt at 7 to 8 years of age and form the midline of the maxilla. The average central incisor is a single rooted tooth which has a crown length of 10.0 mm, a root length of 12.0 mm, and a mesiodistal length of 9.0 mm at its widest point. This tooth is the widest anterior tooth mesiodistally. The labial surface is convex, but less convex than the maxillary lateral incisor. From a facial view, the crown of the tooth appears trapezoidal.

Maxillary Lateral Incisors

The maxillary lateral incisors erupt at approximately 8 to 9 years of age. The average lateral incisor is a single-rooted tooth, which has a crown length of 8.8 mm, a root length of 13 mm, and a mesiodistal width of 6.4 mm at the incisal edge. The maxillary lateral incisor complements the function of the central incisor and resembles that tooth, except crown size and root bulk are smaller. Maxillary lateral incisors can exhibit more variation in tooth form can any other tooth, except the third molar.

Mandibular Central Incisors

The mandibular central incisors erupt at approximately 6 to 7 years of age. The average crown length is 8.8 mm, root length is 11.8 mm, and the mesiodistal diameter is 5.4 mm at the incisal edge. These single-rooted teeth are usually the smallest permanent teeth and the most symmetrical teeth in the mouth.

Mandibular Lateral Incisors

The mandibular lateral incisors erupt at 7 to 8 years of age. The average crown length is 9.6 mm, root length is 12.7 mm, and the mesiodistal diameter is 5.9 mm at the incisal edge. These single-rooted teeth resemble the mandibular central incisors, but are slightly larger in all dimensions.

Canines

Canines are the longest teeth in the mouth. Like incisors, the function of these single-rooted teeth is to cut and tear food. There are four canines in the succedaneous dentition, one located in each quadrant between the lateral incisor and the first premolar. Since these teeth appear at the corners of the mouth when viewed facially, they have a great effect upon appearance and esthetics.

Maxillary Canines

The maxillary canines erupt at 11 to 12 years of age. The average crown length is 9.5 mm, root length is 17.3 mm, and the mesiodistal width is 7.6 mm.

Mandibular Canines

The mandibular canines erupt at 9 to 10 years of age. The average crown length is 10.3 mm, and the root length is 15.3 mm. The mesiodistal width is 7.0 mm.

Premolars

The adult mouth contains eight premolars—four in the upper jaw and four in the lower jaw. These teeth tear food and begin the grinding process and are located between the canines and molars. They succeed the deciduous molars.

Maxillary First Premolars

The maxillary first premolars erupt at 10 to 11 years of age. The average crown length is 8.2 mm, root length is 12.4 mm, and mesiodistal width is 6.9 mm at the incisal edge. The maxillary first premolars have well-defined buccal and lingual cusps. The buccal cusps are about 1.0 mm longer than the lingual cusps. The crowns are shorter than the canines, but from the buccal aspect, look like canines. The mesial surfaces of the teeth at the junction of the crown and root have a concavity. These are the only premolars with two roots.

Maxillary Second Premolars

The maxillary second premolars erupt at 10 to 12 years of age. The average crown length is 7.5 mm, root length is 14.0 mm, and mesiodistal width is 6.8 mm at the incisal edge. The maxillary second premolars act in concert with the maxillary first premolars, and the two teeth resemble each other. The maxillary second premolars have one root as compared with the two roots of the maxillary first premolars, and the cusps of the second maxillary premolars are shorter than those of the first.

Mandibular First Premolars

The mandibular first premolars erupt at approximately 10 to 12 years of age. The average crown length is 7.8 mm, root length is 14.0 mm, and the mesiodistal width is 6.9 mm. These teeth closely resemble the mandibular canines, since the buccal cusps are long and sharp and the lingual cusps are not pronounced. They also resemble the anatomical shape of the mandibular second premolars.

Mandibular Second Premolars

These teeth erupt at age 11 to 12 years. The average crown length is 7.9 mm, root length is 14.4 mm, and the mesiodistal length is 7.1 mm. These teeth appear with a buccal cusp and two smaller lingual cusps.

Molars

Molars perform the grinding job of mastication and reduce food to an appropriate size to swallow. They are the largest teeth in the mouth in terms of bulk. There are 12 molars in the secondary dentition. Each quadrant contains three molars located posterior to the premolars.

Maxillary First Molars

The average crown length of the maxillary first molars are 7.7 mm. These teeth have three roots—two buccal roots of approximately 12 mm length and a palatal root of about 13 mm length. These teeth are wider buccolingually than mesiodistally and are rhomboidal when viewed from the occlusal. There are usually four cusps; however, there is sometimes a fifth cusp, located on the lingual surface, called the cusp of Carabelli. The occlusal surface is separated by a transverse ridge from the mesiolingual to the distobuccal cusps.

Maxillary Second and Third Molars

These teeth supplement the action of the first molars. Second molars are very similar to first molars; the main difference is the lack of development of the distolingual cusps. Third molars often appear as a developmental anomaly with considerable size variation. They are usually not as well developed as second molars and, as a rule, the crowns are smaller and the roots may be fused.

Mandibular First Molars

The average crown length of mandibular first molars is 7.7 mm. There are two roots, one mesial and one distal. Each is approximately 13.5 mm in length. In contrast to maxillary first molars, these teeth are wider mesiodistally than buccolingually. Mandibular first molars usually have five cusps, three buccal and two lingual.

Mandibular Second and Third Molars

The mandibular second and third molars supplement the function of the first molars. Second molars are usually smaller than first molars and have only four cusps. Mandibular third molars vary considerably and are usually not as well developed as second molars. Their crowns generally follow the occlusal pattern of the other mandibular molars, but the roots are often small and not well formed.

Occlusion

Occlusion is the study of how the masticatory system operates. This includes the placement of teeth in the arch, articulation, and the action of the supporting joints and muscles. The goal of oral health care is to maintain or restore the structural and functional harmony consistent with good health and comfort.

Common measurements used to describe occlusion include centric occlusion, centric relation, overjet, and overbite. Centric occlusion occurs at maximum intercuspation (tooth to tooth contact). Centric relation is a point determined when the mandible is in its most retruded position. This measurement is important when centric occlusion cannot be determined accurately as a result of missing tooth structure. Overjet is the horizontal distance and overbite is the vertical distance between upper and lower anterior teeth when teeth are in centric occlusion.

Determining proper occlusion is important in fabricating any dental restoration, since improper occlusion, or malocclusion, can lead to the unbalanced distribution of the forces of mastication and subsequently to more severe dental problems.

The Periodontium

The periodontium consists of those hard and soft tissues that support tooth function. It includes the gingiva, the alveolar bone, the periodontal ligament, and the cementum. The latter three function to attach the tooth to the underlying maxilla or mandible.

The gingiva is the soft tissue that covers the cervical portions of the teeth and the surrounding alveolar bone. It is composed of free gingiva and attached gingiva. The free gingiva extends from the gingival margin of the tooth to the bottom of the gingival sulcus and can be separated from the tooth. The attached gingiva extends until the mucogingival junction, where the alveolar mucosa continues. The gingival margin appears as a wavy path from tooth to tooth, with the gingiva being highest in the interdental spaces. This tissue, which appears interproximally, is the interdental papillae.

The tissue covering the free and attached gingiva is toughened through the process of keratinization and is similar to epidermal tissue. The covering of the alveolar tissue and sulcular tissue is not keratinized and can be more easily damaged.

Each tooth is connected to the underlying alveolar bone through an attachment apparatus. The attachment apparatus consists of the alveolar bone, the periodontal ligament, and the tooth cementum; it supports each tooth by suspending it in a sling mechanism. The periodontal ligament is the tissue enclosing each tooth and connecting the alveolar bone to the cementum. Cementum is a hard material similar to enamel, covering the root surfaces of each tooth. Alveolar bone is similar to bone found elsewhere in the body. However, the condition of this bone is dependent on the function of the tooth it surrounds. If the tooth is under high stress, the alveolar bone tends to become denser, whereas, if the tooth is missing, the bone has a tendency to be resorbed by the body.

A healthy periodontium is essential for the maintenance of oral health. It has become increasingly clear that most tooth loss during the middle and later years is caused by poor periodontal health.

Oral Pathology

Oral pathology is the study of those diseases that affect the components of the oral cavity. The most common pathologies include periodontal disease, caries, and diseases affecting pulpal tissue.

Periodontal Disease

Periodontal disease, or pyorrhea, is one of the most widespread of all oral diseases. The most common periodontal disease is gingivitis, which is an inflammation of the gingiva, believed to be caused by products of microorganisms in plaque. Gingivitis is characterized by red, edematous, tender gingiva, which bleeds easily.

Gingivitis can be localized, involving only a small area, or generalized, involving the entire mouth. It can also be acute or chronic. This disease is prevented, as well as treated, by eliminating plaque through daily brushing and flossing.

Acute necrotizing ulcerative gingivitus (ANUG), also known as trenchmouth, is characterized by ulcerations on the gingiva, particularly on interdental papillae. The diseased tissue appears red and swollen, bleeds easily, and is painful. In some patients, temperature is elevated. The precise etiology of ANUG is unclear, but it appears to be related to physical and mental stress, smoking, and inadequate oral hygiene, which lower overall resistance to infection. This disease is treated by curetting and thoroughly cleaning the affected gingival area. Patients are instructed in proper home care and, if a fever is present, antibiotics may be prescribed.

When periodontal disease affects the alveolar bone, it is called periodontitis. This pathology is usually painless and can result from untreated chronic gingivitis. Periodontal pockets (increased gingival sulcus depth) appear as a result of loss of alveolar bone. This condition is usually treated surgically.

Gingival recession results in an increased exposure of the root of the tooth by an apical movement of the gingiva. Gingival recession can be a sign of periodontal disease caused by improper oral hygiene. However, it is also associated with the normal process of aging. Careful clinical and radiographic evaluation of patients with receding gingiva is important to determine an underlying pathological condition.

Dental Caries

Caries is a disease of the hard tissue of the teeth. In this disease, the inorganic tooth materials are demineralized and the organic tissues are destroyed. Although many years have been spent by researchers in an attempt to discover the exact causes of dental caries, many of the reasons are still unknown. It is known that caries results from an interaction of bacteria, host resistance, and a substrate.

There are several theories to the etiology of caries. A popular theory is called the acidogenic theory. This theory suggests that caries is the result of the activity of acid-producing bacteria. The process occurs as follows: Easily broken down carbohydrates adhere to teeth along with acid-producing bacteria in the form of plaque. The microorganisms cause the breakdown of the carbohydrates, resulting in the production of acids. When acidity in a given area exceeds a certain level, the inorganic tooth matrix is demineralized and the organic matrix destroyed.

A major cause of caries appears to be the refined foods present in daily diets. Refined softened foods tend to be cariogenic. However, occurrence is not the same in all people or groups of people. Different ethnic groups, even within the same area, have different rates of, or predisposition to, the disease. Other contributing factors to host resistance include tooth shape, position, and composition, as well as the chemical composition of the saliva.

Vitamins A and D are especially important to tooth formation. Such minerals as calcium and phosphorus, or their absence in diet, are related to the incidence of caries.

Certain parts of a tooth are more susceptible to dental caries. In general, the caries susceptibility of an area has to do with the difficulty or ease with which the area can be cleansed. Particularly caries-prone areas are pits and fissures on posterior teeth—developmental defects that cannot be cleaned. The proximal surfaces of all teeth are susceptible, specifically at contact, because floss must be used to clean this area. Saliva is a complex fluid the composition of which varies widely from person to person. Even within the same person, daily fluctuation is great. The pH level (i.e., acidity) and the amount of saliva production are also important factors. A decreasing pH level or amount of saliva, or both, is associated with a tendency toward increased caries.

Caries prevention includes local and systemic efforts. Proper oral hygiene and topical application of anticariogenic agents that strengthen the tooth matrix are examples of local measures. Fluoride has been particularly successful in caries prevention and is contained in these topical agents. In addition, fluoride is added to the drinking water of many municipalities. This systemic prophylactic measure has been demonstrated to reduce caries effectively.

Treatment of caries is the mechanical removal of the diseased tissue and appropriate restoration. If caries is left untreated it will dissolve the hard enamel and subsequently affect the softer dentin of the tooth. Here the caries spreads more quickly because the dentin has a higher organic content, which is easier to attack. Left unchecked, the process continues, until the pulp is affected.

Pulpal Diseases

The dental pulp is a highly vascular structure, the primary function of which is the development of dentin, during formation. Once matured, the pulp serves as a thermal sensor, a pain receptor and transmittor, and a supplier of nutrients. There are several causes of pulpal disease including untreated decay, trauma, dental iatrogenic treatment, and exposure to chemical irritants, such as phosphoric acid, silver nitrate, or acrylic monomer.

Pulpal disease can be separated into reversible and irreversible categories.

Hyperemia, a reversible disease, is an excessive accumulation of blood in the pulp causing vascular congestion. Acute pulpitis and chronic pulpitis are examples of irreversible pulpal disease.

Acute pulpitis, or acute inflammation of the pulp, leads to the death of the pulp and is generally very painful. Chronic pulpitis might not cause serious pain, but it can become an acute problem. Root canal therapy is the treatment of choice for irreversible pulpitis.

Developmental Pathologies

In addition to those diseases that affect healthy tooth structure, there are a number of developmental anomalies. Those that affect teeth include anodontia, formation of supernumerary teeth, microdontia, macrodontia, and pathologies occurring during the formation of both enamel and dentin. Andontia, lack of development of teeth, can be either partial or complete. A person can also develop an excess number of teeth; these excessive teeth are called supernumerary teeth. Teeth that are too small (microdontia) or too large (macrodontia) can also develop. Additional disturbances that affect the shape of teeth include germination, fusion, concrescence, and dilaceration. Germination occurs during the attempted division of the tooth bud. Instead of the formation of one complete tooth, two incomplete teeth develop. Fusion occurs when two teeth partially or completely join or fuse, resulting in a single large tooth. If this process occurs after root formation and the cementum of two teeth is joined, it is termed concrescence. Dilaceration refers to the formation of roots with sharp bends or angles. Amologenesis imperfecta refers to anomalies that occur during the formation of enamel, and correspondingly, dentinogenesis imperfecta refers to disturbances occurring during the formation of dentin.

The tongue is also affected by developmental pathologies, including cleft tongue, fissure tongue, geographic tongue, and hairy tongue. A cleft tongue results when fusion of the two halves of the tongue is incomplete. When an abnormal number of grooves or fissures appears on the dorsal side of the tongue it is called a fissured tongue. Benign migratory glossitis occurs when papillae on the tongue lose their surface epithelium. It is also known as geographic tongue because it may appear on different parts of the tongue at different times. A hairy tongue is characterized by an overgrowth (hypertrophy) of the filiform papillae. The tongue appears matted and may discolor having a yellow, brown or possibly black cast. Most of these developmental anomalies of the tongue are not clinically significant and are left untreated.

The most common developmental pathology affecting the lips or palate, or both, is a cleft, which appears as a result of lack of fusion. This condition occurs in approximately one in 800 births. If a cleft significantly interferes with the function of the oral or nasal cavity, surgical correction might be necessary.

Infectious Diseases

Major infectious diseases manifested by clinically apparent symptoms in the oral cavity include syphilis, herpes simplex, aphthous ulcers, chickenpox, and thrush.

Syphilis is a highly contagious disease, usually transmitted through sexual contact. However, the disease can be contracted through direct contact with the oral cavity of a person who is in an infectious stage. During the primary stage, chancres appear primarily on the genitalia, but can also arise on the soft tissues of the oral cavity. During the secondary stage, highly infectious oral lesions called mucous patches appear on the tongue, gingiva, or buccal mucosa. Tertiary syphilis is characterized by a centrally necrotized oral lesion called a gumma.

Herpes simplex, commonly known as herpes or simply as cold sores, is a contagious viral infection characterized by blisterlike lesions that usually appear on the lips, but they are found intraorally as well. Herpes is associated with cases of severe sunburn, trauma, emotional stress, fever, and allergy. The disease is usually left untreated and runs its course in 7–14 days.

Recurring aphthous ulcers are single or multiple intraoral gray lesions surrounded by a reddened area. These lesions are often painful. Causative factors include stress and alcohol. Although treatment is nonspecific, steroid ointments and tetracycline rinses have produced positive responses.

Varicella, commonly known as chickenpox, is a disease of viral origin in which fluid-filled lesions appear on the body. Occasionally, these small lesions occur intraorally.

Mumps, scientifically known as parotitis, involves unilateral or bilateral swelling of the parotid and other salivary glands. Mumps is contagious and is usually found in children; however, adults have been reported to contract the disease.

Moniliasis, or thrush, is an infection caused by the *Candida albicans* fungus. It is characterized by an elevated soft white plaque on the tongue or other oral tissue. Thrush appears most commonly in infants and debilitated persons, but it has become more common in adults as a side effect of antibiotic medication, which tends to decrease other flora normally found in the oral cavity. Treatment is application of an antifungal agent.

Common Oral Pathologies

Other conditions that commonly appear in the oral cavity include Fordyce granules, tori, bruxism, attrition, abrasion, and erosion.

Fordyce granules are a developmental anomaly characterized by elevated sebaceous glands that appear in various sites in the oral cavity. They are small yellowish spots that occur frequently in adults, and rarely in children. Treatment is not necessary, since the granules are not pathologically significant.

Tori are bony protrusions appearing on the palate or mandible. They grow slowly and have no clinical significance unless they interfere with the placement of an oral prosthesis. If interference exists, tori are surgically removed.

Bruxism, the unconscious grinding or clenching of teeth during sleep, can lead to excessive wearing away of tooth structure, as well as bone loss and temporomandibular difficulties. Bruxism differs from attrition, which is the normal physiological process that occurs with aging. Often, bruxism stems from an emotional problem for which treatment can include psychological counseling, as well as the fabrication of protective appliances to be worn during sleep.

Abrasion is the pathological wearing away of tooth structure or soft tissue, or both. This condition usually occurs in the cervical area of a single tooth or of several teeth. Abrasion occurs from excessive or improper toothbrushing or from the use of abrasive toothpastes. This condition is irreversible; further damage can be prevented through patient education.

Erosion is the loss of tooth structure through a chemical process. This pathology usually occurs on labial or buccal surfaces of teeth and can be related to the degree of acidity of saliva.

Tumors of the Oral Cavity

Tumors are areas of swollen tissue often found in the oral cavity. It should be noted, however, that the word tumor does not imply a cancerous or carcinomic lesion. A number of benign tumors frequently occur; those most commonly seen include the following.

Papillomas are benign outward growths of surface epithelium commonly found on tongue, lips, buccal mucosa, gingiva, and palate. Papillomas are surgically removed only if they become uncomfortable to the patient or if they appear in areas that are easily traumatized.

Pigmented nevi, or moles, occur most commonly on the skin, but they are also seen in the oral cavity. Moles are congenital anomalies characterized by brown pigmentation. Removal is recommended if they appear in easily irritated areas or if an observable change in color, size, or shape occurs.

A fibroma or epulis is an overgrowth of connective tissue that can result from infection or irritation. Fibromas grow slowly and are characterized by a change in color. They can occur anywhere in the oral cavity and are usually surgically removed.

Hemangiomas are tumors characterized by a proliferation of blood vessels. They vary widely in size and appear red or blue in color. Hemangiomas usually occur on the skin, lips, or buccal mucosa. They are clinically significant because they can hemorrhage if punctured.

Pyogenic granulomas are inflammatory overgrowths of unknown etiology. They are frequently seen on the gingiva and appear deep red or purple in color. They grow quickly and then remain static. Although painless, most are surgically removed. Pregnancy tumors that are similar in composition often appear during the third month of pregnancy.

Leukoplakia appears as white patches or plaque occurring on mucosal surfaces. Unless infected, it is usually painless. The cause of leukoplakia is unclear, but factors related to its development appear to include tobacco, alcohol, irritations, vitamin deficiencies, and hormonal imbalances. Early diagnosis and histological examination are important, because leukoplakia can precede a malignant condition. Treatment includes elimination of the irritating factors and surgical removal.

Malignant tumors that occur in or around the oral cavity include basal cell carcinoma, epidermoid carcinoma, and melanoma. Basal cell carcinoma occurs on exposed areas of the face and scalp. Characterized by small elevated areas that become ulcerated, it is more prevalent in fair-skinned people. The most likely cause of basal cell carcinoma is overexposure to the sun. This tumor grows slowly and usually does not metastasize (spread). Treatment includes surgical removal and radiation therapy. Prognosis for patients treated for this condition is usually good because of the lack of metastasis.

Epidermoid, or squamous cell, carcinoma is the most common form of cancer of the oral cavity. It can occur anywhere in the oral cavity and can have a different appearance in different areas. Possible causes of this disease include smoking, alcohol, nutritional deficiencies, syphilis, exposure to the sun, and viruses. Treatment for epidermoid or squamous cell carcinoma includes surgical removal, radiation therapy, and chemotherapy.

Melanomas are often fatal neoplasms that usually occur on the skin and oral mucosa. Their appearance is similar to that of pigmented nevi, or moles. Melanomas are uncommon and appear to be caused by trauma or irritation. Treatment is usually radical surgical removal.

Question Section

Directions: Select the number from the figure that illustrates the landmark (bone or structure) in questions 1–21.

Anterior

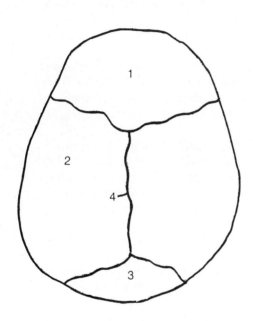

Posterior

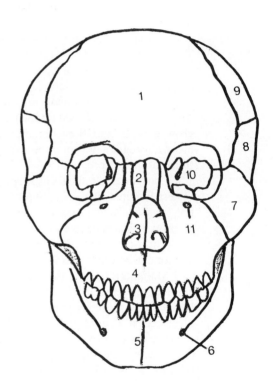

Fig. 11

Fig. 12

Fig. 11:
1. Frontal bone
2. Sagittal suture
3. Parietal bone
4. Occipital bone

Fig. 12:
5. Mental foramen
6. Nasal cavity
7. Orbit
8. Infraorbital foramen
9. Maxillary bone
10. Nasal bone

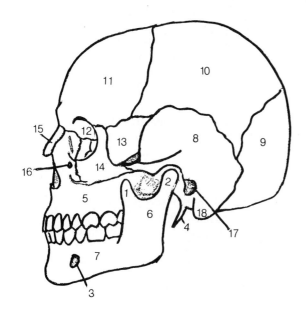

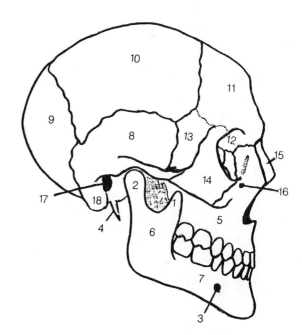

Fig. 13

Fig. 14

Fig. 13:

11. Temporal bone
12. Coronoid process
13. Zygomatic bone
14. Sphenoid bone
15. Ramus of the mandible

Fig. 14:

16. Body of mandible
17. Condylar process
18. Mastoid process
19. External auditory meatus
20. Styloid process
21. Maxillary bone

Directions: Each of the questions or incomplete statements below is followed by four suggested answers or completions. Select the BEST answer in each case.

22. The outer portion of the mandible is composed of
    1. cortical bone
    2. spongy bone
    3. medullary bone
    4. cartilage

23. The type of bone supporting the teeth is called
    1. alveolar bone
    2. cortical bone
    3. periodontal bone
    4. epiphyseal bone

24. If teeth are extracted, the supporting alveolar bone will
    1. be resorbed
    2. form exostosis
    3. become denser
    4. remain the same

25. As a person grows older, the alveolar bone
    1. becomes more brittle
    2. becomes softer
    3. becomes elastic
    4. does not change

26. Foramina are
    1. smooth depressions in bones
    2. protuberances in bones
    3. openings in bone
    4. fossae

27. The maxilla helps form the
    A. orbit
    B. palate
    C. nasal concha
    D. zygomatic arch
    E. ethmoid sinuses
       1. A, B, and D
       2. A, C, and D
       3. B, C, and E
       4. C, D, and E

28. The maxillary tuberosity is located
    1. anterior to the maxillary sinus
    2. posterior to the mandibular third molar
    3. posterior to the maxillary third molar
    4. lateral to the masseter muscle

29. The maxilla does not contact the
    1. frontal bone
    2. zygomatic bone
    3. nasal bone
    4. temporal bone

30. The maxillary sinus is
    1. an air-filled cavity
    2. part of the temporomandibular joint
    3. a fluid-filled pocket
    4. an immovable joint

31. Which tooth is most often located under the maxillary sinus?
    1. the maxillary first molar
    2. the mandibular first premolar
    3. the maxillary central incisor
    4. the maxillary third molar

32. The incisive foramen is located
    1. below the mandibular second premolar
    2. on the hard palate, just behind the maxillary central incisors
    3. on the hard palate, adjacent to the palatal root
    4. below the mandibular central incisors

33. Palatal rugae are
    1. folds of the palatal mucosa
    2. flaps covering taste buds
    3. muscular contractions in the palate
    4. junctions between the hard and soft palate

34. The soft palate is composed of
    1. muscle
    2. bone
    3. cartilage
    4. a combination of muscle and cartilage

35. The uvula is located along the posterior border of the
    1. lingual tonsil
    2. hard palate
    3. soft palate
    4. dorsum of the tongue

36. Which is the most prominent bone making up the skeletal structure of the cheek?
    1. hyoid
    2. vomer
    3. ethmoid
    4. zygomatic

37. The mandible is formed by two bones fusing at the
    1. condyles
    2. ramus
    3. coronoid notch
    4. symphysis

38. The ramus of the mandible contains which structures?
    A. coronoid process
    B. mandibular foramen
    C. mandibular condyle

D. glenoid fossa
E. mental foramen
   1. A, B, and C
   2. B, C, and D
   3. B, D, and E
   4. C, D, and E

39. The body and ramus of the mandible are joined at the
   1. symphysis
   2. angle of the mandible
   3. temporomandibular joint
   4. myelohyoid ridge

40. The following structures pass through the mandibular canal
   A. lingual artery
   B. inferior alveolar artery
   C. inferior alveolar vein
   D. inferior alveolar nerve
   E. mental nerve
      1. A, B, and C
      2. B, C, and D
      3. B, D, and E
      4. C, D, and E

41. The mental foramen is located
   1. below the mandibular central incisors
   2. above the maxillary central incisors
   3. below the mandibular second premolar
   4. posterior to the mandibular third molar

42. Bones that make up the orbit include
   A. ethmoid
   B. lacrimal
   C. zygoma
   D. sphenoid
      1. A, B, and C
      2. A and C only
      3. C and D only
      4. D only
      5. all are correct

43. The articular disc is part of the
   1. orbit
   2. frontal process
   3. hyoid bone
   4. temporomandibular joint

44. The glenoid fossa is located in which bone?
   1. temporal
   2. maxilla
   3. zygomatic
   4. mandible

45. The function of the ligaments of the temporomandibular joint is to
   1. innervate the joint
   2. initiate contraction

   3. limit the movement of the mandible
   4. connect the temporal bone and the maxilla

46. The part of the mandible that does not have muscular attachment is the
   1. myelohyoid ridge
   2. genial tubercles
   3. coronoid process
   4. mandibular notch

47. Which one of the following is not known as a muscle of mastication?
   1. external pterygoid
   2. masseter
   3. myelohyoid
   4. temporal

48. Which muscle attaches to the mandibular condyle?
   1. masseter
   2. internal pterygoid
   3. external pterygoid
   4. temporal

49. Which muscle inserts into the coronoid process?
   1. external pterygoid
   2. internal pterygoid
   3. temporal muscle
   4. masseter muscle

50. Which muscles form a sling around the inferior border of the mandible?
   A. masseter
   B. internal pterygoid
   C. external pterygoid
   D. temporal
      1. A and B
      2. A and C
      3. B and C
      4. C and D

51. A muscle that helps depress the mandible is the
   1. orbicularis oris
   2. myelohyoid
   3. buccinator
   4. superior constrictor

52. Which of the following muscles function to close and retract the jaw?
   A. temporal
   B. masseter
   C. internal pterygoid
   D. external pterygoid
   E. obicularis oris
      1. B and E
      2. A, C, and D

3. A, B, and C
4. all of the above

53. The muscle surrounding the opening of the mouth is the
   1. orbicularis oris
   2. myelohyoid
   3. buccinator
   4. superior constrictor

54. The muscle forming the cheek is the
   1. orbicularis oris
   2. myelohyoid
   3. buccinator
   4. superior constrictor

55. The function of the inferior alveolar nerve is
   1. motor
   2. sympathetic
   3. sensory
   4. parasympathetic

56. After administering an inferior alveolar nerve block, the patient's tongue became numb. Why did this occur?
   1. the tongue is innervated by the inferior alveolar nerve
   2. the lingual nerve was anesthetized
   3. the glossopharyngeal nerve was anesthetized
   4. some of the local anesthetic dropped on the tongue

57. The infraorbital injection is a nerve block for which teeth?
   1. maxillary anteriors
   2. mandibular premolars
   3. maxillary second molars
   4. mandibular incisors

58. The sensory innervation of the maxillary first molars is supplied by the
   1. posterior superior alveolar nerve
   2. middle superior alveolar nerve
   3. both of the above
   4. neither of the above

59. The muscles of mastication are innervated by the
   1. facial nerve
   2. trigeminal nerve
   3. abducens nerve
   4. glossopharyngeal nerve

60. What nerve innervates the buccal gingiva of the mandibular molars?
   1. middle superior alveolar
   2. lingual
   3. long buccal
   4. infraorbital

61. Sensory innervation of the face is transmitted through the
   1. facial nerve
   2. trigeminal nerve
   3. vagus nerve
   4. glossopharyngeal nerve

62. The muscles of facial expression are innervated by the
   1. fifth cranial nerve
   2. seventh cranial nerve
   3. ninth cranial nerve
   4. tenth cranial nerve

63. The sense of smell is carried to the brain by the
   1. optic nerve
   2. facial nerve
   3. olfactory nerve
   4. glossopharyngeal nerve

64. The blood vessel(s) supplying the head with blood is/are the
   1. common carotid arteries
   2. subclavian arteries
   3. pulmonary arteries
   4. inferior vena cava

65. The arteries supplying blood to the mandibular and maxillary teeth are branches of the
   1. internal maxillary artery
   2. common carotid artery
   3. external carotid artery
   4. internal carotid artery

66. The retromolar pad is located
   1. posterior to the maxillary third molar
   2. distal to the last mandibular molar
   3. behind the maxillary central incisor
   4. over the palatine tonsil

67. A frenum is a
   1. muscular attachment
   2. bony attachment
   3. lymphatic connecting tissue
   4. fold of mucous membrane

68. Frena are located
   A. under the tongue
   B. at the junction of the hard and soft palate
   C. in the maxillary labial vestibule
   D. between the maxillary molars
   E. in the mandibular labial vestibule
      1. A, B, and C
      2. A, C, and E
      3. B, D, and E
      4. C, D, and E

69. Tori are
    1. lymphatic tissues
    2. bony protuberances
    3. fibrotic tissues
    4. adipose tissues

70. The side of the nose is called the
    1. tragus
    2. zygoma
    3. ala
    4. vermilion border

71. The vestibule lies between the
    1. buccal gingiva and the cheek
    2. coronoid process and condyle
    3. tongue and the mandible
    4. maxillary teeth and the hard palate

72. The tongue is composed of
    1. smooth muscle
    2. adipose tissue
    3. striated muscle
    4. all of the above

73. Filiform papillae are located on the
    1. buccal mucosa
    2. tongue
    3. floor of the mouth
    4. hard palate

74. In order for taste buds to function, food must be
    1. in solution
    2. in direct contact with the taste bud
    3. either sour or salty
    4. inorganic

75. The pterygomandibular raphe is formed by the meeting of the
    A. external pterygoid muscle
    B. superior constrictor muscle
    C. masseter muscle
    D. buccinator muscle
       1. A and C
       2. B and D
       3. C and E
       4. D and E

76. The tonsils are composed of which type of tissue?
    1. lymphatic
    2. muscle
    3. nerve
    4. adipose

77. The palatine tonsils are located
    1. under the tongue
    2. adjoining the buccal fat pad
    3. on the side of the fauces
    4. on the soft palate

78. Saliva functions in part to
    A. promote the desire for salty foods
    B. begin digestion
    C. lubricate the food bolus
    D. clean the oral cavity
    E. promote plaque accumulation
       1. A, B, and D
       2. B, C, and D
       3. B, C, and E
       4. C, D, and E

79. The major salivary glands are
    A. sublingual gland
    B. parotid gland
    C. submaxillary gland
    D. submandibular gland
    E. Philip's gland
       1. A, B, and C
       2. B, C, and D
       3. A, B, and D
       4. B, C, and E

80. The parotid gland is located
    1. under the tongue
    2. along the inferior border of the mandible
    3. below and in front of the ear
    4. adjacent to the thyroid gland

81. The submandibular gland is located
    1. under the anterior third of the tongue
    2. on the medial surface of the angle of the mandible
    3. opposite the maxillary second molar
    4. in the anterior third of the hard palate

82. The submandibular ducts open
    1. adjacent to the maxillary second molars
    2. next to the palatine tonsils
    3. on both sides of the lingual frenum
    4. at the meeting of the hard and soft palate

83. The parotid ducts open
    1. on both sides of the lingual frenum
    2. on the buccal mucosa opposite the maxillary second molars
    3. adjacent to the palatine tonsils
    4. on the lateral border of the soft palate

84. The first brachial arch gives rise to the
    1. nose
    2. tongue
    3. thyroid gland
    4. mandibular and maxillary alveolar processes

85. Teeth begin to develop
    1. during the sixth week of intrauterine life
    2. at birth

3. 6 weeks after birth
4. 6 months after birth

86. Invagination of the tooth buds results during the
    1. lamina stage
    2. cap stage
    3. bell stage
    4. apposition stage

87. The dental papilla is responsible for development of
    A. dentin
    B. enamel
    C. pulp
    D. root
       1. A and B
       2. A and C
       3. B and D
       4. C and D

88. The dental sac becomes the
    1. pulp
    2. anlage
    3. periodontal membrane
    4. Nasmyth's membrane

89. During which stage of development are dentin and enamel formed?
    1. cap
    2. bell
    3. proliferation
    4. apposition

90. Which part of the tooth forms first?
    1. crown
    2. root
    3. cementum
    4. periodontal ligament

91. Enamel arises from
    1. nerve cells
    2. muscle cells
    3. epithelial cells
    4. connective tissue

92. The pulp of the dentition is derived from the
    1. dental lamina
    2. primordium
    3. dental papilla
    4. enamel cord

93. The cells responsible for the formation of dentin are derived from the
    1. enamel cord
    2. dental papilla
    3. dental sac
    4. dental lamina

94. Which tissue does not have the capacity for growth or repair after the tooth erupts?
    1. enamel
    2. dentin
    3. cementum
    4. pulp

95. The structure that becomes the succedaneous tooth is the
    1. deciduous pulp
    2. permanent tooth anlage
    3. deciduous root
    4. deciduous crown

96. The crowns of anterior teeth are composed of four fused developmental lobes. On which of the following surfaces are the lobes located?
    1. three on the labial and one on the lingual
    2. two on the labial and two on the lingual
    3. one on the labial and three on the lingual
    4. all four on the labial

97. Each developmental lobe on molars is represented by a
    1. fissure
    2. marginal ridge
    3. cusp
    4. groove

98. When a tooth erupts, the root
    1. is fully formed
    2. begins to form
    3. ceases development
    4. partially resorbs

99. The most abundant tissue of the permanent tooth structure is
    1. dentin
    2. enamel
    3. cementum
    4. pulp

100. Secondary dentin
    1. is only in the roots
    2. adjoins the cementum
    3. is a protective mechanism of the tooth
    4. is the first dentin calcified

101. The hardest tissue of the body is
    1. cartilage
    2. enamel
    3. bone
    4. cementum

102. Enamel rods contact the dentinoenamel junction at
    1. oblique angles
    2. acute angles
    3. right angles
    4. obtuse angles

103. Nutrients for the pulp enter and leave the tooth through the

1. apical foramen
2. foramen ovale
3. mental foramen
4. genial tubercles

104. Pulpal tissue consists of
A. ameloblasts
B. cells
C. enamel cuticle
D. connective tissue
E. blood vessels
   1. A, B, and C
   2. B, C, and D
   3. B, D, and E
   4. C, D, and E

105. The cells lining the pulp cavity are
1. ameloblasts
2. odontoblasts
3. cementocytes
4. fibroblasts

106. Painful stimuli are transmitted to the pulp via the
1. enamel
2. dentinal tubules
3. cementoenamel junction
4. periodontal ligament

107. As a person ages, the dental pulp
1. enlarges
2. becomes more fibrous
3. remain the same
4. becomes more cellular

108. The periodontium consists of the
A. pulpal tissue
B. periodontal ligament
C. alveolar process
D. gingiva
E. buccal mucosa
   1. A, B, and C
   2. A, D, and E
   3. B, C, and D
   4. C, D, and E

109. The periodontal ligament lies between the
1. alveolar bone and cementum
2. cementum and dentin
3. enamel and cementum
4. enamel and dentin

110. The proprioceptive mechanism of teeth is derived from
1. temperature receptors in the mouth
2. sensory innervation in the periodontal ligament
3. taste receptors in the mouth
4. pain receptors in the dentin

111. The tooth tissue most closely resembling bone is

1. dentin
2. cementum
3. pulp
4. enamel

112. Keratinization of gingival cells is for
1. color
2. stippling
3. protection
4. proprioception

113. The gingiva is covered with
1. adipose tissue
2. stratified squamous epithelium
3. fibrous tissue
4. alveolar tissue

114. The unattached edge of the gingiva is the
1. free gingiva
2. connected gingiva
3. alveolar mucosa
4. buccal mucosa

115. The gingival sulcus
1. lies between the free and attached gingiva
2. is on the labial surface of anterior teeth
3. lies between the tooth and the internal surface of the free gingiva
4. is coincident with buccal mucosa

116. In a mouth free from periodontal disease, the attached gingiva would appear
1. stippled
2. mottled
3. denuded
4. eroded

117. The interdental papillae is
A. pink
B. triangular shaped
C. located between the teeth
D. stippled
   1. A, B, and C
   2. B and C
   3. B, C, and D
   4. all of the above

118. The level of interproximal alveolar bone is normally
1. higher than buccal bone
2. lower than buccal bone
3. the same as buccal bone
4. none of the above

119. The cells that resorb bone are
1. osteoblasts
2. osteoclasts
3. osteocytes
4. leukocytes

120. The bell-shaped roots of a deciduous molar will surround the
    1. pulpal tissue of a permanent molar
    2. crown of a permanent premolar
    3. mandibular canal
    4. crown of a permanent molar

121. The mesiodistal crown length of which deciduous tooth is longer than the succedaneous tooth that will replace it?
    1. maxillary central incisor
    2. mandibular lateral incisor
    3. maxillary canine
    4. mandibular first molar

122. Exfoliation is the
    1. internal absorption of succedaneous teeth
    2. removal of permanent tooth follicles
    3. shedding of primary teeth
    4. technique used to remove cysts

123. At what age is the last deciduous tooth normally shed?
    1. 9 years
    2. 15 years
    3. 6 years
    4. 12 years

124. The shape of teeth indicates their
    1. buccolingual position
    2. length of service
    3. function
    4. eruption rate

125. A shallow elongated depression in a tooth is called a
    1. groove
    2. valley
    3. line angle
    4. ridge

126. A pit is a
    1. sharp protrusion
    2. circular elevation
    3. sharp, small depression
    4. none of the above

127. Marginal ridges are located on the
    1. occlusal surface
    2. incisal surface
    3. labial surface
    4. buccal surface

128. Mamelons are
    1. grooves in posterior teeth
    2. three small elevations of enamel on anterior teeth
    3. teeth of all mammals
    4. small fractures in permanent teeth

129. The major embrasure is located
    1. on the buccal surfaces of molars
    2. below the cingulum
    3. on the occlusal surfaces of premolars
    4. interproximally between the contact area and the gingiva

130. The minor embrasure functions
    1. as a small cusp
    2. to incise food
    3. to deflect food
    4. to collect food

131. In a multirooted tooth, root canals open into
    1. an occlusal groove
    2. odontoblasts
    3. the pulp chamber
    4. the occlusal foramen

132. A bifurcation exists in which tooth?
    1. central incisor
    2. mandibular second premolar
    3. maxillary first molar
    4. mandibular first molar

133. A trifurcation exists in which tooth?
    1. central incisor
    2. mandibular second premolar
    3. maxillary first molar
    4. mandibular first molar

134. A diastema is
    1. a special diet
    2. a space between adjacent teeth
    3. anterior overlapping
    4. an enlarged tuberosity

135. The clinical crown of a tooth is
    1. always the portion of the tooth above the root
    2. caused by the incomplete fusion of the crown and the root
    3. the portion of the tooth exposed in the mouth
    4. always covered by enamel

136. The anatomical crown and root meet at the
    1. dentoenamel junction
    2. dentocemental junction
    3. cementoenamel junction
    4. attached gingiva

137. The surface of the tooth facing the midline of the mouth is the
    1. mesial
    2. distal
    3. lingual
    4. incisal

138. The surface of the anterior teeth facing the lips is the

1. buccal
2. labial
3. palatal
4. lingual

139. Which teeth have mesial surfaces that contact each other?
    1. central incisors
    2. lateral incisors
    3. first bicuspids
    4. first molars

140. The lingual lobe of an anterior tooth is called a(n)
    1. cusp
    2. lingual depression
    3. anterior elevation
    4. cingulum

141. What protects the interproximal gingival tissue during mastication?
    1. contact areas
    2. buccal contours
    3. lingual contours
    4. palatal contours

142. The facial and lingual contours of teeth protect the
    1. interproximal areas
    2. retromolar pad
    3. facial and lingual gingival tissue
    4. tongue

143. The greatest contour of a deciduous tooth is
    1. the same as a permanent tooth
    2. often located below the gingiva
    3. equal to the greatest width of the roots
    4. all of the above

144. Centric occlusion is
    1. a condition in which teeth are at their maximum intercuspation
    2. the most retruded physiological position of the mandible
    3. the measurement of the horizontal difference between maxillary and mandibular teeth
    4. the side of the mouth to which the mandible is moved

145. Overjet is the
    1. horizontal distance between maxillary and mandibular teeth
    2. coronal length of maxillary anterior teeth
    3. vertical overlap of maxillary and mandibular anterior teeth
    4. labioversion of the mandibular teeth

146. Vertical overbite refers to the

1. horizontal distance between the posterior teeth
2. coronal length of maxillary anterior teeth
3. vertical overlap of the incisal edges of maxillary and mandibular anterior teeth
4. labioversion of mandibular teeth

147. Centric relation is
    1. when teeth are at their maximum intercuspation
    2. the most retruded physiological position of the mandible
    3. the measurement of horizontal difference between maxillary and mandibular teeth
    4. the side of the mouth on which the mandible is moved

148. Mandibular teeth normally occlude
    1. mesial to their maxillary counterparts
    2. distal to their maxillary counterparts
    3. flush with their maxillary counterparts
    4. none of the above

149. If a tooth is extracted, the adjacent teeth
    1. decay very quickly
    2. tend to tilt to fill the space
    3. are not affected
    4. develop deep periodontal pockets

150. The longest tooth in the mouth is the
    1. lateral incisor
    2. central incisor
    3. canine
    4. second molar

151. A distinct characteristic of the maxillary first premolar is the
    1. transverse ridge
    2. lingual pit
    3. mesial fossa
    4. central fossa

152. How many root canals does the maxillary first premolar have?
    1. one
    2. two
    3. three
    4. four

153. The oblique ridge of the maxillary molars connect the
    1. mesiolingual and distobuccal cusps
    2. mesiobuccal and mesiolingual cusps
    3. distobuccal and mesiobuccal cusps
    4. mesiobuccal and distolingual cusps

154. The largest cusp of the maxillary first molar is the

1. distobuccal
2. distolingual
3. mesiobuccal
4. mesiolingual

155. The cusp of Carabelli is sometimes found on what tooth?
     1. maxillary first premolar
     2. maxillary second premolar
     3. maxillary first molar
     4. mandibular second molar

156. The roots of the maxillary first molar are
     A. buccal
     B. palatal
     C. mesial
     D. distal
     E. mesiobuccal
     F. distobuccal
         1. A, B, and D
         2. C, D, and E
         3. B, E, and F
         4. D, E, and F

157. Which tooth usually contacts only one antagonist in the opposing arch?
     1. maxillary central incisor
     2. maxillary lateral incisor
     3. mandibular lateral incisor
     4. mandibular central incisor

158. The smallest permanant tooth in the mouth is the
     1. mandibular central incisor
     2. mandibular lateral incisor
     3. mandibular canine
     4. maxillary lateral incisor

159. Which other tooth most closely resembles the canine?
     1. mandibular first premolar
     2. maxillary first premolar
     3. mandibular second premolar
     4. maxillary second premolar

160. Which tooth is most likely to have three cusps?
     1. mandibular first premolar
     2. maxillary first premolar
     3. mandibular second premolar
     4. maxillary second premolar

161. In normal occlusion, the lingual cusps of the lower molars occlude in the
     1. central fossae of the upper molars
     2. marginal ridges of the upper molars
     3. both of the above
     4. none of the above

162. Which tooth has two buccal grooves?
     1. maxillary first premolar

2. mandibular second molar
3. mandibular first molar
4. maxillary first molar

163. If the mandibular molar is in a retruded position, the occlusion is classified as
     1. mesiocclusion
     2. distocclusion
     3. neutrocclusion
     4. none of the above

164. The smallest cusp of the mandibular first molar is the
     1. mesiolingual cusp
     2. mesiobuccal cusp
     3. distobuccal cusp
     4. distolingual cusp

165. Which tooth has a root containing two canals?
     1. maxillary canine
     2. mandibular first premolar
     3. maxillary second premolar
     4. mandibular first molar

166. The roots of the mandibular second molar are
     A. buccal
     B. palatal
     C. mesial
     D. distal
     E. mesiobuccal
     F. distobuccal
         1. A and D
         2. C and D
         3. D, E, and F
         4. D and E

167. Which tooth most often has fused roots?
     1. mandibular first molar
     2. maxillary first premolar
     3. maxillary first molar
     4. maxillary third molar

Directions: Select the numbered figure that BEST matches the corresponding question.

Questions 168 and 169

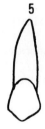 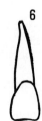 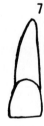 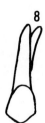

168. Which is the buccal view of the maxillary first premolar?

169. Which is the buccal view of the maxillary canine?

Questions 170 and 171

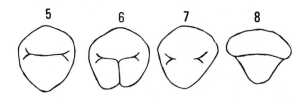

170. Which is the occlusal view of the mandibular second premolar?

171. Which is the occlusal view of the maxillary first premolar?

Questions 172 and 173

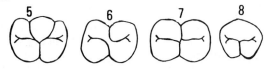

172. Which is the occlusal view of the mandibular first molar?

173. Which is the occlusal view of the maxillary first molar?

Questions 174 and 175

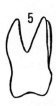 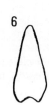 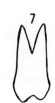

174. Which is the proximal view of the maxillary second premolar?

175. Which is the proximal view of the maxillary first premolar?

Directions: Each of the questions or incomplete statements below is followed by four suggested answers or completions. Select the BEST answer in each case.

176. The study of factors causing disease is
    1. cytology

2. etiology
3. ecology
4. zoology

177. Healing is rapid in the oral cavity because of the abundant
    1. nerve supply
    2. muscle supply
    3. bone supply
    4. blood supply

178. Various causes of pathology in the oral cavity are
    1. detrimental habits
    2. trauma
    3. diet
    4. all of the above

179. Prophylactic refers to
    1. pathogenicity
    2. the cause of the disease
    3. the transmission of bacteria
    4. a preventative measure

180. Atrophy refers to the
    1. varicosity in blood vessels
    2. decrease in size of tissue
    3. amputation of a limb
    4. rejuvenation of tissue

181. The retention of fluids is referred to as
    1. nephritis
    2. syneresis
    3. hemangioma
    4. edema

182. The engorgement of blood is known as
    1. an aneurysm
    2. anemia
    3. hyperemia
    4. cystic lesions

183. Erythema is
    1. a type of oral carcinoma
    2. cryotherapy
    3. redness of the skin
    4. a form of bacteria

184. Symptoms of inflammation are
    A. swelling
    B. pain
    C. shallow depressions
    D. redness
    E. heat
    F. hyperventilation
        1. A, C, D, and E
        2. A, B, D, and E
        3. B, D, E, and F
        4. C, D, E, and F

185. Which condition is the result of defective enamel formation?

1. hypercementosis
2. concrescence
3. dentinogenesis imperfecta
4. enamel hypoplasia

186. Defects in enamel can be caused by
    1. dietary deficiencies
    2. local infection
    3. high fever
    4. all of the above

187. A disturbance occurring during the mineralization of the enamel can result in
    1. denticle formation
    2. hypertrophy of the periodontal membrane
    3. hypocalcified enamel
    4. delayed eruption

188. Mottled enamel is the result of
    1. tetracycline taken by the mother during pregnancy
    2. oral secretion
    3. ingestion of too much fluoride
    4. incorrect tooth brushing

189. Dilaceration refers to
    1. sharp angulations of the root
    2. a fractured crown
    3. a large cingulum
    4. a laceration of the buccal mucosa

190. The physiological wearing away of teeth is called
    1. erosion
    2. abrasion
    3. posterior collapse
    4. attrition

191. Abrasion is the
    1. chemical erosion of the dentinoenamel junction
    2. fracture of cusps of a molar
    3. wearing away of tooth structure by mechanical means
    4. result of defective enamel

192. Which structure is lacking if ankylosis occurs?
    1. bone
    2. periodontal membrane
    3. root
    4. cementum

193. A cleft lip is caused by a lack of fusion between the
    1. frontonasal process and median nasal process
    2. maxillary process and median nasal process

3. maxillary process
4. soft palate and hard palate

194. A supernumerary tooth located between the maxillary central incisors is called a(n)
    1. odontoma
    2. incisive cyst
    3. ectopic eruption
    4. mesiodens

195. Which teeth are most often impacted?
    1. canines
    2. lateral incisors
    3. first premolars
    4. third molars

196. The tooth most often congenitally missing is the
    1. maxillary central incisor
    2. mandibular first molar
    3. maxillary canine
    4. mandibular third molar

197. Aging will bring on which of the following changes in the oral cavity?
    A. gingival recession
    B. decrease in the size of the tongue
    C. decrease in the size of the pulp chamber
    D. increase in the number of taste buds
    E. attrition
       1. A, B, and C
       2. A, C, and E
       3. B, D, and E
       4. C, D, and E

198. Tic douloureux is a pathological condition of which cranial nerve?
    1. I
    2. V
    3. VII
    4. X

199. A muscle spasm is
    1. the tearing of a muscle
    2. hypertrophy of muscle tissue
    3. a sudden contraction of muscle tissue
    4. the hyperextension of a joint

200. The unconscious grinding of teeth is called
    1. bruxism
    2. abrasion
    3. granulation
    4. kinesiology

201. An open bite refers to a condition wherein
    1. there are no posterior teeth
    2. there are spaces between teeth in the same arch
    3. the anterior teeth do not contact
    4. the teeth contact only during mastication

202. The ability to ward off disease is known as
    1. infection
    2. host resistance
    3. postponement
    4. the autogenic ability

203. An antibody is
    1. an autoimmune disease
    2. part of the body's defense system
    3. an enzyme
    4. none of the above

204. Bacterial invasion of the circulatory system is referred to as
    1. hyperemia
    2. bacteremia
    3. toxemia
    4. granuloma

205. A recurrent viral infection in the mouth is
    1. pyogenic granuloma
    2. herpes simplex
    3. aphthous ulcer
    4. thrush

206. An oral fungal infection is
    1. herpes
    2. aphthous ulcer
    3. thrush
    4. a melanoma

207. Symptoms of acute necrotizing ulcerative gingivitis (ANUG) might include
    A. ulcerations on the gingiva
    B. bleeding gums
    C. headaches
    D. elevated temperature
        1. A, C, and D
        2. A, B, and C
        3. B, C, and D
        4. A, B, and D

208. Osteomyelitis is a disease process that might affect the
    1. temporal muscle
    2. mandible
    3. fifth cranial nerve
    4. salivary glands

209. What disease causes swelling of the parotid glands?
    1. gingivitis
    2. measles
    3. mumps
    4. scarlet fever

210. A salivary stone is called
    1. tartar
    2. a salivary nodule
    3. a sialograph
    4. a sialolith

211. Salivary flow may affect the
    1. eruption sequence of primary teeth
    2. shape of the uvula
    3. type of food desired
    4. caries rate

212. Salivary flow is affected by
    1. thoughts
    2. diet
    3. drugs
    4. all of the above

213. Caries can be controlled by
    1. chemical means
    2. nutritional means
    3. mechanical means
    4. all of the above

214. Stains can be caused by
    A. drugs
    B. oral flora
    C. milk
    D. smoking
    E. toothpaste
        1. A, B, and D
        2. B, C, and D
        3. B, C, and E
        4. C, D, and E

215. Calculus forms
    1. on the clinical crown
    2. on enamel
    3. on root surfaces
    4. all of the above

216. The most effective means of preventing periodontal disease is
    1. dietary
    2. mechanically
    3. chemically
    4. using antibiotic therapy

217. Pulpal reaction to irritants can result in
    1. secondary dentin formation
    2. fibrosis of the pulp
    3. death of the pulp
    4. all of the above

218. Hormonal changes can affect the
    1. periodontium
    2. formation of a mucocele
    3. fluoride uptake of permanent molars
    4. all of the above

219. Neoplasm refers to
    1. tissue dysplasia
    2. a malignant growth
    3. a new growth
    4. an allergic reaction

220. Benign refers to

1. aplasia of the buccal mucosa
2. desquamation of the oral mucosa
3. a lesion composed of normal tissue
4. ulcerative lesions on the tongue

221. White areas in the mouth are called
   1. leukoplakia
   2. serous nodules
   3. Fordyce's granules
   4. edema

222. Which of the following are examples of benign tumors?
   A. desquamative gingivosis
   B. lipoma
   C. periodontosis
   D. fibroma
   E. papilloma
      1. A, B, and D
      2. B, C, and E
      3. B, D, and E
      4. C, D, and E

223. Leukemia is a disease of
   1. nerve tissue
   2. muscle tissue
   3. cartilage tissue
   4. blood tissue

224. The spreading of cancer to different sites in the body is called
   1. metastasis
   2. toxemia
   3. peritonitis
   4. carcinoma

225. Cancer is definitively diagnosed by
   1. color reagents
   2. microscopic slides
   3. tactile senses
   4. radiographs

Answers and Explanations

1. **1**

2. **4**

3. **2**

4. **3**

5. **6**

6. **3**

7. **10**

8. **11**

9. **4**

10. **2**

11. **8**

12. **1**

13. **14**

14. **13**

15. **6**

16. **7**

17. **2**

18. **18**

19. **17**

20. **4**

21. **5**

22. **1** The outer part of the mandible is composed of cortical bone. This bone is extremely dense and hard and accounts for the strength of the mandible. The cortical bone will not permit the infiltration of anesthetics and therefore, block anesthesia must be used in the mandibular arch.

23. **1** The bone that supports the teeth is called the alveolar bone. Other names for alveolar bone are cancellous or medullary bone. Fibers of the periodontal membrane are inserted into the part of the alveolar bone known as the lamina dura.

24. **1** The formation and maintenance of alveolar bone is dependent on tooth formation and eruption. If a tooth is missing due to lack of formation, the supporting alveolar bone will not form. If a tooth is removed, the supporting bone will not function as such, and the body will resorb it.

25. **1** As a person ages, the alveolar bone becomes harder and more brittle. This factor is important when considering surgical and orthodontic procedures in older patients.

26. **3** Foramina are openings or holes in bone. They permit the entrance and exit of blood vessels and nerves.

27. **1** The maxilla helps form the orbit, palate, zygomatic arch, and nose.

28. **3** The maxillary tuberosity is a bony structure located posterior to the maxillary third molar. It is the distal extension of the alveolar ridge.

29. **4** The maxilla does not contact the temporal bone. The maxilla has four processes: the frontal, zygomatic, palatine, and alveolar.

30. **1** The maxillary sinus is an air-filled cavity the functions of which are to lighten the skull, warm and moisten the inhaled air, filter the inspired air, and add resonance to the voice.

31. **1** The teeth most often found below the maxillary sinus are the maxillary second premolars, first molars, and second molars. Inflammation of the maxillary sinus (sinusitis) can result when these teeth are percussed.

32. **2** The incisive foramen is located just behind the maxillary central incisors. Through this opening pass the nerves that transmit the sensory innervation of the anterior palate.

33. **1** Palatal rugae are composed of folds of palatal mucosa. They extend from the suture line laterally in the anterior third of the hard palate.

34. **1** The soft palate is composed of several muscles. The muscles contract during swallows and seal the nasal pharynx, thereby preventing the movement of food and liquid into the nasal cavity.

35. **3** The uvula is the small projection located along the posterior border of the soft palate. It is muscular in composition and functions to close off the nasopharynx in swallowing.

36. **4** The zygomatic bone is the most prominent facial bone and is also called the cheekbone.

37. **4** The mandible is formed by two bones that fuse shortly after birth at the symphysis, a slight elevation between the mandibular central incisors,

extending from the alveolar bone to the inferior border of the mandible.

38. **1** The ramus of the mandible contains the coronoid process, mandibular foramen, mandibular condyle, sigmoid notch, and oblique ridges.

39. **2** The ramus and the body of the mandible join at the angle of the mandible. Normally the angle is 100 degrees; if it is more obtuse, a class III malocclusion usually occurs.

40. **2** The mandibular canal contains the inferior alveolar artery, vein, and nerve. These structures supply the needs of the mandibular teeth, bone and the anterior gingiva.

41. **3** The mental foramen is located below the mandibular second premolar. The vessels and nerves that enter and leave the foramen supply the vasculature and innervation to the soft tissue in the anterior portion of the mandible.

42. **5** The bones that comprise the orbit containing the eye are the ethmoid, lacrimal, zygoma, and sphenoid.

43. **4** Components of the temporomandibular joint are the glenoid fossa, a depression in the temporal bone; the glenoid tubercle, an anterior protuberance of the glenoid fossa that helps limit the anterior movement of the mandible; the articular disc, fibrocartilage between the glenoid fossa and the mandibular condyle; the mandibular condyle, the bony protuberance in the posterior superior part of the mandibular ramus; and capsular and temporomandibular ligaments.

44. **1** The glenoid fossa is located in the temporal bone.

45. **3** The functions of the ligaments of the temporomandibular joint are to limit movement of the joint, enclose the joint, and secrete synovial fluid.

46. **4** The mandibular notch, the area between the coronoid process and the condyle, has no muscular attachments.

47. **3** The myelohyoid is not considered a muscle of mastication. The muscles of mastication are the masseter, internal pterygoid, external pterygoid, and temporal.

48. **3** The external pterygoid muscle originates in the greater wing of the sphenoid and the external pterygoid plate; it inserts into the head of the condyle and the articular disc. Simultaneous contraction of the two external pterygoids results in protrusion and opening of the mandible. If one external pterygoid contracts, lateral movement of the mandible results.

49. **3** The temporal muscle is a broad, fan-shaped muscle that originates in the temporal fossa. The muscle extends forward and downward under the zygomatic arch and inserts into the coronoid process and along the anterior border of the mandibular ramus. When this muscle contracts, the pull is in an upward and posterior direction, closing the mandible.

50. **1** The masseter and the internal pterygoid form a sling around the mandible. The masseter originates along the zygomatic arch and inserts on the lateral inferior border of the angle of the mandible. The internal pterygoid originates on the external pterygoid plate and inserts on the medial inferior border of the angle of the mandible. Both muscles function to elevate the mandible.

51. **2** Muscles that help open the mouth are the myelohyoid, external pterygoid, geniohyoid, and digastric.

52. **3** Closing the jaw is the function of the temporal, masseter, and internal pterygoid muscles. The external pterygoid muscle aids in opening the jaw. The obicularis oris is a muscle of facial expression.

53. **1** The orbicularis oris is the muscle that surrounds the mouth. It functions to close the lips, press the lips against the teeth, and protrude the lips.

54. **3** The buccinator muscle forms the cheek; it functions during mastication to place and hold food between the teeth.

55. **3** The inferior alveolar nerve is a branch of the mandibular nerve and is sensory to the lower teeth, lower lip, chin, and some gingival tissue. It enters the mandible canal and divides at the mental foramen into the mental and incisive nerves.

56. **2** The lingual nerve is located close to the injection site of the inferior alveolar nerve; it is therefore subjected to the same anesthetic as the inferior alveolar nerve.

57. **1** The infraorbital injection will anesthetize the anterior and middle superior alveolar nerves. These nerves supply sensory innervation to the maxillary anterior teeth, maxillary premolars, and the mesial buccal root of the maxillary first molar. This injection is used when inflammation prevents infiltration anesthesia.

58. **3** The innervation of the maxillary first molar is the middle superior alveolar nerve for the mesiobuccal root and the posterior superior alveolar nerve for the palatal and distal buccal root.

59. **2** The muscles of mastication are all innervated by the mandibular branch of the trigeminal nerve.

60. **3** The buccal gingiva in the mandibular molar area is innervated by the long buccal nerve, also known as the buccinator. This nerve is a branch

of the mandibular nerve. Dental procedures requiring the painful manipulation of the mandibular buccal mucosa require the operator to anesthetize this nerve.

61. **2** Sensory innervation of the face is derived from the trigeminal nerve. The innervation is divided into the mandibular nerve, which innervates the lower face; the maxillary nerve, which innervates the mid face; and the ophthalmic nerve, which innervates the upper face and skull areas.

62. **2** The muscles of facial expression are innervated by the seventh cranial nerve, the facial nerve. This nerve passes through the parotid gland. A misplaced inferior alveolar block injection into the parotid gland might anesthetize this nerve and cause temporary facial paralysis.

63. **3** The sense of smell is transmitted to the brain by the first cranial nerve, the olfactory nerve.

64. **1** The blood vessels that supply blood to the head are the right and left common carotid arteries.

65. **1** The internal maxillary artery supplies blood to the maxillary and mandibular teeth by branching into the inferior alveolar artery, the posterior superior alveolar artery and the infraorbital artery; the latter branches into the middle alveolar artery and the anterior superior alveolar artery.

66. **2** The retromolar pad is an oval soft tissue elevation located on the mandibular ridge posterior to the last molar. This is a landmark when deciding the distal extension of a removable prosthesis.

67. **4** A frenum is a fold of mucous membrane.

68. **2** Frena are located between the upper mucous membrane and the gingiva located between the upper central incisors; the lower mucous membrane and the gingiva located between the lower central incisors; and the mucous membrane on the floor of the mouth and the underside of the tongue. If the lingual frenum is short, the tongue is limited in movement, and the patient is known as tongue tied.

69. **2** Tori are bony protuberances or exostoses. They are most frequently located on the hard palate or the lingual surface of the mandible in the premolar area. Tori become a problem if a prosthesis is to be constructed over them. If they are enlarged, they can be surgically removed.

70. **3** The side of the nose, adjoining the nostrils, is known as the ala. A line drawn between the ala of the nose and the tragus of the ear parallels the maxillary teeth and is used as a guide when setting artificial teeth.

71. **1** The vestibule is a potential space located between the labial mucosa of the cheek and lips and the buccal and labial gingiva. Removable prostheses often extend into the vestibule.

72. **3** The tongue is composed of striated, or voluntary, muscle. The musculature is divided into intrinsic muscles, concerned with the shape of the tongue, and extrinsic muscles, concerned with moving the tongue to different areas of the mouth.

73. **2** The mucous membrane of the dorsum of the tongue contains the following papillae: fungiform, filiform, foliate, and vallate.

74. **1** In order for taste buds to function, food must be in solution. Taste buds are spread over the tongue and are especially numerous around the vallate papillae. The basic tastes are sweet, sour, salty, and bitter.

75. **2** The pterygomandibular raphe is a fibrous band formed by the meeting of the buccinator and superior constrictor muscles. The raphe extends from the pterygoid hamulus to the myelohyoid line of the mandible.

76. **1** The tonsils are composed of lymphatic tissue. The three pairs of tonsils are the palatine, lingual, and nasopharyngeal.

77. **3** The palatine tonsils are located on the side of the fauces. Children have larger tonsils than adults. This tissue is readily examined during a routine oral survey; the most common pathological condition of tonsils makes them appear swollen and spotted with small abcesses.

78. **2** Saliva functions to begin the process of digestion, excretion, and lubrication of the food bolus, to clean the oral cavity, and to kill bacteria.

79. **1** The sublingual, parotid, and submaxillary glands are the major salivary glands. The submandibular gland is considered a minor salivary gland, and the Philip's gland is not related to oral secretions.

80. **3** The parotid gland, located below and in front of the ear, becomes enlarged when a person has the mumps.

81. **2** The submandibular gland is located on the medial surface of the mandible at the angle of the mandible. The third major salivary gland is the sublingual gland, which is located under the tongue.

82. **3** The submandibular ducts (Wharton's) open in small elevations on both sides of the lingual frenum.

83. **2** The parotid ducts (Stensen's) open on the buccal mucosa opposite the maxillary second molars. To decrease salivary flow a cotton roll may be placed in the maxillary fold to press against the orifice of the duct.

84. **4** The first brachial arch gives rise to the mandible, parts of the maxilla, the muscles of mastication, the lower lip, and parts of sphenoid bone.

85. **1** Teeth begin to develop at 6 weeks of intrauterine life. The initial stage is the formation of tooth buds by the downward proliferation of cells from the dental lamina.

86. **2** Invagination of the tooth bud results in the cap stage. The cap stage is a continuation of the proliferation of the enamel organ and the dental papilla.

87. **2** In approximately the tenth week in utero, the dental papilla forms. This will develop into the dentin and pulp.

88. **3** The dental sac becomes the periodontal membrane and the cementum.

89. **2** It is during the bell stage that cells of the developing tooth differentiate into ameloblasts and odontoblasts and begin to deposit the enamel and dentin matrices respectively.

90. **1** The first part of the tooth to be formed is the crown. It is not until the enamel and dentin have reached the future cementoenamel junction that root formation begins.

91. **3** Enamel is derived originally from the dental lamina, which is made up of epithelial cells. The epithelial cells proliferate to form the enamel organ, which then differentiates into ameloblasts which form the enamel.

92. **3** The pulpal tissue is derived from mesenchymal cells, which proliferate to become the dental papilla. The dental papilla then differentiates to form the dental pulp.

93. **2** The odontoblasts are derived from the dental papilla. The stimulus for this formation is the differentiation of the ameloblasts by the enamel organ.

94. **1** The enamel-forming cells, ameloblasts, are no longer present after the tooth erupts. The enamel organ, which contains the ameloblasts, becomes Nasmyth's membrane, which covers the crown and is destroyed by abrasion when the tooth erupts.

95. **2** The structure that becomes the succedaneous tooth is the permanent tooth germ anlage. This structure begins to form during the cap stage and is located lingual to the developing tooth buds derived directly from the dental lamina.

96. **1** Four developmental lobes fuse to form the crowns of the anterior teeth. Three lobes fuse to form the labial surface and one lobe forms the cingulum on the lingual surface.

97. **3** Each developmental lobe on molars is represented by a cusp. The mandibular first molar is formed by the fusion of five developmental lobes while the mandibular second molar is formed by the fusion of four developmental lobes.

98. **2** The onset of the eruption process occurs when the tooth begins to move toward the oral cavity and is completed when the tooth is in functional occlusion. Eruption begins with the formation of the root.

99. **1** The most abundant tooth tissue is dentin. Dentin is a living tissue maintained by the pulp. The tooth is capable of forming additional dentin by odontoblastic activity.

100. **3** Secondary dentin is slowly and continuously deposited throughout the vital life of the tooth. If an irritant is present, the odontoblasts respond by quickly depositing secondary dentin, known as reparative secondary dentin, to protect the tooth.

101. **2** The hardest and most brittle tissue of the body is enamel.

102. **3** Enamel rods usually contact the dentino-enamel junction at right angles. The rods run a straight course to the surface of the crown, an important factor when considering cavity design.

103. **1** Nutrients for the pulp enter and leave the tooth through the apical foramen. The apical foramen is most often located near, but not at, the anatomic apex of the root.

104. **3** The pulpal tissue consists of cells (odontoblasts and fibroblasts), connective tissue (fibers and intercellular material), blood vessels, lymphatic vessels, and nerve fibers.

105. **2** Odontoblasts line the pulp cavity of all vital teeth. These cells have initially produced the dentin and are capable of producing more dentin throughout the vital life of the tooth.

106. **2** Painful stimuli are transmitted to the pulp via odontoblastic processes located in the dentinal tubules. The odontoblastic processes are stimulated by a disruption of the lymphatic fluid that fills the dentinal tubules.

107. **2** As a person ages, the dentinal pulp decreases in size and in cell number while increasing in fibrous components.

108. **3** The periodontium consists of the periodontal membrane, the alveolar bone, the gingiva, and cementum.

109. **1** The periodontal ligament lies between the cementum and the alveolar bone. It is made up of collagenous fibers, some of which are embedded in the cementum, and some of which are embedded in the alveolar bone.

110. **2** The proprioceptive mechanism of teeth is controlled by receptors located in the periodontal ligament. The receptors transmit information about the position of the teeth to the central nervous system, which can react by opening the mouth. Other important proprioceptive receptors are located in the fibrous capsule of the tem-

poromandibular joint and the muscles of mastication.

111. **2** Cementoblasts form cementum and become cementocytes, which maintain the cementum. This process is analogous to that of osteoblasts and osteocytes.

112. **3** Keratinization of the attached gingiva and the mucosa of the palate provides protection to the underlying tissue from the trauma of mastication.

113. **2** The gingiva is covered with stratified squamous epithelium.

114. **1** The edge or cuff of the gingiva not attached to the tooth is the free gingiva. The gingival papilla is the interdental extension of the free gingiva.

115. **3** The gingival sulcus is bordered by the tooth, the internal surface of the free gingiva, the gingival attachment, and the oral cavity.

116. **1** Healthy attached gingiva has an "orange peel" or stippled effect.

117. **1** The interdental papilla is pink, triangular and located between the teeth. The interdental papilla is free gingiva, not attached gingiva, thus it would not appear stippled.

118. **1** The level of interproximal bone is normally higher than either the buccal or lingual plates of bone. This bone level follows the contour of the cementoenamel junction of the teeth.

119. **2** Osteoclasts are multinucleated cells that resorb bone. When orthodontically moving teeth, osteoclastic activity resorbs the bone ahead of the tooth, while osteoblastic activity deposits bone behind the tooth.

120. **2** The bell-shaped roots of the deciduous molars surround the crowns of the permanent premolars and give the deciduous molars the stability they require to function.

121. **4** The mesiodistal crown length of the deciduous molars is longer than the premolars that will replace them. All other succedaneous teeth are larger than their deciduous counterparts.

122. **3** Exfoliation is the shedding of primary teeth. This is an active process that occurs between the ages of 6 and 12 and is caused by the resorption of the roots of the primary teeth.

123. **4** The last deciduous teeth to be shed are the deciduous second molars. This usually occurs between 11 and 12 years of age.

124. **3** The anatomical form of a tooth indicates its function: incisors cut, cuspids grasp and tear, bicuspids grasp and shred, and molars grind.

125. **1** A groove is an elongated depression formed when two developing lobes fuse.

126. **3** A pit is a sharp, small depression usually found at the junction of two fissures. A fissure is a developmental defect caused by the incomplete fusion of developing lobes.

127. **1** Marginal ridges are elevations of enamel forming the mesial and distal borders of the occlusal surface of posterior teeth. There are also marginal ridges on the lingual surface of anterior teeth forming the lateral borders of the teeth.

128. **2** Mamelons are three small elevations of enamel on the incisal edge of anterior teeth. Each elevation represents part of a developmental lobe. Mamelons are quickly worn away by use shortly after the tooth erupts.

129. **4** Embrasures are formed when two teeth contact. The major embrasure is located between the contact area and the gingiva. The interdental papilla is situated in the major embrasure.

130. **3** The minor embrasure is located interproximally above the contact area. It functions to deflect food, thereby preventing the impaction of food interproximally.

131. **3** The root canals of multirooted teeth open into the pulp chamber. The chamber has a floor, walls, and roof. The contents of the chamber are removed when performing either a pulpotomy or pulpectomy.

132. **4** A bifurcation is the space between roots of teeth that have two roots. Teeth that have bifurcations are the mandibular first and second molars and the maxillary first premolar.

133. **3** A trifurcation is the space between the roots of teeth that have three roots. The maxillary molars are teeth with three roots.

134. **2** A diastema is a space between adjacent teeth. It most frequently exists between the maxillary central incisors. A diastema can be created by the movement or drifting of teeth, caused by the lack of supporting bone.

135. **3** The anatomical crown is the portion of the tooth above the cementoenamel junction. The clinical crown will be larger than the anatomical crown if there is gingival recession beyond the cementoenamel junction. The clinical crown will be smaller than the anatomical crown if the gingiva is above the cementoenamel junction.

136. **3** The cementoenamel junction is also known as the cervical line.

137. **1** The surface of the tooth that faces the midline is the mesial surface. The surface that is the farthest from the midline is the distal surface.

138. **2** Anteriorly, the surface of the teeth facing the lips is the labial surface. Posteriorly, the surface of the teeth facing the cheek is the buccal surface. The surface of the upper teeth facing the palate is

the palatal surface. The surface of the lower teeth facing the tongue is the lingual surface.

139. **1** The upper and lower central incisors are the only teeth that have mesial surfaces in contact with each other.

140. **4** Anterior teeth are formed by the fusion of four developmental lobes. Three form the labial portion of the tooth, and one forms the lingual lobe known as the cingulum.

141. **1** Contact areas serve two functions: to protect the interproximal gingival tissue during mastication and to stabilize the dental arches preventing mesial or distal movement of the teeth.

142. **3** The theory that the gingiva is protected by tooth contour and tooth alignment is known as the soft tissue protection theory.

143. **2** The greatest contour of deciduous teeth is often located below the gingiva. This is an interesting fact, since the soft tissue protection theory is violated, yet normally the gingiva in children is healthy.

144. **1** When the teeth are at their maximum intercuspation, in an unstrained fashion, they are in centric occlusion.

145. **1** Overjet, also known as horizontal overbite, is the horizontal distance between the incisal edges of the maxillary and mandibular anterior teeth when they are in occlusion.

146. **3** Vertical overbite refers to the vertical overlap of the incisal edges of the maxillary and mandibular anterior teeth when the teeth are in occlusion.

147. **2** The most retruded physiological position of the mandible is the glenoid fossa in the centric relation.

148. **1** Mandibular teeth normally occlude mesial to their maxillary counterparts. In the absence of this relationship, malocclusion results.

149. **2** If a tooth is lost, the adjacent teeth tend to tilt and extrude to fill the available space. Teeth will move into areas of least resistance.

150. **3** The longest tooth in the mouth is the canine. The great length accounts for the stability of the tooth, which makes it an excellent abutment of prosthetic appliances. The canine is often referred to as the cornerstone of the mouth.

151. **3** A distinct characteristic of the maxillary premolar is the mesial fossa or concavity. Gingival recession and bone loss sufficient to expose the fossa in the oral cavity make it difficult to keep the area clean.

152. **2** The maxillary first premolar usually has two roots, buccal and palatal, as well as two root canals.

153. **1** The oblique ridge of the maxillary molar connects the mesiolingual and distobuccal cusps. The ridge can be so prominent that the occlusal groove pattern appears to be separated into a mesial and distal part. This is important in cavity preparation.

154. **4** The largest cusp of the maxillary first molar is the mesiolingual cusp. The smallest cusp is the distolingual cusp.

155. **3** The cusp of Carabelli is the fifth cusp sometimes present on the palatal surface of the mesiolingual cusp of the maxillary first molar. The cusp is nonfunctional.

156. **3** The roots of the maxillary first molar are the palatal (the largest root), mesiobuccal, and distobuccal. The roots form a tripod type of support; this accounts for the great stability of the tooth.

157. **4** The mandibular central incisor and the maxillary third molars are the only teeth that contact one antagonist in the opposing arch.

158. **1** The mandibular central incisor is the smallest permanent tooth in either arch.

159. **1** Although the mandibular first premolar has two cusps, the lingual cusp is small and nonfunctional. The shape of the buccal cusp is known as caniniform.

160. **3** The mandibular second premolar usually has three cusps: one buccal cusp, molariform in shape, and two small lingual cusps.

161. **4** In normal occlusion, the lingual cusps of the mandibular molars and the buccal cusps of the maxillary molars do not contact the fossae of their antagonists. The cusps that contact the fossae of their antagonists are the buccal cusps of the mandibular molars and the lingual cusps of the maxillary teeth.

162. **3** The mandibular first molar has three buccal cusps and two buccal developmental grooves: the mesiobuccal and distobuccal. These grooves are formed when the three buccal developmental lobes fuse. Incomplete fusion leads to increased caries susceptibility.

163. **2** If the mandibular first molar is in a retruded position the occlusion is classified as distoocclusion or class II malocclusion. Mesiocclusion or class III malocclusion is the classification given when the mandibular first molar is in a protruded position.

164. **3** The mandibular first molar has five cusps, the smallest of which is the distobuccal. This cusp is about one half the size of any of the other cusps. This is the only tooth where five cusps are regularly found.

165. **4** The mesial root of the mandibular first molar contains two root canals: mesiobuccal and mesio-

lingual. Each canal usually has its own apical foramen.

166. **2** The roots of the mandibular molars are the mesial and distal roots. The roots of the first molar are usually spread wider than the roots of the second molar. The anatomy of these roots is an important consideration when selecting teeth as abutments and when treating bifurcation involvements in periodontics.

167. **4** Third molars often have fused roots.

168. **8**

169. **5**

170. **6**

171. **5**

172. **5**

173. **6**

174. **6**

175. **7**

176. **2** The science that studies the cause and origin of disease is etiology. Definitive treatment for most diseases is dependent on knowing their etiology.

177. **4** Healing is rapid in the oral cavity because of the abundant blood supply. If the tongue is injured it will heal faster than other injured oral structures, because it has a larger blood supply than do other oral structures. The excellent blood supply also protects the oral tissue from infection from oral surgical procedures although the mouth is a sea of potential pathogens.

178. **4** Various etiologies of pathology in the oral cavity are habits, diet, heredity, temperature, trauma, chemical, bacterial, viral, and fungal.

179. **4** Prophylactic means preventing disease. Examples of prophylactic measures are the use of penicillin to prevent heart complications in patients with a history of rheumatic fever; prophylactic odontotomy, a technique that eliminates pits and fissures and thereby reduces the chance of caries in these areas; and the use of fluoride to decrease enamel solubility.

180. **2** Atrophy refers to a decrease in size of normal tissue caused by a decrease in the size or number of cells. Atrophy can be caused by normal aging or by pathological causes: disuse, circulation, or pressure. Hypertrophy is an increase in cell size.

181. **4** The retention of fluid in a specific area of the body is known as edema. It is often related to circulatory changes or allergies.

182. **3** The engorgement of blood is known as hyperemia. This reaction occurs during inflammation and accounts for the redness and heat in the affected area.

183. **3** Erythema is an abnormal redness of the skin attributable to inflammation, x-ray treatment, or a disease process.

184. **2** Symptoms of inflammation are redness caused by the dilation of blood vessels, heat caused by dilation of blood vessels, swelling caused by fluids leaving the blood vessels and accumulating in the area, pain caused by pressure of fluids on sensory nerves, and impairment of function.

185. **4** Enamel hypoplasia is a condition that results from defective enamel formation. The enamel is usually pitted or grooved across the crown as a result of the disturbance of the ameloblasts during the enamel matrix formation.

186. **4** Some causes of defects in enamel are dietary deficiencies, local infection, high fever, trauma, and drugs.

187. **3** A disturbance during the mineralization of the enamel matrix can result in enamel hypocalcification. This condition often occurs with enamel hypoplasia; the causes of the two conditions are the result of the same etiology.

188. **3** Mottled enamel is the result of a disturbance during tooth formation due to the ingestion of excess fluoride. The enamel has a brown opaque appearance. The treatment is usually for cosmetic reasons and may range from fillings to full coverage.

189. **1** Dilaceration refers to a sharp angulation of the root. It is usually caused by trauma during root formation. There is no treatment necessary for the condition; if, however, root canal therapy or extraction is necessary, complications can arise.

190. **4** Attrition is the physiological wearing away of the occlusal and proximal surfaces of teeth associated with aging. This process occurs in both the primary and permanent dentition. Excessive attrition can be caused by bruxing and other oral habits.

191. **3** Abrasion is the mechanical wearing away of tooth structure by a foreign body. The most common cause is toothbrushing with a stiff bristle brush using an abrasive dentifrice. Other causes are habits such as pipe smoking and holding other objects habitually between the teeth.

192. **2** Ankylosis is the direct attachment of the tooth to bone with no intervening periodontal membrane. It occurs most frequently in deciduous molars. Causative factors include trauma, infection, or external resorption. Treatment, if it is a deciduous tooth, is the surgical removal of the tooth, which will then permit the permanent tooth to erupt. If a permanent tooth is ankylosed, no treatment is necessary, but problems can arise if the tooth is extracted.

193. **2** A cleft lip is a defect below the ala of the nose

on one or both sides. It is caused by the lack of fusion between the maxillary process and the median nasal process. A cleft palate is the lack of fusion along the median line of the palate. It can vary from a cleft of part of the soft palate to a cleft of the entire soft and hard palate.

194. **4** The most common supernumerary tooth is a mesiodens, located between the maxillary central incisors. The second most common supernumerary tooth is the maxillary fourth molar.

195. **4** An impacted tooth is one that is physically prevented from erupting into the oral cavity. The most commonly impacted tooth is the third molar. The second most commonly impacted tooth is the maxillary canine.

196. **4** The tooth most frequently congenitally missing is the third molar. The mandibular second premolar and the maxillary lateral incisors are also frequently congenitally missing.

197. **2** Aging results in varying amounts of gingival recession and a decrease in the size of the pulp chamber. The contents of the pulp become more fibrous and less cellular. There is also attrition of incisal edges and occlusal surfaces of the teeth.

198. **2** Tic douloureux is a pathological condition of the fifth cranial nerve. It is associated with trigger zones on the face that, when stimulated, set off an excruciating pain, usually lasting a few seconds. The cause of this disease is unknown, but it could be related to the proximity of blood vessels to the trigeminal nerve.

199. **3** A muscle spasm is a sudden involuntary contraction of muscle tissue. The tissue can remain contracted for an extended period of time, or it can alternate with periods of relaxation.

200. **1** The unconscious grinding of teeth is called bruxism. Some possible causes are occlusal descrepancies and psychological factors associated with tension release.

201. **3** An open bite refers to an orthodontic problem wherein the anterior teeth do not contact each other. The etiology may be a habit such as thumb sucking or tongue thrusting. The treatment may include discontinuance of the habit and orthodontic intervention.

202. **2** The ability to ward off disease is known as host resistance; it can be natural, such as elements in saliva that decrease the caries rate, or acquired, such as the decrease in tooth solubility caused by the incorporation of fluoride into the tooth.

203. **2** Antibodies are proteins that are part of the body's defense system. They are produced in response to a foreign body, an antigen. Immunity, the ability of the body to resist infection, depends on the formation of antibodies.

204. **2** Bacterial invasion of the circulatory system is referred to as bacteremia. This type of infection usually involves the whole body and is known as a systemic infection.

205. **2** Herpes simplex is the virus that causes recurrent sores in the oral cavity. The disease is initiated by an attack of primary herpes, which is contagious in young children. The lesions of primary herpes are widespread throughout the mouth. Subsequent attacks are usually associated with single lesions. There is no known specific treatment for the lesion, which takes about 14 days to heal.

206. **3** Thrush, or moniliasis, is caused by the fungus *Candida albicans*. This organism is normally found in the oral cavity; an imbalance attributable to nutritional problems or antibiotic therapy is responsible for its overgrowth and subsequent disease state.

207. **4** Symptoms of ANUG include ulcerations on the gingiva, bleeding gums, and elevated temperature. Headaches are not often associated with ANUG.

208. **2** Osteomyelitis is an inflammation of bone that can result from a periapical infection. The disease is either chronic or acute. Treatment is removal of the causative agent, antibiotic therapy, and drainage in acute stages.

209. **3** Mumps usually causes the inflammation and swelling of the parotid glands. The patient has fever and chills and might find it difficult to open the mouth.

210. **4** A salivary stone is known as a sialolith. If the stone blocks the duct of a salivary gland, the gland may swell due to the backup saliva. A sialograph is the radiograph used to help diagnose the problem. The treatment is the removal of the stone by manipulation or surgery.

211. **4** The flow, consistency, and chemical composition of saliva affect the caries rate. Xerostomia, a decrease in salivary flow, increases the caries rate.

212. **4** Salivary flow is affected by drugs, lack of salivary gland formation, x-irradiation, nutrition, and even thoughts.

213. **4** Caries can be controlled chemically (fluoride), nutritionally (decreasing the consumption of refined carbohydrates), and mechanically (removing plaque from the teeth every 24 hours).

214. **1** Stains are classified as extrinsic, which are removable by prophylaxis, or intrinsic, which are part of the tooth structure. Stains are caused by drugs, chromogenic bacteria, smoking, and problems in tooth formation.

215. **4** Calculus will form on any structure upon which plaque will form in the oral cavity. The process of calculus formation is the deposition of

salts from either the saliva or serum in the plaque matrix.

216. **2** Periodontal disease is an inflammatory disease that begins at the gingiva and progresses to destroy the alveolar bone supporting the teeth. The cause of disease is primarily bacterial plaque. Many other factors contribute to the disease, such as diet, occlusal problems, dentistry, and endocrine problems. To date the most effective means of preventing periodontal disease is the mechanical removal of the bacterial plaque at least once a day.

217. **4** Pulpal reaction to irritants can result in secondary dentin formation or inflammation, which can lead to microabscess formation, fibrosis, or death of the pulp.

218. **1** Hormonal changes affect the periodontium. Examples of endocrine changes in the mouth are pregnancy gingivitis, increased rate of bone loss in diabetes, swelling of the gingiva during the menstrual cycle, and accelerated rate of eruption caused by hyperthyroidism.

219. **3** Neoplasm refers to a new growth that will not disappear when the etiology is removed. Neoplasms are classified as benign or malignant. Malignant tumors are life threatening and will result in the death of the host if they are not removed.

220. **3** Benign refers to tumors (neoplasms) composed of normal tissue. They are named according to their tissue of origin with the suffix "oma." These lesions are dangerous if they are located in areas wherein their physical presence, pressure by growth, or creation of hypersecretion is damaging. This can occur in the brain, trachea, or endocrine glands, as well as other parts of the body.

221. **1** A white patch in the oral cavity is called leukoplakia. The cause is a chronic irritant, such as smoking or rubbing by the sharp edge of a fractured tooth. Some leukoplakic areas undergo changes and become a carcinoma.

222. **3** Examples of benign tumors are lipoma, an outgrowth of fatty tissue; fibroma, an outgrowth of fibrous tissue; and papilloma, an outgrowth of surface epithelium.

223. **4** Leukemia is a disease of white blood cells. Manifestations of the disease appear in the oral cavity as spontaneous hemorrhage, poor healing, and gingival enlargement.

224. **1** Metastasis is the spreading of cancer to different sites in the body. The most frequent malignant oral tumor is squamous cell carcinoma, which metastasizes through the lymphatic system.

225. **2** The definitive diagnosis of cancer is made by removing a piece of the lesion (a biopsy) and studying it under a microscope.

Bibliography

Dahlberg, A. *Dental Morphology and Evolution,* Chicago and London: University of Chicago Press, 1971.

Fuller, J.L. and Denehy, G.E. *Concise Dental Anatomy and Morphology,* Chicago and London: Yearbook Medical Publishers, Inc., 1977.

Goss, C.M. *Gray's Anatomy,* 29th ed. Philadelphia: Lea & Febiger Publishers, 1973.

Graber, T.M. *Orthodontics,* 3rd ed. Philadelphia: W. B. Saunders Co., 1972.

Greep, R.O. and Weiss, L. *Histology,* 3rd ed. New York: McGraw-Hill Inc., 1973.

Kraus, B.S.; Jordan, R.E.; and Abrams, L. *Dental Anatomy and Occlusion,* Baltimore: Williams & Wilkins Co., 1969.

Orban, B. *Oral Histology and Embryology,* 9th ed. St. Louis: The C. V. Mosby Co., 1980.

Robbins, S.L. and Angell, M. *Basic Pathology,* 3rd ed. Philadelphia: W. B. Saunders Co., 1981.

Scopp, I.W. *Oral Medicine,* 2nd ed. St. Louis: The C. V. Mosby Co., 1973.

Shafer, W.G.; Howe, M.K.; and Levy, B.M. *Textbook of Oral Pathology,* 3rd ed. Philadelphia: W. B. Saunders Co., 1974.

Wheeler, R.C. *An Atlas of Tooth Form,* 4th ed. Philadelphia: W. B. Saunders Co., 1969.

Wheeler, R.C. *Dental Anatomy, Physiology and Occlusion,* 5th ed. Philadelphia: W. B. Saunders Co., 1974.

3

Radiology

Course Synopsis

Introduction

In 1895, Wilhelm Conrad Roentgen, a professor of physics in Germany, found that experiments with a cathode ray tube produced a glowing reflection on a special screen opposite to the tube.

The ray that caused the glowing was called an x-ray by Dr. Roentgen. He discovered that these x-ray beams are produced whenever fast-moving electrons strike another substance. In 1896, Dr. Otto Walkoff, a dentist in Germany, made the first dental use of an x-ray beam by radiographing a lower premolar; the exposure time was 25 minutes, as opposed to the current exposure time of tenths of a second.

Several others made contributions to the use of x-rays. In 1898, Dr. Edmund Kells began to use x-ray beams in dentistry, while William Rollins, an inventor from Boston, advocated caution in the use of this radiation.

Through the diligent work of leaders in the field, and advanced technology, x-ray films have become an important and sophisticated diagnostic tool in medicine and dentistry.

Properties

X-rays have certain special properties. They travel in straight lines and cannot be seen in the visible light spectrum. They have short wavelengths, and consequently high energy, which gives them penetrating power to travel through objects. They can also darken a photographic plate. The penetration power and photographic ability of the x-ray beam makes it useful as a diagnostic tool for medicine and dentistry. However, x-rays affect living tissue and should be used with caution, and only when necessary.

In addition to being useful for diagnostic purposes in medicine and dentistry, high doses of concentrated x-rays on human tissue are used to destroy areas of neoplastic cells (tumors) in the battle against cancer.

X-Ray Production

Knowledge and an understanding of x-ray production are critical for the proper exposure of radiographs. The dental x-ray machine houses a tube in which x-rays are produced when high-energy electrons strike a plate. Basic components of an x-ray tube are necessary for the production of x-rays. In the tube, the tungsten filament provides the source of electrons. This filament is located at the cathode, the negatively charged side of the x-ray tube. Turning on the x-ray machine heats the tungsten filament, and an electron cloud forms around it. The number or density of electrons in the cloud is controlled by the milliamperage (mA). A high-amperage (current) low-voltage system is used to generate a large number of electrons. These electrons are subsequently attracted to the target at the anode (the positive side of the x-ray tube) by a voltage difference between the anode and cathode. The stream of electrons crossing the tube, called the cathode ray, strikes the target (focal spot), and x-rays as well as heat are produced (see Fig. 15).

Since the target and the filament have different electrical needs to produce the electron cloud and create the difference in potential for the cathode ray, each x-ray unit contains two transformers. A stepup transformer for the target increases the voltage from 110 volts to a range of 50,000–100,000 volts (50–100 kvp), and a step-down transformer for the filament decreases the voltage to 3–5 volts.

All x-rays generated are not equal. Some have high energy and others do not. Lower energy rays, those with longer wavelengths, are not useful because they have a lower penetration power and represent a radiation hazard. An aluminum disk 2–2.5 mm thick filters out the less penetrating rays before they leave the x-ray machine, while letting the more penetrating rays through.

Since the film to be illuminated is approximately 1 1/4 × 1 5/8 inches, the spread or divergence of the x-ray beam must be controlled. Otherwise, areas peripheral to the targeted area would be exposed and would increase patient exposure. This process, called collimation, is accomplished by a lead diaphragm located within the x-ray tube, which limits the size of the x-ray beam.

Three parameters are controlled by the operator of an x-ray unit:

1. Quality (penetrating power) of the x-ray beam, expressed as kilovoltage (kvp)
2. Quantity (number) of x-rays produced, expressed as milliamperage (mA)
3. Length of time the x-rays are produced, expressed as exposure time

The exposure time is usually the only parameter that is varied within a dental office. Suitable penetrating power for dental x-rays ranges from 50 to 100 kvp, and the required quantities of x-rays are produced in the 5–15-mA range.

Radiographic Exposures

The property of tissues of varying densities to absorb different amounts of the x-rays passing through them produces the film records (radiographs) of internal structures of the body.

The number of x-rays that hit the film determines the degree of blackening, or density, of the radiograph. Areas and structures that are denser, such as bone and metallic restorations, absorb more x-rays. Therefore, few x-rays reach the film, making the film appear radiopaque (white) in these areas. Structures and areas that are less dense, such as pulp chambers and sinus cavities, appear radiolucent (black) on radiographs.

The range of shades from white to black, including all shades of gray, is called contrast. Low-contrast radiographs are produced from high kilovoltage; these films contain more shades of gray and are therefore more diagnostic. It is also important to minimize the degree of distortion in radiographs. Minimum distortion can be accomplished by meeting three criteria:

1. Only the most parallel rays strike the object, and subsequently the film.
2. A minimum distance is maintained between the object and the film.
3. The object and the film are parallel to each other.

However, these criteria present problems. A lengthy focal-film distance (FFD) is necessary for the most parallel rays to reach the object.

The inverse-square law, which relates energy and distance, demonstrates that large focal-film distances (FFDs) require very high levels of energy. Therefore, an

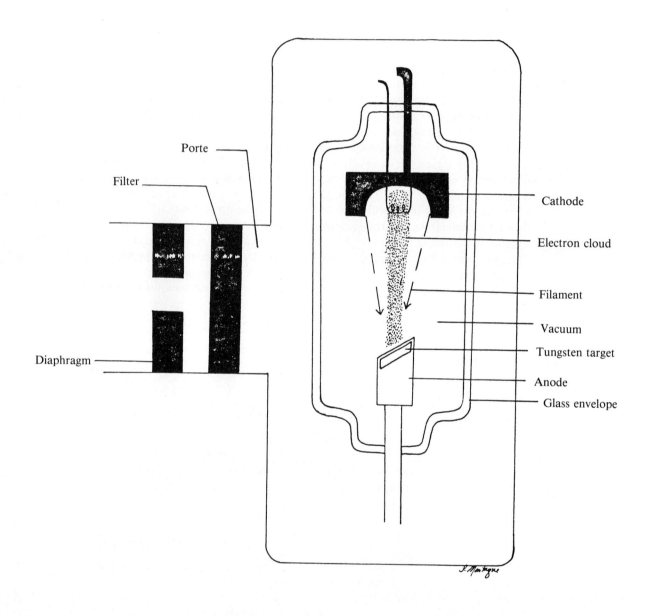

Fig. 15. Diagram of x-ray head.

increased FFD necessitates increased exposure, resulting in increased radiation to the patient.

The most commonly used FFDs in dentistry are 8, 12, and 16 inches.

The maintenance of a minimum distance between the object and the film (object-film distance) and parallelism between the object and the film are two criteria that compromise each other. The anatomy of intraoral structures prevents the film from being parallel to the object, and hence be as close as possible to the object (see Fig. 16).

Techniques of Intraoral Radiography

Two techniques are used to take a series of radiographic films: paralleling and bisecting the angle.

The *paralleling technique* is based on the principle that the object (tooth) and the film are parallel to each other, and the central ray is directed perpendicular to both (see Fig. 17).

Increased object-film distance results in loss of image detail, which is compensated for by using a 16-inch FFD. Advantages and disadvantages to the paralleling technique are as follows:

Advantages

1. The image formed on the film will have dimensional accuracy.
2. Owing to minimum distortion, periodontal bone height can be accurately diagnosed.
3. On maxillary molar projection, there is little or no root superimposition.

Disadvantages

1. Intraoral film-holding devices must be used. These devices can be difficult to work with and uncomfortable for the patient.
2. Some patients have anatomical features, such as low palatal vaults, which prevent proper placement of film.
3. The use of a 16-inch FFD necessitates an increase in exposure time.

In the *bisecting-the-angle technique,* an imaginary line is identified that bisects the angle formed by the long axis of the tooth and the film; the central ray is directed perpendicularly to the imaginary line. This technique uses an 8-inch FFD (see Fig. 18). Advantages and disadvantages to the bisecting-the-angle technique are as follows:

Advantages

1. Shorter exposure times can be used because there is a shorter FFD.
2. The use of the patient's finger for holding the film eliminates the need for holding devices.
3. Anatomical features usually do not interfere with film placement.

Disadvantages

1. The image projected on the film is dimensionally distorted in varying degrees.
2. True alveolar bone height can be misinterpreted.
3. The use of an 8-inch FFD results in divergent rays; therefore, the image is not an optimum reproduction of the object.
4. The patient's finger is exposed to ionizing radiation.

The Film Packet

Dental intraoral radiographs come in various sizes. Three common sizes are adult size, pedodontic size, and narrow interior film. There are also larger occlusal films and longer bite-wing films.

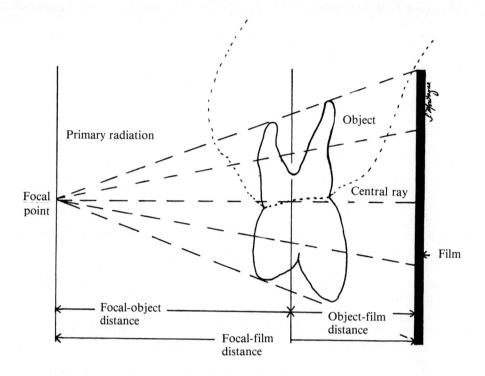

Fig. 16. Relationship among focal point, object, and film.

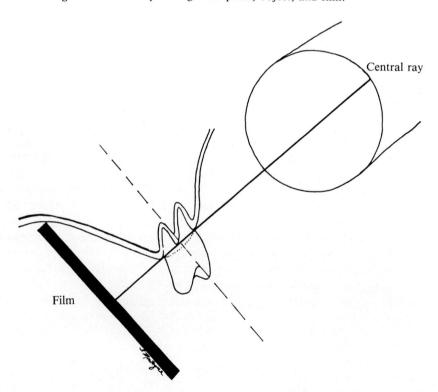

Fig. 17. Central ray, tooth, and film packet in parallel-angle technique of intraoral radiography.

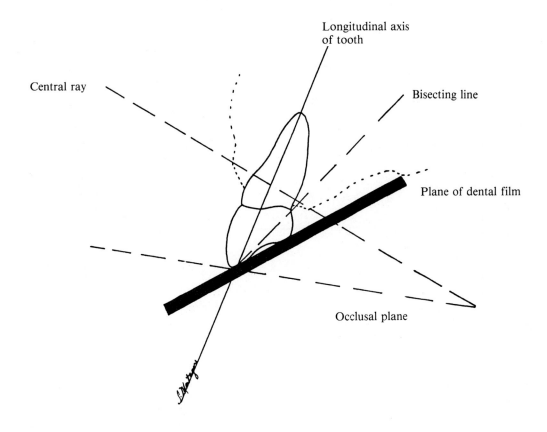

Fig. 18. Bisecting-the-angle technique of intraoral radiography.

The film packet must be moisture and light resistant, flexible, and easy to open in the darkroom. The packet contains a waterproof outer covering, black paper, the film, and a piece of lead foil that absorbs any unused radiation. The foil backing also serves to reduce background scatter and thereby prevents film fogging (see Fig. 19).

The film itself is composed of a silver halide emulsion, covered by gelatin on a cellulose acetate film. The size of the silver halide crystals determines the film speed, or sensitivity. This film speed affects the amount of radiation and the length of time (milliamperes) required to produce an image on the film. Faster films have larger crystals and therefore require fewer milliamperes. However, films with larger crystals give poorer definition or detail on a film. Slower films, which have smaller crystals, give more detail, and require more milliamperes.

Film speed is designated by the American National Standards Institute (ANSI) by letter groups A–F, with speed increasing incrementally with the alphabet. Fast films D–F are used because they require less radiation exposure to the patient and the definition or detail that is sacrificed is minimal.

Dental films should always be stored in a lead-lined container or compartment. Films that are outdated, or affected by undesired radiation or light, become fogged, compromising their diagnostic value.

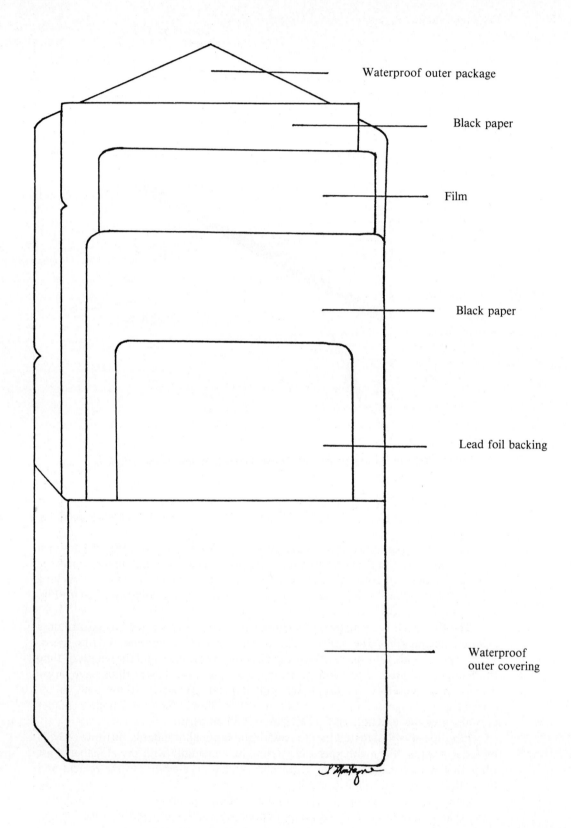

Fig. 19. Dental film packet.

The Full Mouth Series

A full mouth series of radiographs for an adult with a full complement of teeth is usually composed of at least 14 periapical films and four bite-wing films. Periapical films show the entire tooth and the supporting alveolar bone. They are used to diagnose bone and root pathology and to provide information on tooth formation and eruption.

Bite-wing films show upper and lower teeth in occlusion. The full roots of the teeth are not visible on the film. Bite-wing films are useful in identifying recurrent decay, proximal decay, the proximal gingival marginal fit of restorations, and periodontal bone loss.

The following projections constitute a typical full series for a patient with a complete dentition:

Maxillary Periapicals
   Right and left central and lateral incisors
   Right and left canines
   Right and left premolars
   Right and left molars
Mandibular Periapicals
   Central and lateral incisors
   Right and left canines
   Right and left premolars
   Right and left molars
Bite-wings
   Right and left premolars
   Right and left molars

Regardless of whether the paralleling or bisecting-the-angle technique is used, certain procedures and rules must be followed:

1. Seat the patient with head positioned so that the occlusal plane of the jaw being radiographed is parallel to the floor and the midsagittal plane is perpendicular to the floor.
2. Remove any eyeglasses or removable prosthetic appliances.
3. Drape the patient with a leaded lap apron which extends from the neck past the genital area.
4. Turn the knob to the desired exposure time before placing the film in the patient's mouth. (A chart listing the desired exposure times for each area to be radiographed should be posted near the machine.)
5. After an exposure is made, remove the film from the patient's mouth. Dry the film and place it in a lead-lined container.
6. Never place films, either exposed or unexposed, within an operatory where exposures are made.
7. Follow a definite order when taking a full series. Do not shift from area to area.

   A suggested sequence is as follows:
1. Maxillary right projections
2. Maxillary left projections
3. Bite-wings (right, then left)
4. Mandibular right projections
5. Mandibular left projections

   If the bisecting-the-angle technique is used, the following rules are followed:
1. The patient holds the maxillary films with the thumb.
2. The patient holds the mandibular films with an index finger.
3. The central ray is perpendicular to the plane of the film packet.

4. The film should extend evenly 1/8–1/4 inch below/above the incisal or occlusal edges of the teeth.
5. The central ray is aimed at the center of the film packet.

If the paralleling technique is used, bite-wings are taken the same way as in the bisecting-the-angle technique. The major difference between periapical film positioning in the paralleling technique and the bisecting-the-angle technique is the angle formed by the film and the long axis of the tooth. In the bisecting–the–angle technique, the film is held as close as possible to the tooth being radiographed. In the paralleling technique, the film is held with a holding device so that it is parallel to the long axis of the tooth (usually ½–1 inch from the tooth). (See Tables I and II for details of a suggested full series using the bisecting-the-angle techniques and paralleling, respectively.)

The Edentulous Full Series

The edentulous full series usually consists of 14 periapical films. Bite-wing films are not taken. The projections are as follows:
1. Maxillary central and lateral incisors
2. Maxillary right and left canines
3. Maxillary right and left premolars
4. Maxillary right and left molars
5. Mandibular central and lateral incisors
6. Mandibular right and left canines
7. Mandibular right and left premolars
8. Mandibular right and left molars

When taking an edentulous full series, the following modifications are necessary:
1. Replace the occlusal plane with the crest of the edentulous ridge.
2. Increase the vertical angulation.
3. Decrease the exposure time.

The edentulous series is important in diagnosing pathological conditions, such as cysts and abscesses, and in locating retained root tips and impacted teeth.

The Pedodontic Full Series

The composition of a pedodontic series differs with the age of the child and the size of the mouth. The following film sizes are commonly used:
1. 7/8 × 1 3/8 inches for 5-year-olds
2. 15/16 × 1 9/16 inches anterior and 1 1/4 × 1 5/8 inches posterior for 6-9-year-olds

A typical pedodontic series consists of 12 projections:
1. Maxillary central and lateral incisors
2. Maxillary right and left canines
3. Maxillary right and left premolars and molars
4. Mandibular central and lateral incisors
5. Mandibular right and left canines
6. Mandibular right and left premolars and molars
7. Right premolar and molar bite-wing
8. Left premolar and molar bite-wing

Common Errors in Exposure of a Full Mouth Series of Radiographs

Table III lists errors commonly made in the exposure of a full mouth series, as well as the reasons for these errors:

Table I

Suggested Full Series: Bisecting-the-Angle Technique

Projections	Film Position	Vertical Angulation	Direction of the Central Ray
Maxillary right and left central and lateral	Held vertically; central and lateral incisors are centered	+50°	Below the midpoint of the nares
Maxillary right and left canine	Held vertically; canine is centered	+50°	The base of the lateral nasal grooves
Maxillary right and left premolars	Held horizontally; premolars are centered	+40°	The most anterior part of the cheekbone
Maxillary right and left molars	Held horizontally; second molar is centered	+30°	Through the zygomatic arch
Right and left premolar bite-wing	Bite tab is placed on occlusal surfaces of the first and second premolars; patient bites on tab	+10°	The center of the bite tab
Right and left molar bite-wing	Bite tab is placed on occlusal surface of the second molar; patient bites on tab	+10°	The center of the bite tab
Mandibular central and lateral incisors	Held vertically; centrals are centered	−20°	The depression in the face just above the chin
Mandibular right and left canines	Held vertically; canine is centered	−20°	The root of the canine
Mandibular right and left premolars	Held horizontally; premolars are centered	−15°	The metal foramen
Mandibular right and left molars	Held horizontally; second molar is centered	−5°	The roots of the molars

Table II

Suggested Full Series: Paralleling Technique

Projections	Film Placement	Vertical Angulation	Direction of the Central Ray
Maxillary right and left central and lateral	Held vertically; central and lateral incisors are centered; parallel to long axis of the tooth	Central ray is perpendicular to the film packet	Central ray is aimed at the center of the film
Maxillary right and left canine	Held vertically; canine is centered; parallel to long axis of the tooth	Central ray is perpendicular to the film packet	Central ray is aimed at the center of the film
Maxillary right and left premolars	Held horizontally; premolars are centered; parallel to long axis of the tooth	Central ray is perpendicular to the film packet	Central ray is aimed at the center of the film
Maxillary right and left molars	Held horizontally; second molar is centered; parallel to long axis of the tooth	Central ray is perpendicular to the film packet	Central ray is aimed at the center of the film
Right and left premolar bite-wing	Bite tab is placed on occlusal surfaces of the first and second premolars; patient bites on tab	+10°	Central ray is aimed at the center of the bite tab
Right and left molar bite-wing	Bite tab is placed on occlusal surface of the second molar; patient bites on tab	+10°	Central ray is aimed at the center of the bite tab
Mandibular central and lateral incisors	Held vertically; central incisors are centered; parallel to long axis of the tooth	Central ray is perpendicular to the film packet	Central ray is aimed at the center of the film
Mandibular right and left canines	Held vertically; canine is centered; parallel to long axis of the tooth	Central ray is perpendicular to the film packet	Central ray is aimed at the center of the film
Mandibular right and left premolars	Held horizontally; premolars are centered; parallel to long axis of the tooth	Central ray is perpendicular to the film packet	Central ray is aimed at the center of the film
Mandibular right and left molars	Held horizontally; second molar is centered; parallel to long axis of the tooth	Central ray is perpendicular to the film packet	Central ray is aimed at the center of the film

Table III

Errors in Exposure of Full Mouth Series of Radiographs

Common Error	Reasons
Elongation (most common error)	Too little vertical angulation; occlusal plane not parallel to the floor; film not against tissue; poor film placement
Foreshortening	Too much vertical angulation; poor chair position
Cone cutting (clear film, curved line)	Beam not aimed at center of film
Film reversal or herringbone effect	Film placed in mouth backward
Film placement	Film not placed far enough in the patient's mouth
Sagittal plane orientation (occlusal surfaces appear because patient has leaned over; elongation and distortion)	Plane not perpendicular to the floor
Overlapping	Incorrect horizontal angulation (central ray is not perpendicular to the center of the film)
Crescent-shaped marks (black lines)	Overbent films; cracked emulsion
Light films (underexposed)	Incorrect milliamperes (too low) or time (too short); cone not apporoximating the patient's face; incorrect focal film distance (FFD)
Dark films (overexposed)	Incorrect milliamperes (too low) or time (too long)
Double exposure	Film used twice
Fogged films	Exposure to radiation other than primary beam
Artifacts	Failure to remove prosthestic appliances, earrings, or eyeglasses
Clear films	Unexposed

Supplementary Diagnostic Radiographic Techniques

The following instances will not permit a standard full series to provide all the information necessary to make an accurate diagnosis:
1. Areas inaccessible to typical intraoral film need to be visualized
2. Buccolingual dimensions need to be established
3. Large pathologies need to be diagnosed
4. Patient is unable to accommodate the x-ray or refuses an intraoral film

Consequently, additional types of radiographic aids are required in making a differential diagnosis.

Occlusal Films

Radiographic films made of the maxilla and mandible are larger films (2 1/4 × 3 inches) used to determine the buccolingual dimensions of impacted teeth and to locate salivary stones. Table IV lists the features of making occlusal films.

Table IV

Occlusal Films

Arch	Film Packet Placement	Direction of Central Ray
Maxillary	On occlusal surfaces of maxillary teeth; patient bites down on film packet	Perpendicular to the film packet; cone is 2–4 inches away from face
Mandibular	On occlusal surfaces of mandibular teeth; patient bites down on film packet	Beneath the mandible; perpendicular to the film packet cone is 2–4 inches away from face

Extraoral Films

Extraoral films are radiographs taken with the film outside the patient's mouth. The size of these films varies from 5 × 7 inches, to 8 × 10 inches, to 5 × 12 inches. These films are held in cassettes that perform the same function as the film packet. Most cassettes are metal, but lightweight plastic cassettes are used when taking a panoramic radiograph. Intensifying screens in the cassettes are used to intensify the radiation and therefore decrease the exposure time. Table V describes features of extraoral films.

Table V

Extraoral Films

Type of Film	Area Visualized
Lateral skull	Whole skull pathological survey
Anterior–posterior	Anterior–posterior plane of skull fracture survey
Water's view	Sinuses

Lateral oblique of the mandible	One side of mandible, usually for third molar impactions
Temporomandibular joint (TMJ)	TMJ in various positions
Cephalometric (usually a lateral skull plate)	Identifies anthropometric landmarks essential to orthodontic diagnosis

Innovations in radiography have led to the ability to take a film of the complete upper and lower jaw simultaneously. This procedure is accomplished by using a panoramic x-ray unit. In essence, the patient's head is fixed and the x-ray tube and film focus and rotate around the patient's head. As a result, a continuous picture is produced on a single film. Advantages and disadvantages of panoramic radiography include the following:

Advantages

1. Areas not seen on a routine full mouth series are shown.
2. Both upper and lower teeth are shown on one film.
3. Less patient cooperation is required.
4. Gagging is eliminated.
5. Less time is required.
6. The patient is exposed to minimum amounts of radiation.

Disadvantages

1. The radiograph is not as diagnostic as are individual films for caries or bone height.
2. Images of teeth are enlarged.
3. Overlapping occurs in the premolar area.
4. Anterior teeth are difficult to see when they have pronounced inclinations.

The Darkroom

A latent image exists on the film after it is exposed in the patient's mouth. The energized silver halide crystals must be processed through chemical reactions in order for the latent image to become a visible image. This developing process occurs in the darkroom.

The darkroom is a separate room used specifically for processing exposed radiographs. The following components and requirements are essential:

1. No light leaks (films out of their holders are light sensitive)
2. Safelight (usually a 10- or 15-watt bulb with a red filter placed about 3–4 feet from the working surface)
3. Developing tank: three compartments
   a. developer (usually on the right)
   b. wash
   c. fixer
4. Timing device
5. Thermometer (in developing solution)
6. Rack on which to place films
7. Clean working surface
8. Sink (for cleaning tanks)
9. View box
10. Storage space

Before developing films, all solutions should be stirred to ensure that the solutions are homogeneous and that the temperatures are equalized. The date, the number of films, the rack number or letter, and the patient's name and chart number should be recorded on the radiographic information sheet. Failure to maintain accurate records or to process films correctly will result in unnecessary radiation to the patient, because radiographs will have to be retaken.

The Development Process

Under safelight conditions, each film should be carefully unwrapped and placed on the film rack. The development process for films is then accomplished in five steps:

1. *Developing:* The developing solution is a basic solution of Elon or metal hydroquinone that reduces the energized silver halide crystals to silver. The silver is precipitated on the film base and appears black (radiolucent). Since this precipitation process is dependent on the concentration and temperature of the development fluid, the radiograph is very sensitive to both the length of time in the developer and the temperature of the solution. The optimum time–temperature relationship is 4 1/4 minutes at 68°F.

2. *Washing:* The developed film is then washed for approximately 20 seconds. Washing stops the developing stage and removes any remaining developing solution that might contaminate the fixer.

3. *Fixing:* The fixing solution is an acidic solution that contains sodium thiosulfate and sodium sulfite, which removes the unexposed (or unenergized) silver halide crystals from the emulsion and preserves the picture. Potassium aluminum is also contained in the solution for the purpose of shrinking and hardening the film. Radiographs must be placed in the fixer for a minimum of 10 minutes, since inadequate fixation will cause the films to turn brown.

4. *Washing:* Films must be placed in running water for at least 20 minutes. This final wash ensures removal of the fixing solution from the emulsion.

5. *Drying:* Films must be dried in a dust-free, clean area; either by air drying or machine drying.

Table VI lists common errors made in the darkroom.

Table VI

Common Mistakes in the Darkroom

Error	Causes
Record keeping	Racks not labeled
Fogged film	White light leak; faulty safelight
Underdeveloped film	Incorrect time (short) and temperature (cold); expended solutions (weak solutions)
Overdeveloped films	Incorrect time (long) and temperature (hot)
Developer cut-off (top of film is clear straight line)	Solutions too low
Clear films (emulsion washed away)	Films left in wash (running rinse water) for more than 24 hours
Stained film	Sloppy or dirty working surface
Scratched film	Racks hit; fingernails too long
Brown films	Films have not had adequate fixation
Torn emulsion	Films touching or overlapping while drying
Static marks (multiple black linear streaks)	Static electricity caused by friction
Lost films	Films not placed carefully in rack

Automatic Processing

In recent years, automatic processing equipment has become available that permits films to be carried on a series of rollers from solution to solution. The appropriate time–temperature relationship is set and dry films emerge in approximately 5 minutes. These machines save time; however, they require periodic cleaning, and solutions must be changed regularly.

Steps for Mounting Radiographs

1. Separate the films into three piles.
   a. *Anterior periapicals:* the teeth are shown on the film vertically (up and down)
   b. *Posterior periapicals:* the teeth are shown on the film horizontally (across)
   c. *Bite-wings:* the crowns of both the upper and lower teeth are shown on the film (the roots are not visible)
2. View the anterior films with the dot facing outward (labial mounting). Separate the maxillary films from the mandibular films. They can be identified by referring to anatomical landmarks.
3. Mount the anterior periapical films. The incisal edges of the maxillary anteriors are to be facing downward. The incisal edges of the mandibular anteriors are to be facing upward (This is the same position as the teeth in the mouth.)
4. View the posterior films with the dot facing outward. Separate the mandibular films from the maxillary films.
5. Mount the posterior periapicals. The occlusal surfaces of the maxillary teeth are to be facing downward. The occlusal surfaces of the mandibular teeth are to be facing upward.
6. View the bite-wing films with the dot facing outward.
7. Mount the bite-wings. The bite-wings should match with the crowns of the periapical films directly above.
   Figure 20 presents a sample array of a full mouth series of radiographs.

Checking the Mounted Radiographs

1. Are all the dots facing outward?
2. Are all the incisal and occlusal surfaces facing in the proper direction?
3. Do the radiographs on the right side match? (Refer to restorations, missing teeth, impactions, and crown and root shape.)
4. Do the radiographs on the left side match?
5. Do the bite-wings match with the crowns of the periapical films?
6. Are there any discrepancies (a film that appears inappropriate in the series)?

Landmarks to Facilitate Mounting

1. The slight curve upward from the cuspid area toward the molar area, formed by the occlusal (biting) surfaces of the teeth.
2. The upward curve of bone at the end of the mandibular arch.
3. The appearance of the area behind the maxillary molars (shadows formed) as compared with the appearance of the area behind the mandibular molars (definate shape of the mandible).
4. The root difference between maxillary and mandibular teeth.
5. Root tips which usually curve toward the distal.
6. The mental foramen in the lower bicuspid area.

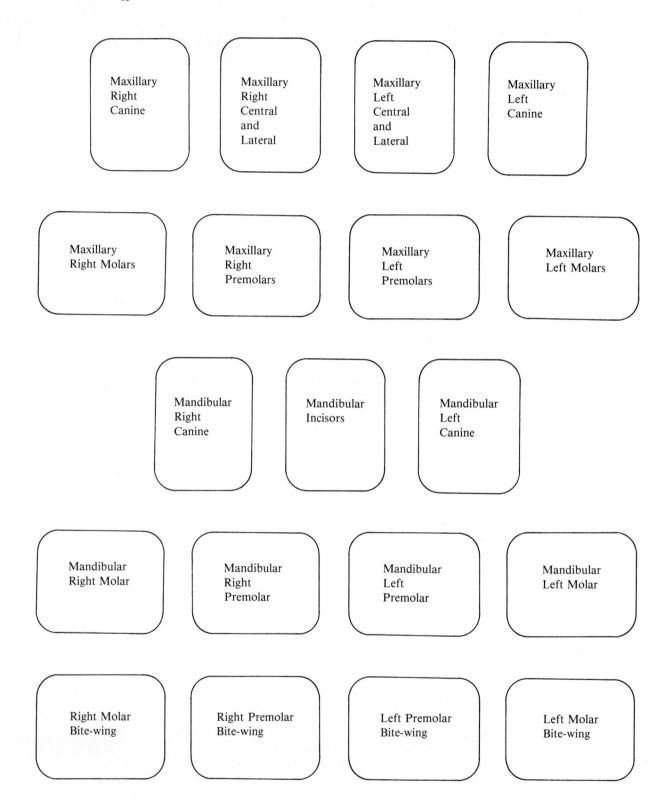

Fig. 20
Sample Mounting of Full Mouth Series

7. The mandibular canal in the lower jaw.
8. The differing bone densities in the mandibular and maxillary arches.
9. The difference in size of anterior teeth (mandibular anterior teeth are smaller than the maxillary anterior teeth).
10. The darkened area (maxillary sinus is radiolucent) usually visible above and between the roots of the maxillary bicuspid and molar areas.
11. The white lines (floor and walls of the cavities and sinuses) visible on the maxillary arch.
12. Maxillary first bicuspids usually have two roots, whereas mandibular bicuspids have one root.
13. Mandibular first and second molars usually have two divergent curved roots with bone clearly visible between them. This is particularly true of the first molar. Maxillary molars have three roots: two buccal and one palatal. The large palatal root obscures the intraradicular bone.

Distinguishing the Right from the Left

1. The dot (bubble or elevation) on the film packets should be placed facing the surfaces of the teeth.
2. If the distal anatomic surfaces of the teeth are to the right, when the dot is outward, the film is on the left side. If the distal surfaces are to the left, the film is on the right side.
3. If it is a maxillary view, the crowns of the teeth should be placed in the mount with their incisal or occlusal surfaces pointed downward. If it is a mandibular view, the incisal or occlusal surfaces should be pointed upward.

Radiation Protection

Radiation has been a well-researched and popular topic. Dental auxiliaries and dentists must be aware of potential hazards in order to protect themselves and patients, and to allay the fears that many patients have over the dangers associated with dental x-ray films.

When a dental radiograph is taken, many of the x-rays do not strike the film. Some x-rays are absorbed by the tissues adjacent to the film packet. There is no doubt that overexposure to radiation is dangerous. It is therefore the responsibility of the dentist and dental auxiliaries to expose the patient to a minimum amount of radiation.

A well-calibrated x-ray unit will disseminate about 1 rem per second. An average full mouth series will expose the patient to a local body dosage of approximately 3 rems. Doses that cause reddening of the skin would have to be as high as 250 rems in a two-week period, which would be equivalent to approximately 80 full series during that period.

Radiation exposure to the patient is minimized by the following procedures:
1. Follow federal regulations and guidelines when purchashing x-ray units.
2. Periodically check x-ray machines for leakage.
3. Check machines to ensure that filters and collimators are properly placed.
4. Drape patients with leaded lap aprons.
5. Use fast-speed film.
6. Employ the use of lead-shielded, open-ended cones, which reduce scattered radiation.
7. Avoid retakes.

Radiation exposure to the operator is minimized by the following steps:

1. Stand at least 6 feet away or behind a lead shield, or both.
2. Do not hold the film for a patient during an exposure.

No working areas should be in the direct line of the x-ray machine. As a further precaution, all personnel should wear film badges that periodically monitor dosages. Workers who follow radiation safety measures should receive no unnecessary exposure to radiation.

Question Section

Directions: Each of the questions or incomplete statements below is followed by four suggested answers or completions. Select the BEST answer in each case.

1. X-rays are made up of
   1. electrons
   2. neutrons
   3. photons
   4. protons

2. The generation of x-rays requires
   A. electrons
   B. heating of the cathode
   C. a target
   D. a lead screen
   E. cooling of the cathode
      1. A, B, and C
      2. A, B, and D
      3. B, D, and E
      4. C, D, and E

3. The portion of the target that is struck by electrons is called the
   1. principal point
   2. end point
   3. photon point
   4. focal spot

4. Milliamperage controls
   1. the speed with which electrons move from cathode to anode
   2. cooling of the anode
   3. heating of the anode
   4. heating of the cathode

5. The cathode is a filament composed of
   1. gold
   2. silver
   3. tungsten
   4. copper

6. Collimation of the primary beam
   1. dictates the contrast of the final radiograph
   2. decreases the exposure time
   3. restricts the shape and size of the beam
   4. makes the primary beam more difficult to connect

7. The lead diaphragm determines the size and shape of the
   1. electron cloud
   2. film used
   3. x-ray beam
   4. all of the above

8. Proper collimation for the film size and target–film distance will
   1. increase the kvp
   2. decrease the wavelength
   3. decrease the radiation received by the patient
   4. increase the wavelength

9. The penetrating power of x-rays depends on
   1. kvp
   2. mA
   3. film speed
   4. focal-film distance

10. The size of the collimated beam for intraoral radiology measured at the patient's skin is
    1. 1.5–1.75 inches
    2. 2.0–2.25 inches
    3. 2.75–3.0 inches
    4. 3.25–3.5 inches

11. Filtration of the x-ray beam protects the patient by
    1. eliminating all radiation from the x-ray head
    2. eliminating weak wavelength x-rays from the x-ray beam
    3. eliminating short wavelength x-rays from the x-ray beam
    4. decreasing exposure time

12. The most penetrating x-rays have
    1. low frequencies
    2. soft rays
    3. long wavelengths
    4. short wavelengths

13. If the mA is increased while the kvp and the exposure time are kept constant, the resulting films will
    1. be lighter
    2. be darker
    3. remain the same
    4. have a herringbone pattern

14. The x-ray at the center of the primary beam is called
    1. cathode ray
    2. secondary ray
    3. restricted beam
    4. central ray

15. The housing of the x-ray tube is
    1. copper
    2. plastic
    3. tungsten
    4. glass

16. As the target–film distance is increased, there is
    1. more chance of elongation
    2. more chance of overlapping
    3. more chance of foreshortening
    4. less distortion

17. Overlapping is a result of
    1. incorrect vertical angulation
    2. incorrect horizontal angulation
    3. excessive bending of the film
    4. all of the above

18. After a film is exposed, the target–film distance is doubled. The exposure time necessary to obtain a second film of equal density to the first film is
    1. the same as the first film
    2. twofold
    3. threefold
    4. fourfold

19. Which cells are most sensitive to x-rays?
    1. muscle
    2. nerve
    3. sperm
    4. epithelial

20. Which cells are least sensitive to x-rays?
    1. ova
    2. blood
    3. sperm
    4. nerve

21. The first sign of x-ray dermatitis is
    1. loss of hair
    2. purulent exudate
    3. erythema
    4. pain

22. Scatter radiation is a type of
    1. secondary radiation
    2. primary radiation
    3. stray radiation
    4. none of the above

23. The lead foil in the x-ray film packet is used to
    A. stop unused radiation
    B. tell the front of the film from the back
    C. prevent film fogging
    D. decrease operator's radiation exposure
       1. A and D
       2. A and C
       3. B and C
       4. C and D

24. The quality, or penetrating power, of secondary radiation is
    1. more than that of primary radiation
    2. less than that of primary radiation
    3. the same as that of primary radiation
    4. unrelated to that of primary radiation

25. If a radiograph remains in the developing solution too long, the film will be
    1. lighter
    2. darker
    3. lighter only if the temperature is increased
    4. unaffected because time is not a factor

26. Two films are developed for the same length of time but at different temperatures. The film developed at the higher temperature will be
    1. lighter
    2. darker
    3. the same
    4. a herringbone pattern

27. Film fog can occur if there is
    1. a light leak in the darkroom
    2. bending of the film
    3. reversal of the film
    4. extremely thick bone

28. Films not fixed for a long enough period of time will appear
    1. to have black lines running through them
    2. to be brittle
    3. to have a brown tint
    4. white

29. Film is washed after removing it from the developing solution to
    1. remove any debris on the film
    2. speed up the developing process

3. stop the developing process
4. remove the precipitated silver salts

30. For the developing chemicals to work, the solution must be
   1. acidic
   2. neutral
   3. basic
   4. none of the above

31. Fixing the film
   1. removes the unaffected silver salts
   2. removes the affected silver salts
   3. softens the film
   4. peels the emulsion from the film base

32. The fixing solution is
   1. acidic
   2. neutral
   3. basic
   4. first basic, then neutral after dilution

33. Reticulation is
   1. cracking of the film emulsion
   2. an electric charge in the developing solution
   3. a latent image
   4. caused by excess radiation

34. The optimum time–temperature relationship for processing dental radiographs is
   1. 74°F for 4½ minutes
   2. 68°F for 6 minutes
   3. 50°F for 5 minutes
   4. varied according to manufacturer's specifications

35. The panoramic radiograph is not diagnostic for
   1. caries detection
   2. general survey
   3. confirmation of mandibular fractures
   4. detection of impacted wisdom teeth

36. Bite-wing radiographs are useful in helping to determine
   1. interproximal caries
   2. proximal bone height
   3. fit of crowns
   4. all of the above

37. The raised button on the radiograph aids in
   1. processing
   2. drying
   3. mounting
   4. determining film speed

38. The radiograph film is covered with an emulsion of
   1. silver bromide salts
   2. cellulose

3. silver acetate
4. potassium bromide

39. Film speed is determined by the
   1. amount of silver bromide salt
   2. thickness of cellulose acetate base
   3. size of the silver bromide crystal
   4. side of the film exposed

40. The best technique for reducing the radiation exposure to both patient and operator is the use of
   1. an automatic timer
   2. fast film
   3. thinner films
   4. a thicker cellulose acetate base

41. To visualize the two roots on the maxillary first premolar, the central ray should be directed
   1. perpendicular to the buccal surface
   2. perpendicular to the lingual surface
   3. toward the occlusal surface
   4. slightly from the mesial or distal surface

42. The most radiolucent structure of a tooth is the
   1. enamel
   2. dentin
   3. cementation
   4. pulp chamber

43. The most radiopaque structure of a tooth is the
   1. enamel
   2. dentin
   3. cementation
   4. pulp chamber

44. The chemicals used in processing solutions are dissolved in
   1. cellulose acetate
   2. distilled water
   3. a thick emulsion
   4. potassium bromide

45. The operator must avoid
   1. stray radiation
   2. secondary radiation
   3. the primary beam
   4. all of the above

46. If an unexposed film is processed, it will appear
   1. white
   2. black
   3. blue
   4. clear

47. Secondary radiation emanates from the
   1. patient's mouth

2. exposed film
3. closed end of cone
4. all of the above

48. To avoid gonadal exposure to x-rays, which of the following should be used?
    1. higher kvp
    2. a lead apron
    3. finer detailed film
    4. increased vertical angulation

49. When radiographs are taken of a pregnant patient
    1. periapical rather than bite-wing films should be taken
    2. bite-wing rather than periapical films should be taken
    3. the patient should be treated as all other patients
    4. as few films as possible should be taken

50. Who should hold the film in a patient's mouth if he or she is unable to do so?
    1. the dentist
    2. the assistant
    3. a friend or relative
    4. the receptionist

51. When exposing a radiograph, the operator should stand
    1. at least 6 feet from the x-ray head
    2. 2 feet to the right of the primary beam
    3. any distance in back of the x-ray head
    4. 4 feet in front of the patient

52. The maximum whole body dose considered permissible to those who work with radiation is
    1. 0.1 rem/week
    2. 1 rem/week
    3. 10 rems/week
    4. 100 rems/week

53. The greatest danger to the operator is
    1. the central ray
    2. secondary radiation
    3. the primary x-ray beam
    4. all of the above are of equal danger

54. Which characteristic of x-rays makes them both beneficial and hazardous?
    1. they destroy tissue
    2. they cause embolisms
    3. they use the body's heat
    4. they cause large fatty deposits to form

55. A technique used to measure the operator's exposure to radiation is
    1. to check the color of the operator's fingers

2. for the operator to wear a radiation film badge
3. the frequency of stomach pains
4. to multiply the number of films the operator has exposed by 0.1 rem

56. A constant source of radiation is
    1. strontium 90
    2. natural elements
    3. the sun
    4. all of the above

57. The amount of radiation a person receives
    1. begins anew each day
    2. is cumulative only on the skin
    3. is cumulative in the entire body
    4. none of the above

58. Maximum protection of the patient requires that the x-ray beam pass through a(n)
    1. plastic closed-ended cone
    2. shielded open-ended cone
    3. water filter
    4. oil filter

59. Small silver halide crystals on the film result in
    A. more radiation to the patient
    B. better detail
    C. slower film
    D. faster film
    E. film fogging
       1. A, B, and C
       2. A, B, and D
       3. A, C, and E
       4. B and D

60. Occlusal films are used to determine
    1. mesiodistal orientation of a tooth
    2. buccolingual orientation of a tooth
    3. the presence of anterior caries
    4. none of the above

61. Intensifying screens
    1. are used in intraoral films
    2. decrease exposure time
    3. create additional x-rays
    4. fuse with the film

62. Which extraoral film is used to visualize the sinus?
    1. lateral oblique film
    2. lateral skull film
    3. Water's film
    4. posterior–anterior film

63. The principle used in panoramic radiography is
    1. long cone
    2. laminagraphy

3. horizontal curvature
4. panoramography

64. The temperature of the radiographic processing solutions is adjusted by
    1. individual heaters
    2. chemical interaction
    3. a temperature-adjustable water bath
    4. gas heaters

65. Which type of film cannot be used intraorally?
    1. bite-wing
    2. occlusal
    3. periapical
    4. none of the above

66. Periapical films
    1. show the entire tooth
    2. show the supporting structure of the tooth
    3. come in various sizes
    4. all of the above

67. The occlusal plane of the arch being radiographed should be
    1. perpendicular to the floor
    2. parallel to the floor
    3. at an angle of 45 degrees to the floor
    4. at an angle of 30 degrees to the floor

68. The ala–tragus line is parallel to the floor when taking
    1. maxillary periapical films
    2. bite-wings
    3. maxillary occlusal films
    4. all of the above

69. When using the bisecting the angle technique
    1. the central beam is perpendicular to the floor
    2. the central beam is perpendicular to the tooth
    3. the central beam is perpendicular to the line bisecting the angle formed by the tooth and film
    4. the central beam is perpendicular to the cheek

70. When using the paralleling technique
    1. the film is parallel to the tooth
    2. the film always touches the tooth
    3. you must use an 8-inch plastic cone
    4. all of the above

71. Film racks should be
    1. clean and dry
    2. numbered and lettered
    3. neither of the above
    4. both of the above

72. Light films will result from

A. underdeveloping
B. overdeveloping
C. underexposure
D. overexposure
E. underfixing
F. overfixing
    1. A, C, and F
    2. B, C, and F
    3. A and C
    4. A, B, and F

73. Dark films will result from
A. underdeveloping
B. overdeveloping
C. underexposing
D. overexposing
E. overfixing
    1. A, C, and E
    2. B, D, and E
    3. B and C
    4. B and D

74. Firm placement of the film will help prevent
    1. overlapping
    2. foreshortening
    3. gagging
    4. elongation

75. Periapical films should extend beyond the occlusal plane
    1. 1/8 inch
    2. 1/4 inch
    3. 3/8 inch
    4. 1/2 inch

76. If a film is exposed on the wrong side, the result will be
    1. darker films
    2. no image at all
    3. no effect
    4. a herringbone pattern

77. X-rays are most effectively stopped by
    1. a vacuum
    2. tungsten
    3. copper
    4. lead

78. Blurred films can result from
    1. incorrect vertical angulation
    2. movement of the patient
    3. increased kvp
    4. old film

79. The usual number of films in a complete dentulous radiographic survey is
    1. 10
    2. 18
    3. 24
    4. 26

80. After the films are removed from the fixer, they are washed for
    1. 5–10 minutes
    2. 11–19 minutes
    3. 20–30 minutes
    4. 1 hour

81. In the paralleling techniques, a device used to hold the film in the patient's mouth is
    1. the patient's finger
    2. a bite block
    3. a second film
    4. all of the above

82. Elongation is caused by
    1. insufficient vertical angulation
    2. too much vertical angulation
    3. insufficient horizontal angulation
    4. excessive bending of the film

83. Foreshortening is caused by
    1. insufficient vertical angulation
    2. too much vertical angulation
    3. insufficient horizontal angulation
    4. excessive bending of the film

84. Cone cutting results from the central ray
    1. not being aimed at the center of film
    2. having incorrect horizontal angulation
    3. having insufficient vertical angulation
    4. being eliminated from a closed plastic cone

85. Black lines across the film may be the result of
    1. cone cutting
    2. double exposure
    3. excessive bending
    4. underexposure

86. Proper patient positioning for intraoral films requires the sagittal plane be
    1. parallel to the floor
    2. perpendicular to the floor
    3. parallel to the central ray
    4. perpendicular to the central ray

87. If the sagittal plane of the patient's head is positioned incorrectly, the result might be
    1. overlapping
    2. elongation
    3. darker films
    4. all of the above

88. Exposure time is determined by
    A. kvp
    B. mA
    C. the patient's weight
    D. vertical angulation
    E. the area being radiographed
       1. A, B, and D

2. A, B, and E
3. A, D, and E
4. B, C, and D

89. When seating the patient for a radiograph, the operator should
    1. tell the patient what is being done
    2. have the patient remove eyeglasses
    3. have the patient remove intraoral removable appliances
    4. all of the above

90. Vertical angulation in the bisecting technique for the same radiograph can differ in patients because of
    1. the size of the teeth
    2. anatomical differences
    3. gagging
    4. age

91. A latent image is
    1. an image taken with a long exposure
    2. found on only fast films
    3. composed of energized silver halide crystals
    4. a very light image on the developed film

92. Which of the following conditions cannot be identified radiographically?
    A. herpetic lesions
    B. periodontitis
    C. salivary stones
    D. frena
    E. root tips
       1. A and B
       2. A and D
       3. C and D
       4. C and E

93. Exposure of a radiograph on a child
    1. requires less time than an adult
    2. requires more time than an adult
    3. requires the same time as an adult
    4. should never be attempted

94. The strength of the safelight permitted in the darkroom depends on the
    1. size of the film
    2. light tightness of the room
    3. sensitivity of the film
    4. tooth being radiographed

95. Extraoral films are
    1. more sensitive to light than intraoral films
    2. less sensitive to light than intraoral films
    3. just as sensitive to light as intraoral films
    4. not sensitive to light

96. How often should the processing solutions be changed?

1. each week
2. every 3-4 weeks
3. every 5-6 weeks
4. every 7-8 weeks

97. The thermometer used to measure the temperature of the processing solutions is located
    1. in the developer
    2. in the wash water
    3. in the fixer
    4. above the processing solutions

98. The best way to dry processed films is to
    1. place them on paper towels
    2. hang them suspending the films in the air
    3. place them in envelopes
    4. place them flat on the counter

99. Extraoral films are placed in rigid frames called
    1. film frames
    2. skull plates
    3. jaw plates
    4. cassettes

100. Extraoral films are used
    1. to help diagnose fractures
    2. when a patient cannot open his or her mouth
    3. to help visualize pathological conditions of the sinus
    4. all of the above

101. A logical sequence for a full mouth survey of a patient with a complete dentition is
    1. upper arch, bite-wings, lower arch
    2. upper arch, lower arch, bite-wings
    3. bite-wings, lower arch, upper arch
    4. none of the above

102. Radiographs of edentulous portions of a patient's mouth
    1. are unnecessary
    2. should be exposed only on request of the patient
    3. should be exposed routinely
    4. should be exposed only if the entire arch is edentulous

103. If the end of the x-ray cone approximates the tip of the patient's nose, the operator is exposing a radiograph of the
    1. maxillary cuspid
    2. maxillary central incisors
    3. mandibular incisors
    4. maxillary bicuspid

104. The best sequence for exposing maxillary radiographs is
    1. central incisors, right cuspid, left cuspid
    2. central incisors, right cuspid, right bicuspid
    3. central incisors, right bicuspid, right cuspid
    4. central incisors, right molar, right bicuspid

105. The developing solution
    1. should always be left open
    2. should always be covered
    3. should be covered only when films are being developed
    4. could be left covered or uncovered

106. Films left overnight in the fixer
    1. will be clear
    2. will be too dark to read
    3. will not be affected
    4. will disintegrate

107. During processing when can radiographs safely be exposed to light?
    1. after development
    2. after the first wash
    3. after being placed in the fixer
    4. after the final wash

108. A patient claims that she gags easily. The operator should
    1. begin taking films in the anterior and work posteriorly
    2. ask the patient to hold her breath before each exposure
    3. have her rinse with mouthwash
    4. all of the above

109. Cephalometric radiographs are used in which area of dentistry?
    1. operative
    2. pedodontics
    3. orthodontics
    4. periodontics

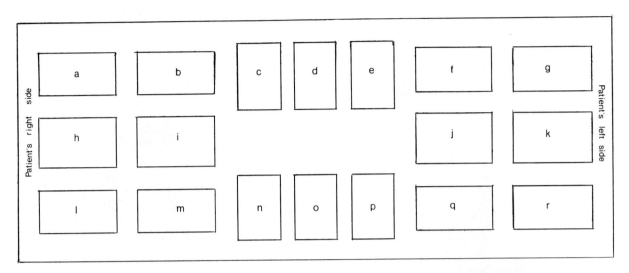

Fig. 21

Directions: Figure 21 is a mount for radiographs with each space assigned a letter. Select the correct placement for each of the radiographs which follow. The bubble or raised dot on each film is toward you.

Questions 110 to 151

110.
1. m
2. r
3. j
4. g

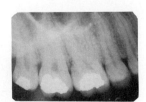

111.
1. c
2. d
3. o
4. q

112.
1. h
2. l
3. a
4. f

113.
1. p
2. o
3. e
4. n

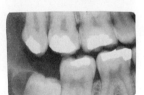

114.
1. a
2. b
3. f
4. g

115.
1. h
2. i
3. j
4. k

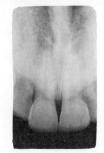

116.
1. c
2. d
3. e
4. p

117.
1. a
2. b
3. f
4. g

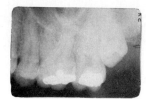

118.
1. c
2. d
3. e
4. o

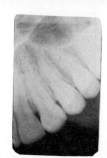

119.
1. h
2. i
3. j
4. k

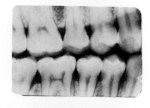

120.
1. c
2. d
3. e
4. p

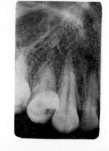

121.
1. h
2. i
3. j
4. k

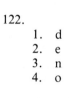

122.
1. d
2. e
3. n
4. o

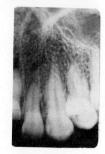

123.
1. c
2. d
3. o
4. p

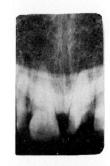

124.
1. l
2. m
3. q
4. r

125.
1. c
2. e
3. n
4. p

126.
1. c
2. e
3. n
4. p

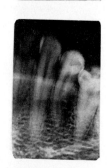

127.
1. m
2. b
3. f
4. g

128.
1. m
2. b
3. q
4. j

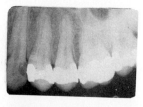

129.
1. h
2. i
3. j
4. k

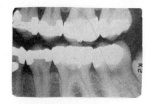

130.
1. c
2. e
3. n
4. p

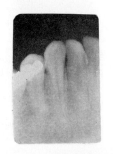

131.
1. a
2. m
3. r
4. f

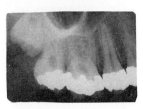

132.
1. b
2. i
3. f
4. g

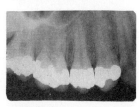

133.
1. l
2. m
3. f
4. r

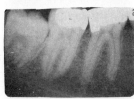

134.
1. j
2. b
3. m
4. g

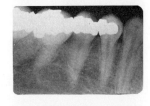

135.
1. i
2. j
3. a
4. h

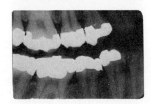

136.
1. b
2. j
3. l
4. m

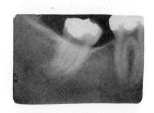

137.
1. f
2. k
3. m
4. q

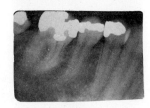

138.
1. a
2. f
3. j
4. l

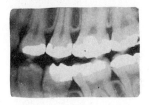

139.
1. i
2. k
3. l
4. r

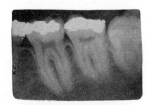

140.
1. c
2. d
3. o
4. p

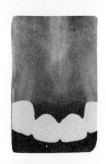

141.
1. c
2. e
3. n
4. p

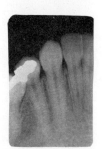

142.
1. b
2. g
3. h
4. q

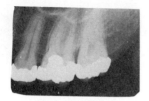

143.
1. c
2. e n
3. n
4. p

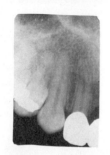

144.
1. h
2. i
3. j
4. k

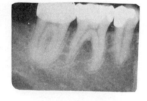

145.
1. l
2. m
3. q
4. r

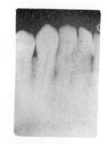

146.
1. c
2. e n
3. n
4. p

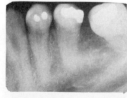

147.
1. b
2. f
3. i
4. q

148.
1. a
2. g
3. k
4. l

149.
1. c
2. e n
3. n
4. p

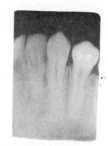

150.
1. b
2. g
3. j
4. m

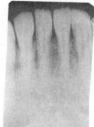

151.
1. d
2. e o
3. o
4. p

Directions: Select the numbered answer that BEST identifies the error in radiographic technique.

Questions 152 to 161

152.

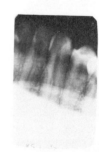

1. cone cutting
2. incorrect vertical angulation
3. incorrect horizontal angulation
4. incorrect film placement

153.

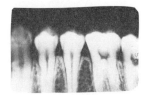

1. cone cutting
2. incorrect vertical angulation
3. incorrect horizontal angulation
4. incorrect film placement

154.

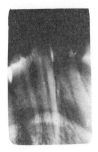

1. cone cutting
2. incorrect vertical angulation
3. incorrect horizontal angulation
4. incorrect film placement

155.

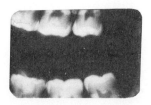

1. cone cutting
2. incorrect vertical angulation
3. incorrect horizontal angulation
4. incorrect film placement

156.

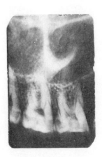

1. cone cutting
2. incorrect vertical angulation
3. incorrect horizontal angulation
4. incorrect film placement

157.

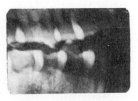

1. incorrect horizontal angulation
2. film is reversed
3. underexposed
4. none of the above

158.

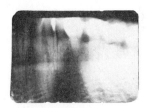

1. incorrect horizontal angulation
2. film is reversed
3. underexposed
4. none of the above

159.

1. incorrect horizontal angulation
2. film is reversed
3. underexposed
4. none of the above

160.

1. incorrect horizontal angulation
2. film is reversed
3. underexposed
4. none of the above

161.

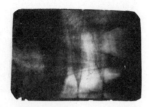

1. incorrect horizontal angulation
2. film is reversed
3. underexposed
4. none of the above

Answers and Explanations

1. **3** X-rays are made up of bundles of energy called photons. Photons of x-ray frequency are capable of penetrating objects.

2. **1** The sequence of events that leads to x-ray generation is first heating the cathode to produce an electron cloud. The density of the cloud produced depends on the milliamperge (mA). Second is the creation of an electric potential between the cathode and anode (target). The speed of the crossing depends on the kilovolt (kvp). Third, the collision of the electrons with the anode produces x-rays (photons).

3. **4** The portion of the target struck by the electrons is called the focal spot. Heat produced when electrons strike the focal spot must be dissipated or the x-ray tube might become damaged.

4. **4** The milliamperage controls the heating of the cathode and thereby the density of the resultant electron cloud. Increasing the mA will result in a denser cloud and an increase in the number of x-rays produced.

5. **3** The cathode is composed of a tungsten filament surrounded by a molybdenum focusing cup. The anode is composed of a tungsten target set inside a copper core.

6. **3** Collimation of the primary beam restricts its size and shape so it coincides as closely as possible with the size and shape of the film. As the collimated beam approaches the size of the film there is an increased possibility of cone cutting.

7. **3** The lead diaphragm determines the size and shape of the x-ray beam as it leaves the x-ray head. The distance between the target and the film will determine the size of the beam at the film.

8. **3** Proper collimation of the primary beam results in a beam that closely approximates the size and shape of the film. This decreases the patient's exposure to radiation.

9. **1** The kvp determines the penetrating power of the x-ray beam. Increasing the kvp increases the electrical potential between the cathode and anode. This increases the force driving the electrons from the cathode to the anode which results in an increase in the penetrating power of the resulting x-ray beam. Dental radiology uses 45–95 kvp.

10. **3** Collimation limits the diameter of the x-ray beam to 2.75–3.0 inches at the patient's skin.

Ideally the x-ray beam should be just as large as the film being used.

11. **2** Filtration is the passing of the x-ray beam through an aluminum disk to eliminate the longer, weaker wavelength x-rays. Longer wavelength x-rays, also known as soft x-rays, do not have penetrating power and could be absorbed by the patient's cheek.

12. **4** The most penetrating x-rays have short wavelengths and high frequencies. They are called hard x-rays.

13. **2** Increasing the mA increases the electron density and subsequently the quantity of the resulting x-rays. An increase in the quantity of x-rays will result in more x-rays affecting the film, and subsequently darker film.

14. **4** The x-ray at the center of the primary beam is called the central ray.

15. **4** The housing of the x-ray tube is a glass envelope. The glass is lead lined except where the x-rays leave the tube.

16. **4** As the target–film distance increases, there is less distortion because the x-rays are more parallel as they strike the object and film. If the target–film distance is increased, the exposure time must be increased to obtain a properly exposed film.

17. **2** Overlapping occurs if the central ray is not parallel to the proximal contacts in the horizontal plane. If overlapping occurs parts of adjacent teeth are superimposed on each other and the films cannot be used diagnostically.

18. **4** When the target–film distance is doubled, the exposure time must be increased fourfold to maintain equal film density. This is an example of the inverse-square law of radiation, which states that radiation intensity is inversely proportional to the square of the distance.

19. **3** Sperm cells are the most radiosensitive cells listed. Cells that undergo active division are the most radiosensitive. The following is a list of cells ranked according to their radiosensitivity:
    sperm and ova
    blood cells
    epithelial cells
    connective tissue cells
    nerve cells
    muscle cells

20. **4** See answer **19**.

21. **3** The initial sign of x-ray dermatitis is erythema (reddening).

22. **1** Scatter radiation is a type of secondary radiation created when the primary beam passes through an object.

23. **2** The lead foil in the x-ray film packet serves several puposes; it stops the radiation which passes through the film, prevents fogging of the film by stopping secondary radiation behind the film from hitting the film and adds body to the film.

24. **2** The penetrating power of primary radiation is greater than the penetrating power of the resulting secondary radiation produced. When the primary beam strikes an object it gives up some energy and the resultant secondary radiation has less energy and less penetrating power.

25. **2** The longer film remains in the developer the more silver halide will precipitate and therefore the darker the film will become.

26. **2** Higher temperature will cause an increase in the precipitation of the silver halide, resulting in a darker film.

27. **1** Film fog appears as dull gray finish on the processed film. Some causes are light leak in the darkroom, old film, or exposure of film to secondary or stray radiation.

28. **3** Film not fixed for a long enough period of time (about 10 minutes) will have a brown tint. Radiographs may be read after a short period of fixing (wet reading) but must be returned to the fixing solution to ensure complete removal of the unaffected silver bromide crystals.

29. **3** The film is washed after it is removed from developer and before it is put in the fixer in order to wash off the developing solution and stop the developing process. Washing also removes all chemicals from the film so the fixing solution is not contaminated.

30. **3** In order to develop films the developing solution must have a basic pH. The following chemicals make up the developer: hydroquinone, an oxidizing agent which gives the film contrast; Elon, another oxidizing agent to give film detail; sodium sulfite, a preservative to lengthen the life of the solution; sodium carbonate, to make the solution basic; potassium bromide, to make the aforementioned chemicals act selectively; and distilled water, the medium in which the chemical activity takes place.

31. **1** Fixing the film removes the unaffected silver salts. Areas in which these salts are removed will appear lighter in the final film. Fixing also rehardens the emulsion.

32. **1** The fixing solution is acidic. The following chemicals make up the fixer: sodium thiosulfate, which dissolves undeveloped silver salts; alum, to shrink and harden the gelatin emulsion; sodium sulfate, a preservative against oxidation; acetic acid, to increase action of the preservative; and distilled water, the medium in which the chemical activity takes place.

33. **1** Reticulation is the cracking of the film emulsion due to large temperature differences between the processing solutions.

34. **4** The optimum time–temperature for processing films varies with manufacturer's specifications.

35. **1** The panoramic x-ray is used for general surveys, confirmation of fractures, determination of the position of third molars, and where intraoral techniques cannot be used.

36. **4** Bite-wing films are used for diagnosis of interproximal caries, visualizing the height of interproximal bone and determining the proximal adaptation of restorations.

37. **3** The button or dot is used to orient the films when mounting. All films should be oriented with the button in the same direction when mounting.

38. **1** The radiograph is a cellulose acetate base thinly covered on both sides with a gelatin emulsion of silver bromide salts.

39. **3** Film speed is determined by the size of the silver bromide crystals. Larger crystals produce faster film. Faster film requires less total radiation for exposure. Film speed ranges from A to F; F is the fastest.

40. **2** The best technique to decrease radiation exposure is to use the fastest film possible.

41. **4** The maxillary first bicuspid has two roots which lie beside each other in a buccal palatal orientation. To radiographically separate the roots, which may be necessary in root canal therapy, the horizontal angulation should have the central beam slightly mesial or distal to the ideal angulation. The ideal horizontal angulation, with the central ray perpendicular to the buccal surface, would cause the roots to be superimposed on one another.

42. **4** The most radiolucent structure listed is the pulp chamber. Radiolucency depends on the density of an object. The less dense an object, the more radiolucent it is and the darker it will appear on radiographs.

43. **1** The most radiopaque structure of a tooth is the enamel. The denser a structure the more radiopaque it is and the lighter it will appear on a radiograph.

44. **2** The chemicals used in processing solutions are dissolved in distilled water. Other types of water

contain chemicals that can interfere with the proper processing of radiographs.

45. **4** The operator must avoid all radiation. He or she is most frequently exposed to secondary radiation.

46. **4** When a film is placed in the fixing solution unaffected (or unprecipitated) silver bromide crystals are removed. Therefore, the emulsion of an unexposed film will be completely removed and the film will be clear.

47. **4** Secondary radiation is radiation resulting from the interaction of the primary beam and any object it contacts.

48. **2** To prevent gonadal exposure to x-rays, the patient should wear a lead apron. X-rays will not pass through lead; therefore, the gonadal tissue, which is very sensitive to radiation, will be protected.

49. **4** Embryos have a considerable amount of immature rapidly dividing cells susceptible to changes from radiation; therefore, as few x-rays as possible of pregnant women should be taken.

50. **3** To keep the operator's exposure to radiation to a minimum a rule of never holding film in a patient's mouth must be observed. Assistants and receptionists must abide by the same rule. It is best to ask a friend or relative to hold the film if it is necessary.

51. **1** In order to be protected from secondary radiation, the operator should stand at least 6 feet away from the x-ray head when exposing film.

52. **1** Maximum whole body dose considered permissible is 0.1 rem/wk (100 mR/week). Ideally, the operator should receive zero occupational radiation.

53. **2** The most frequent type of radiation to which the operator is exposed is secondary radiation and it is therefore the greatest danger.

54. **1** The characteristic of x-rays that makes them both beneficial and hazardous is their ability to destroy tissue. Radiation is used in medicine both as a diagnostic tool and to intentionally destroy certain tissue (such as carcinomas).

55. **2** An easy way to tell the amount of radiation one is receiving is to wear a radiation film badge. The badge is worn for a period of time after which the radiation exposure can be measured. If the occupational dose is too high, measures must be taken to correct the problem.

56. **4** Daily doses of radiation are received from strontium 90 (from atomic explosions), natural elements in the earth (e.g., uranium), and the sun.

57. **3** The amount of radiation a person receives is cumulative in the entire body; therefore, people working with x-rays should take proper precautions to decrease their exposure.

58. **2** Maximum protection of the patient requires that the x-rays pass through a shielded open ended cone. X-rays passing through a closed short cone produce scatter radiation.

59. **1** Small silver halide crystals on the film result in a slow film that requires a long exposure time but results in a radiograph with fine detail. Slow film does not offer a sufficient increase in diagnostic value over fast film to justify its use.

60. **2** An occlusal film is used to tell the buccolingual orientation of an object, as a survey film for an edentulous patient and as an extraoral film in special instances.

61. **2** Intensifying screens decrease exposure time of extraoral radiographs by creating an illuminating pattern of the object through which the x-ray has passed. The illuminating pattern continues to expose the film after the radiation exposure has stopped.

62. **3** Waters' film is an extraoral film used to help visualize the sinus. Extraoral films are large films which are positioned beside the patient's face. They are used to visualize large portions of the skull, mandible, or maxilla.

63. **2** The principle used in panoramic radiography is laminagraphy. Laminagraphy is the focusing of the x-ray beam at a point which will appear on the resulting film. Other objects in the beam's path are out of focus and do not appear on the radiograph.

64. **3** The temperature of the processing solution is usually adjusted by immersing containers of the processing solution in a temperature-adjustable water bath.

65. **4** All the listed types of film can be used intraorally.

66. **4** Periapical films are used to show the entire tooth and the supporting structures. They come in three sizes: small for children, regular for adults, and narrow for anterior teeth.

67. **2** When positioning the patient the occlusal plane of arch being radiographed should be parallel to the floor.

68. **4** The ala-tragus line is parallel to the floor when taking maxillary periapical films, bite-wing films, and the maxillary occlusal films.

69. **3** The bisecting-the-angle technique requires that the central ray be perpendicular to the line bisecting the angle formed by the film and the tooth.

70. **1** The paralleling technique requires that the film be parallel to the tooth and that a 16-inch cone be used.

71. **4** X-ray racks should contain enough clips to hold a full series of films, be numbered or lettered for patient identification, and be clean and dry so as not to contaminate the processing solutions or affect the films.

72. **3** Light films may result from underexposing (not enough radiation reaches the film because of insufficient quantity or insufficient exposure), underdeveloping (insufficient amounts of affected silver halide are precipitated; this can be caused by cold developing solution or keeping the films in the developing solution too short a period of time) or overwashing resulting in lighter films because affected silver halide crystals will be washed off.

73. **4** Dark films can result from overexposure (too much radiation contacts the film because of an increase in the quantity of radiation or the exposure time) or overdevelopment (more silver halide crystals are precipitated if the developing solution is too warm or if the films are left in the solution too long).

74. **3** Firm placement of the film will help prevent gagging by avoiding movement of the film over gag-sensitive areas of the palate.

75. **1** The periapical films are extended 1/8 inch beyond the occlusal surface or incisal edge. The resulting film should also show 3 mm beyond the root apex.

76. **4** A herringbone pattern results if the film is exposed when it is reversed in the patient's mouth. This pattern is caused by the radiation passing through the lead foil, which has this pattern. The resultant film is light and cannot be used for diagnostic purposes.

77. **4** X-rays are most effectively stopped by lead; however, all matter will attenuate x-rays to varying degrees.

78. **2** A blurred film will result if the patient moves while dental film is being exposed.

79. **2** The full mouth series of a dentulous person is composed 18 to 20 films. An 18-film series would consist of films of the maxillary and mandibular central and lateral incisors, right and left canines, right and left premolars, right and left molars, and bite-wings of the right and left premolars and right and left molars.

80. **3** After fixing, the film is washed for 20–30 minutes and then dried. If the films are washed too long they will become lighter because some of the precipitated silver bromide will wash off. If the films are not washed long enough some residue from the fixer may remain and the films will have a brown tint.

81. **2** Devices used to hold the film in the paralleling technique include bite blocks and hemostats.

82. **1** Elongation can be caused by insufficient vertical angulation, improper positioning of the patient's head, or improper film placement.

83. **2** Foreshortening can be caused by too much vertical angulation, improper positioning of the patient's head, or improper film placement.

84. **1** Cone cutting is caused by the central ray not being aimed at the center of the film. This results in part of the film not being exposed to radiation.

85. **3** Black lines across the film are indicative of excessive bending that has cracked the emulsion.

86. **2** The sagittal plane of the patient's head should be perpendicular to the floor. The vertical angulation on the x-ray head is based on this position.

87. **2** If the sagittal plane is incorrect, there will be a problem with vertical angulation. Two problems associated with vertical angulation are elongation and foreshortening.

88. **2** The exposure time is determined by: the mA, the kvp, the density of the bone and structures the primary beam must pass through, the film speed, and the focal (target) film distance.

89. **4** When seating the patient for a radiograph, the operator should inform the patient what will occur and ask the patient to remove eyeglasses and/or intraoral removable prostheses.

90. **2** Vertical angulation may be altered from patient to patient depending on anatomic structure differences such as the height of the vault of the palate.

91. **3** The latent image is not truly an image but a potential image composed of energized silver halide crystals. The latent image will become a visible image after processing the exposed film.

92. **2** Soft tissue conditions cannot be identified radiographically unless they are lesions within hard tissues; therefore, herpetic lesions and frena cannot be identified radiographically. A soft tissue lesion, such as a granuloma, within bone will appear radiographically radiolucent compared with its more radiopaque surrounding.

93. **1** Less time is necessary for radiographic exposures on children because the tissues the radiation must pass through are not as dense as those of adults.

94. **3** The strength of the safelight in the darkroom is dependent on the film sensitivity. The faster the film the more light sensitive the film, and therefore the less the strength of the safelight.

95. **1** Extraoral films are more light sensitive than are intraoral films.

96. **2** The processing solutions should be changed at least every 3–4 weeks, depending on usage. The solutions lose strength through exposure to air, heavy usage, and contamination.

97. **1** The thermometer used to measure the temperature of the processing solutions is located in the developing solution. The temperature of the developer will determine how long the films will be kept in this solution. Until a temperature equilibrium is reached the water bath is warmer than the developing solution. If the thermometer was kept in the water bath, the resulting films, developed before equilibrium was reached, would be underdeveloped.

98. **2** The processed films should be dried by suspending them in air. A fan may be used to speed up the drying process; however, the films should not be allowed to touch each other or anything else until they are dry.

99. **4** Extraoral films are sheets of film placed in rigid metal-plastic frames called cassettes. To decrease the amount of radiation needed for an exposure the cassette usually contains an intensifying screen.

100. **4** Extraoral films are used to help visualize fractures, pathological conditions of the sinus, the temporomandibular joint, the position of impacted teeth and large pathological lesions. They are also used when a patient cannot open his or her mouth.

101. **1** A logical sequence for a full mouth survey is one where the patient's position is changed as infrequently as possible. First the maxillary periapical radiographs and bite-wings are taken with the ala–tragus line parallel to the floor. Then the patient's head position is altered so that the occlusal plane of the mandibular teeth is parallel to the floor, and mandibular radiographs are exposed.

102. **3** Radiographs of edentulous areas should be exposed routinely to check for any pathology in the area (e.g., retained root tips, foreign bodies).

103. **2** When the end of the cone approximates the tip of the patient's nose a radiograph of the patient's central incisors is being exposed. The vertical angulation is about +50°.

104. **2** The best sequence for maxillary radiographs is to begin with film easy for the patient to hold and continue in a sequence which will avoid any possible omissions. The best choice is to begin with the central incisors and continue posteriorly on one side and then repeat the pattern on the other side.

105. **2** Developing solution has an affinity for oxygen. Therefore, if it is left uncovered, the chemicals will oxidize and lose their strength.

106. **3** Films cannot be overfixed and can be left in the fixer indefinitely.

107. **3** It is safe to expose radiographs to light after they have been placed in the fixer. The radiographs can be read at this time and then placed back into the fixer to complete the processing.

108. **4** The gag reflex can be stifled by having the patient use mouthwash, hold his or her breath, use film-holding devices, and/or use distractions such as holding a leg in the air until the muscles become fatigued.

109. **3** Cephalometric films are extraoral films used in orthodontics to relate anatomic landmarks of the mandible and maxilla to the rest of the skull.

110. **2**

111. **3**

112. **3**

113. **4**

114. **2**

115. **1**

116. **2**

117. **4**

118. **3**

119. **2**

120. **1**

121. **4**

122. **2**

123. **2**

124. **4**

125. **3**

126. **4**

127. **3**

128. **3**

129. **4**

130. **3**

131. **1**

132. **1**

133. **1**

134. **3**

135. **1**

136. **3**

137. **3**

138. **3**

139. **4**

140. **2**

141. **3**

142.	2	147.	4	152.	1	157.	1
143.	1	148.	1	153.	4	158.	1
144.	1	149.	4	154.	2	159.	2
145.	1	150.	2	155.	4	160.	3
146.	3	151.	3	156.	4	161.	4

Bibliography

Barr, J.H. and Stephens, R.G. *Dental Radiography,* Philadelphia: W. B. Saunders Co., 1980.

Eastman Kodak Company. *X-rays in Dentistry,* Rochester, N.Y.: 1977.

Frommer, H.H. *Radiology for Dental Auxiliaries,* 3rd ed. St. Louis: The C. V. Mosby Co., 1982.

Langland, O.E. and Sippy, F.H. *Textbook of Dental Radiography,* Springfield, Ill.: Charles C Thomas Publishers, 1978.

Manson-Hing, L.R. *Fundamentals of Dental Radiography,* Philadelphia: Lea & Febiger Publishers, 1979.

O'Brien, R. *Dental Radiography: An Introduction for Dental Hygienists and Assistants,* 4th ed. Philadelphia: W. B. Saunders Co., 1982.

Wolf, D. *Essentials of Dental Radiology for Dental Assistants and Hygienists,* 2nd ed. Englewood Cliffs, N.J.: Prentice-Hall Inc., 1980.

Wuehrmann, A. and Manson-Hing, L.R. *Dental Radiology,* 5th ed. St. Louis: The C. V. Mosby Co., 1981.

4

Dental Materials

Course Synopsis

Introduction

Dental materials include a wide range of natural and prepared substances used in the delivery of oral health care. Auxiliaries play an essential role in the preparation, manipulation, and delivery of these materials. Consequently, understanding the factors that affect the materials and the uses and proper manipulation of different materials enable auxiliaries to function more effectively.

Gypsum Products: Plaster and Stone

Gypsum products are used in dentistry to form casts and dies that are positive reproductions of patients' hard and soft oral tissues. These materials can also be used intraorally as impression materials for taking full denture impressions or soldering registrations for casting. However, intraoral use of gypsum products is diminishing, since other materials can give equal accuracy and detail and are easier to use intraorally.

Plasters and stones are made by grinding gypsum under high temperatures (230°–250°F) to drive off part of the water of crystallization. This process is called calcining. The main constituent of all plasters or stones is calcium sulfate hemihydrate; the degree of refinement of the calcium sulfate hemihydrate is contingent on whether plaster or stone is desired. Particles in plaster are more irregular and spongy, whereas stone has more dense particles in more crystalline forms. The difference in particle shape between plasters and stones reflects the difference in properties. Plasters are not as strong as stones, although both are easy to manipulate.

Stone can be further classified into class I and II stones. Class I stone contains more regular particles and is mainly used for pouring casts. Class II stone, also known as improved stone, contains a greater number of random-shaped particles and as a result is a harder material. Improved stone is primarily used to make dies.

Gypsum products set exothermically, that is, heat is released. The amount of water mixed with the plaster or stone is very important and is expressed as the water to powder (w/p) ratio. For example, the more water added, the longer the setting time and the weaker the result. Setting time is also affected by the length and speed of mixing. The longer and more rapid the mix, the shorter the setting time. Setting time can be accelerated or retarded by using chemical additives. Sodium tetraborate (Borax) will retard setting time, whereas adding salts, such as sodium chloride, in small quantities will accelerate the set.

Accurate models demand that gypsum products, when set, not change their shape; consequently, the dimensional stability of these products is important. Improper manipulation can cause changes in dimension that can result in an inaccurate model from an accurate impression.

Plasters and stone are mixed in a flexible rubber bowl with a stiff spatula. A premeasured amount of water is added to the gypsum product. One difficulty encountered with mixing is the incorporation of air bubbles. These bubbles, however, can be removed by using an automatic vibrator and vibrating the mix until no more bubbles come to the surface. The mix can then be poured or shaped as needed.

Dental Cements

Cements in dentistry are used as luting agents for temporary and permanent restorations and orthodontic bands, as temporary restorations, and as thermal insulators for the pulp under metallic restorations. Varnishes and liners, also included under the classification of cements, are used in thin layers on the dentin to prevent irritating chemicals from reaching pulpal tissues. They are also used as sedative material.

Zinc phosphate cement (ZOP) is a powder/liquid system. The powder is composed of zinc oxide and magnesium oxide, and the liquid contains phosphoric acid, water, and a small amount of aluminum phosphate.

Zinc phosphate cements are high in acidity and can cause pulpal damage if not mixed properly. As is true of all cements, they are soluble in oral fluids and will not adhere to tooth structure under moist conditions.

Advantages of ZOP are its malleability and high compressive strength. Setting time can also be controlled, thereby providing the dentist with the flexibility to use the material for the desired purpose.

ZOP is mixed on a dry, cool glass slab. Drops of the liquid are placed on the slab and small increments of powder are incorporated. The material is mixed over a large area with a small metal spatula. This process, called slaking, is continued until the cement becomes as thick as desired for the function (e.g., thinner for cementation of restorations and thicker for bases under restorations). Setting time, if desired, can be delayed up to nine minutes.

Zinc oxide–eugenol (ZOE) is usually dispensed in a powder/liquid system. The powder is composed of zinc oxide, which can contain a small amount of fillers and zinc salts and the liquid is eugenol (oil of cloves).

This cement has a sedative effect on the pulpal tissues and is used to ameliorate pain from toothaches. ZOE is easy to manipulate and setting can be controlled by accelerators, decreasing moisture, or altering the powder/liquid ratio. ZOE has low compressive strength and is highly soluble in oral fluids; consequently, it is not used in final restorations.

ZOE is mixed by adding the powder to the liquid in small amounts and vigorously spatulating the mix on the oil-impervious pad or glass slab until the desired thickness is obtained. As with all cements, the more powder used, the stronger the material. By adjusting the amount of powder added, setting time can be delayed up to 10 minutes.

ZOE also comes in a strengthened form, reinforced with ethopybenzoic acid (EBA). It is a powder/liquid system that is easy to manipulate, flows readily under pressure, and has a long working time. It achieves adequate strength only if there is a high powder–liquid ratio. The material is mixed on a glass slab, and powder is added to the liquid. The mix is then spatulated vigorously under pressure for 2 minutes in order to achieve fluidity. Setting time is 7–13 minutes. This material can be used to cement castings permanently.

Polycarboxylate cement, also referred to as carboxylate and polyacrylate is a powder/liquid system used for luting or insulating pulpal tissue. The powder consists mainly of zinc oxide with some magnesium oxide and aluminum oxide; the liquid contains polyacrylic and organic acids in an aqueous solution. This cement is not irritating to pulpal tissue, has a relatively low solubility in oral fluids, and adheres best to clean enamel. One disadvantage is its short working time (maximum 3½ minutes) and setting time (5–8 minutes).

Polycarboxylate cement can be mixed on paper or glass. When mixed on a cool glass slab, however, working time is increased. Premeasured powder is incorporated into the liquid in large quantities and is spatulated quickly until homogeneous.

Varnishes and liners are used to insulate pulpal tissue. Varnish is a coating material, consisting mainly of a natural gum, or a synthetic resin in an organic solvent solution. Varnishes block irritating chemicals contained in restorative materials (amalgam or bases) from entering the dentinal tubules and affecting the pulp.

The technique for using varnish involves dipping a cotton pledget into the varnish, removing the excess, and coating the walls of the cavity. Two thin coatings should be applied to cover all surfaces completely. Setting time is 15–20 seconds.

Calcium hydroxide is a liner available in liquid/paste or paste/paste form. The paste hardens and forms a thin layer over the dentin; it stimulates the formation of secondary dentin, which acts as additional protection for the pulp. It also forms a barrier against irritants from marginal leakage of restorative materials. This material must only be used on dentin, since placement on enamel walls of cavity preparations can contribute to marginal leakage of final restorations as a result of its high degree of solubility in oral fluids.

Direct Restorative Materials

Direct restorative materials are used to replace tooth structure which has been naturally or mechanically removed. These materials are classified into restorative materials used for anterior teeth and those used in the posterior area of the mouth.

Direct anterior restorative materials have been created to esthetically replace lost tooth structure. Gold foil, rarely used on anterior teeth in the Western world, is the only exception.

Silicate cement is an anterior restorative material supplied in a powder/liquid form. The silicate powder is a glass product, containing silica, aluminum, sodium or calcium phosphate, calcium fluoride, and sodium–aluminum fluoride. The liquid is a phosphoric acid solution containing phosphoric acid, aluminum and zinc phosphates, and water. The powder of the silicate material is manufactured by a complex process of fusing the glass particles into a manipulative form. Silicate cements are anticariogenic because of the active fluorides in the cement. However, they are no longer widely used because they have a high degree of solubility, abrasion, and dehydration in oral fluids, which tend to reduce the life of the restoration. In addition, if silicate cements are improperly mixed, the resulting high acidity can cause pulpal damage.

A glass slab (cooling of the slab will lengthen the setting time) must be used with a cement spatula that is not stainless steel. The premeasured powder is incorporated into the liquid in large portions in less than 60 seconds. A puttylike mix will result. In order to seal the dentinal tubules and protect the pulp, a layer of varnish must be applied before the silicate material is placed in the cavity preparation. Using a matrix, insertion should be quick and should take place under dry conditions. It is recommended that varnish or petroleum jelly be placed over the exposed surfaces of the restoration immediately after insertion, to prevent dehydration and discoloration.

Composite materials are used for the same purposes as silicates and acrylics. In addition, composite can be used to correct anomalies of enamel development and other esthetic problems and to bond orthodontic brackets. Composites contain a monomer or an aromatic dimethacrylate (most commonly BIS-GMA), an accelerator, organic peroxide, and a filler, such as quartz or glass. Catalysts that quicken setting time vary according to the system used. These systems include self-curing, ultraviolet light curing, and visible light curing. Composite is moderately strong and can be easily manipulated; however, it can be abraded and lose its finish easily.

If the composite is a paste/paste self-curing system, it is mixed by placing equal portions of catalyst and base on a small mixing pad. Different sides of double-ended plastic spatulas are used to avoid contaminating the materials. The two pastes are incorporated into a homogeneous mixture. The composite is then inserted into the preparation and is held in place with a celluloid matrix. Etching enamel walls with phosphoric acid before insertion improves retention and diminishes marginal leakage.

Direct gold restorations are used in many areas of the oral cavity. The use of gold is costly, time consuming, and often unesthetic and, as a result, is diminishing. Direct gold restorative materials come in several forms: gold foil, mat gold, powdered gold, and mat gold–calcium alloy, also referred to as electroloy. Manipulation varies slightly from one type to the next; the type of gold chosen is dependent on individual preference.

Working the gold into the preparation is facilitated by the malleability, ductility, and welding ability of the material. It adapts to the walls of a preparation very well, making recurrent caries formation less likely than with other materials. Gold foil does not corrode or tarnish. The time involved in condensation of a gold foil restoration is extensive, since the material must be condensed layer by layer (cold welded), and as a result it can present difficulties for the patient.

In order for the gold to be pure (without moisture or the presence of ammonia used in manufacturing) each particle of gold must be annealed before it is placed into the cavity preparation. This process can be done on an annealing tray placed over a flame or on a hot plate. After the gold particle (e.g., pellet, powder) has been annealed, it is then placed into the correct spot by the dentist and condensed into the preparation. After adequate condensation the restoration is polished.

Acrylic resins are polymeric restorative materials used in anterior teeth. The resins come in a powder and liquid form. The liquid is a monomer comprising methyl methylacrylate (hydroquinone), an accelerator, and an organic sulfonic acid. The powder is a polymer of polymethyl methacrylate, benzoyl peroxide (a catalyst), and metal oxides. The material has an ability to withstand fracture and is available in a wide range of shades. Disadvantages include a low resistance to wear and inability to prevent recurring caries. In addition, the restoration can change shape over time and alternately expands and contracts; this results in an exchange of fluids in the margins, the process known as percolation.

There are two techniques of applying direct acrylic resins to a tooth preparation: brush or nealon, and bulk techniques. In the brush technique, liquid and powder are placed into separate dappen dishes. A sable brush is dipped into the liquid and then into the powder, and the acrylic bead is then placed into the tooth preparation. This method is repeated until the tooth is fully restored. In the bulk technique, powder and liquid are mixed in a single dappen dish until a doughlike consistency is obtained. The mix is placed in the tooth preparation with a plastic instrument and is held in place with a matrix until it is set.

Dental amalgam (amalgam), a combination of mercury with a silver–tin alloy containing small amounts of copper and zinc, is the material of choice for approximately 75% of all dental restorations. Each constituent of the material adds properties to the final product. Silver adds strength and decreases flow. Tin tends to reduce expansion, but it also reduces strength. Zinc acts as a deoxidizer. Copper improves strength and hardness. Mercury wets the alloy particles and chemically reacts with the alloy to begin the hardening process.

Mercury in liquid form is mixed with the metallic alloy which is produced in powder, chips, or spheres. This process is termed trituration. Trituration can be either manual, mixed with a mortar and pestle, or mechanical, vibrated in an amalgamator. Premeasured and premixed capsules that eliminate proportioning and handling the materials are available to use in amalgamators. The resulting amalgam is plastic and can be inserted, condensed, and carved easily in the cavity preparation.

Undertrituration or overtrituration diminishes the properties of amalgam. Undertriturated amalgam becomes crumbly and is difficult to manipulate. Its strength is also diminished. Overtriturated amalgam is runny in consistency and is difficult to manipulate.

Amalgam is widely used for its high compressive strength, relative inexpensiveness, ease of manipulation, and tendency to reduce marginal leakage. A major disadvantage of dental amalgam is mercury toxicity. Mercury is highly toxic to humans, and either direct contact with the metal or inhalation of its vapors can result in pathologies ranging from minor irritability to death.

Premeasured capsules eliminate direct contact with free mercury and as a result are becoming increasingly popular as a preventive measure. Additional disadvantages include low tensile or flexing strength and low edge strength.

Impression Materials

Impression materials are used in dentistry to obtain accurate, detailed negative images of hard and soft oral tissues. There are two major categories of impression materials, elastic and plastic, which can be further subdivided into chemosetting and thermosetting. Elastic materials are capable of being deformed under stress and returning to their original shape after setting. These materials are divided into two groups: hydrocolloids, including reversible and irreversible, and elastomers, including polysulfide, silicone, and polyether.

Hydrocolloids

Reversible or agar hydrocolloid is a thermoelastic material in which an impression is recorded through the physical change of agar from a sol to a gel. Agar hydrocolloid is packaged in tubes and is composed of 80–85% water, 12–15% agar, a small percentage of sodium tetraborate (Borax), which adds strength, and 2% potassium sulfate, which enhances proper setting. The material is prepared by placing it in a water bath at 212°F. It is stored at 150°F in a second bath. Before the impression is taken, it is placed in water-cooled trays and immersed in a third conditioning bath to bring the material to a tolerable temperature for the oral tissues.

Agar hydrocolloids are extremely accurate materials and are used for final impressions to make models for the fabrication of partial dentures, crowns, bridges, and inlays. The material has a low tear strength and the potential for high-dimensional change resulting from imbibition (the taking up of water). To minimize dimensional distortions, the impression should be poured immediately.

Irreversible or alginate hydrocolloid is a material that produces an impression through the process of chemical change. Mixing the soluble sodium alginate, which also contains calcium sulfate, with water results in the formation of an insoluble calcium alginate gel. Trisodium phosphate in the powder acts as a retardant, permitting more working time. The remaining ingredients include diatomaceous earth, which acts as a filler, a complex fluoride compound, which helps create adequate surface strength for the gypsum model materials, a coloring agent, and flavor additives.

The material is manipulated by first placing the powder, measured in scoops, into a rubber mixing bowl. A measured amount of room temperature (70°F) water is then added and the mix is spatulated in a whipping motion until a homogeneous sol is formed. The temperature of the water is extremely important, since higher temperatures shorten working and setting times. The mix is immediately placed in a fitted perforated or rim-locked tray.

Alginate is not as accurate in recording fine detail as other impression materials (e.g., reversible hydrocolloids), and as a result it is used to take impressions for study models used in diagnosis and the fabrication of orthodontic appliances and night guards. The material can be used to take final impressions for partial dentures. Alginate is easy to manipulate, in addition to being inexpensive. It has a low tear strength and is not dimensionally stable because of syneresis (loss of water) and imbibition. These impressions should be poured immediately.

Elastomers

Elastomers are elastic impression materials manufactured from synthetic rubber and appearing soft and rubberlike when set.

Polysulfide impression material, also known as mercaptan, produces an impression through the chemical process of polymerization, which is the chemical reaction whereby single units (monomers) link to form larger units (polymers). The material is supplied in two tubes of paste. One tube, the base, contains the basic reactive substance, a low-molecular-weight polysulfide polymer, and fillers. The other tube, the accelerator, contains lead peroxide and sulfur, which actually cause the vulcanization reaction that forms a longer-chain rubber material.

The material is mixed by spatulating equal lengths of base and accelerator on a paper pad for 45–60 seconds. The material, homogenized in color, is then placed in a preformed custom or stock tray and inserted into the patient's mouth. The material sets in about 6–8 minutes and is very accurate. It is used to take final impressions for models on which crowns, bridges, inlays, and partial dentures are fabricated. The material's disadvantages are its offensive smell, staining ability and inconsistent setting time which is shortened by increased temperature and humidity.

Silicone impression material is similar to polysulfide material in many ways. It sets via a polymerization reaction in 6–8 minutes and is supplied in two tubes (a base and a catalyst). It is carried to the mouth in the same type of tray as polysulfide and is used for the same purposes. The base, a paste, contains a polymer, dimethylsilocaine, and an organic filler. The catalyst, usually a liquid, contains an octoate that initiates the reaction. The base is dispensed onto a paper pad and the catalyst is added. The material is spatulated for about a minute until a homogeneous color results. Its color and odor are among its advantages, while its disadvantages include a shorter shelf-life than that of other impression materials. Silicone is also available in a putty/wash system. The putty is mixed with a liquid catalyst. The putty contains up to 70% fillers as compared with the 45% of the regular-bodied silicone. After the putty has set, a "wash" material (a fluid silicone base mixed with the same liquid catalyst) is smoothed over the putty impression and placed over the teeth. This process results in an accurate, detailed impression.

Polyether impression materials are the third impression material in the elastomeric group and are similar to polysulfide and silicone in their polymerization reaction. However, when polyether is used, the impression can be recorded in a single step without a second wash impression. The material is supplied in two tubes; the base contains a polyether polymer and the accelerator is a sulfonic acid ester. The materials are dispensed in equal lengths onto a paper mixing pad and spatulated for about 45–60 seconds until a homogeneous color is attained. Setting time is 2½–3 minutes. Polyether materials are highly accurate and are used for the same purposes as other elastic impression materials. A factor to be considered when using these materials is the difficulty of removing set impressions from the patient's mouth.

Plastic Impression Materials

Impression materials categorized as plastic are those that are unable to return to their original shape after deformation. They are model plastic (compound), dental wax, zinc oxide–eugenol paste, and impression plaster. The latter two are sometimes subclassified as rigid materials.

Thermal modeling plastic or dental compound is a material that produces an impression through a physical change of shape at a specific temperature. It is comprised of various thermoplastic resins, waxes, fillers, and coloring agents. Thermal modeling plastics are used to take preliminary impressions for full or partial dentures and for final impressions of single crown preparations. When denture impressions are desired, wafers or cakes are used; when single crown impressions are desired, sticks are used. Dental compound has low thermal conductivity and should be heated slowly and evenly. When preparing the material for a preliminary impression, it should be softened in a water bath at 130°F until it can be kneaded. The compound should not remain in the water for too long a period, because some of the necessary ingredients dissolve and a grainy material results. Similarly, when stick compound is warmed over a flame it should be heated in a manner that prevents melting or dripping in order to maintain suitable flow properties. The materials are impressed against the mouth tissues while still warm and flowing (113°F). By the time the material reaches mouth temperature (98.6°F), it exhibits very little flow. Corrective washes (or final impressions) are taken over denture impressions.

Waxes are thermoplastic materials that come in many forms and are used for various procedures. They are categorized into three groups: pattern waxes, processing waxes, and impression waxes.

Pattern waxes are used to form the patterns from which metal or resin restorations are cast. Examples of pattern waxes are inlay wax, used to produce patterns for inlays, crowns, and pontics, and casting wax, used to create the pattern for the metal framework of a removable prosthesis.

Processing waxes are waxes used in the laboratory. Examples include boxing wax used to prepare gypsum models, sticky wax used to reattach plaster impressions, and periphery wax used to adjust trays to the appropriate size.

Impression wax manufactured in various arch shapes is used when taking full denture impressions. Examples include corrective impression wax used to record or fill specific areas of impressions made from other materials when minute detail is desired, and bite wax and wafer impression wax used to record occlusal registration.

These dental waxes are composed of a combination of materials which form organic polymers. Ingredients include resins, oils, fat, gums, pigments, and natural and synthetic waxes.

ZOE can be used as an impression material as well as a cement. When used for impressions, ZOE functions as a final wash and is inserted into a preliminary impression tray. It is most often used for full denture impressions in a preformed tray. The material is dispensed in a paste/paste system and mixed on oil impervious paper. Initial setting time is approximately 3–6 minutes, and final set ranges from 10 to 15 minutes. Setting time can be accelerated using a zinc acetate salt or a drop of water. Although the material is dimensionally stable, ZOE impression paste can irritate oral tissues because of its eugenol constituent, which can cause burning or stinging.

Plasters are also used as impression materials. They are most often used to record the position of prepared teeth in soldering fixed bridges. Setting accelerators are added to regulate setting time and control dimensional stability. Plaster has limited use as an impression material because it can lock into intraoral undercuts; consequently, it must be fractured and reassembled outside the mouth. Elastomeric impression materials provide similar accuracy without the disadvantage of the difficulty of removal and consequently are used more frequently.

Cast Restorations

Often, in a severely deteriorated tooth that is missing a considerable amount of structure direct filling materials such as amalgam cannot be used because they would be unable to withstand masticatory forces; rather, stronger cast restorations are fabricated.

The use of pure metal in dentistry is quite limited; the most commonly used materials are combinations of two or more metals, known as alloys.

Gold alloys are cast into inlays, crowns, bridges, and partial denture frameworks. The base metal alloys, such as cobalt chromium, are used in constructing partial denture frameworks.

Casting gold alloys can contain gold, silver, copper, palladium, platinum, and zinc. The properties of gold alloys are affected by changing the percentage of the components. The increased cost of gold has brought about the use of many alloys containing lower proportions of gold. In addition, more nonprecious alloys are being used as substitutes. The properties that each constituent of the gold alloy adds to the final casting are as follows: Gold resists tarnish and corrosion and contributes ductility and malleability to the alloy. Silver reduces the deep yellow color of gold and red tint of copper, by its natural gray color. Copper increases the strength and hardness of the alloy and generally reduces the melting point. Platinum increases the strength, hardness, and resistance to tarnish and corrosion. Like silver, it also helps whiten the color. Palladium increases the melting point, hardens the compound, and whitens the alloy. Zinc acts as a scavenger, reacting with any oxides first, and increases the castibility of the alloy. It also reduces the melting point.

Gold alloy materials are classified according to gold content and hardness, which correlates to material strength. There are four types of dental gold alloys. Type I alloys are soft and are used for simple inlays. Type II alloys are harder and can be used for two- and three-surface inlays and are the most common alloys used for operative procedures. Type III are alloys used for fixed prostheses. Type IV alloys are extra hard and are used for denture frameworks. The objective of the casting procedure is to provide an accurate metallic duplication of missing tooth structures. The first procedure in the casting of an inlay or a crown is the preparation of a wax pattern. This pattern is carved directly on the prepared tooth or on a die representing a reproduction of the tooth and prepared cavity. If the pattern is made in the tooth itself, the technique is termed direct. Similarly, if the pattern is made on a die, the technique is termed indirect.

The wax pattern forms the outline of the mold into which the molten gold alloy is cast. It is therefore imperative that the pattern accurately represent the missing tooth structure.

After the pattern is removed from the prepared cavity, it is attached to a sprue former. The sprue former provides an ingate into the investment through which the molten alloy can enter the mold. The size of the sprue former depends on the type and size of the pattern, the type of casting machine used, and the dimensions of the flask or ring in which the casting is made.

The wax pattern is then surrounded by a gypsum material known as investment. The investment serves as a binder to hold the other ingredients together and provides rigidity. Since gold alloy contracts upon setting, expansion of investment is desirable for compensation. The setting expansion or thermal expansion can be controlled by altering the proportion of water in the investment mix. Thus, the appropriate amount of expansion to compensate for the shrinkage of gold can be attained.

After the investment has hardened for at least 30 minutes, the sprue former is removed and the sprue, if it is plastic or wax, is left in the investment. The casting ring containing the invested pattern is heated slowly to the temperature at which the maximal thermal expansion of the investment is obtained (usually 700°C or 1292°F), and the wax pattern is eliminated by the heat. The investment should be heated for at least 1 hour. After the casting temperature has been attained, the casting can be made.

After the casting has been completed, when the metal is dull red, the ring is immersed in water. The casting is brushed free of debris; however surface film may make the casting appear dark. A process called pickling, that is, heating the discolored casting in a 50% solution of hydrochloric acid, removes the film. The casting can then be fit and finished.

Soldering is the process of joining metals and is used in dentistry to join parts of a bridge during assembly; to increase bulk on inlays and crowns to establish proper contact areas; to join wrought metal parts to removable partial dentures; and to join orthodontic appliances.

The intermediary alloy, solder, has a lower melting temperature than the metals being joined and is used as the filler material. The solder should ideally have a strength equal to the metals being joined and a matching color. In addition, it must not corrode or tarnish in the oral environment.

Porcelain

Dental porcelain is a highly esthetic material widely used in final restoration. It is highly compatible with oral tissues and is resistant to abrasion. It is used in the fabrication of artificial teeth in dentures, for crowns, and as a veneer fused to metal copings. Porcelains are classified by the temperature at which they mature. All are made of particles of feldspar and quartz. The feldspar serves as a matrix for the quartz, and the quartz is a strengthener and filler.

Porcelain is highly resistant to the forces of compression but also highly susceptible to bending forces. Consequently, restorations and tooth preparations must be designed to deemphasize exposure to unnecessary bending forces in the oral cavity.

Porcelain is produced as a powder that is mixed with water to form a pastelike substance that can be molded or condensed into the desired shape. The substance is then fired in a furnace and is subsequently glazed to polish the surface and improve the strength of the restoration. It is important to use minimum amounts of water to avoid shrinkage during the condensation or firing processes.

The finished restoration can then be placed into the mouth. Restorations totally fabricated from porcelain are used primarily in the anterior portion of the mouth. When used for posterior restorations, the material is fused to a cast alloy coping which fits the prepared tooth or teeth. This type of restoration emphasizes the esthetic qualities of porcelain while diminishing its disadvantages.

Synthetic Resins

Synthetic resins are nonmetallic compounds that can be molded into many forms for commercial use. Often synthetic resins are components of clothing, appliances, and many other products found in the home and the workplace. Recently, synthetic resins have begun to have wide use in dentistry. Originally, they were used to replace denture bases because they were lighter and more esthetic than the older vulcanite materials. Recent research and refinement have led to the increased use of this material.

Synthetic resins are either thermoplastic or thermosetting. The thermoplastic resins can be molded without chemical change that uses heat and pressure. Thermosetting resins undergo a chemical change called polymerization during the molding process. This process sometimes happens with the addition of heat but in some products, accelerators, and catalysts are used to begin the polymerization process.

Acrylic resin (methyl methacrylate), a thermal setting resin, is widely used in dentistry. The acrylic resin in a liquid form (monomer) is mixed with a powder (polymer). Polymerization occurs through a series of progressive chemical reactions, in four phases. The acrylic resin progresses from the sandy stage to the sticky stage, to a doughlike material, and finally to a stiff or solid stage.

Denture bases are made from acrylic resins because of the material's dimensional stability, esthetic appearance, ability to absorb shock, and weight. Self-curing acrylic resins can be worked and set at room temperature and are often used to repair dentures that have broken. Acrylic resins are also used to rebase and reline dentures. Because the oral tissues on which the dentures rest change with time, dentures must sometimes be adapted to accommodate these changes. When dentures are rebased, the old base is used as an impression tray. The former base is replaced with one made from a new impression. The same teeth are used for the new base.

When minor changes occur in the oral tissues, a denture can be relined, rather than rebased. The existing base is used to take an impression, and the appropriate amount of acrylic is added to accommodate the changes.

Acrylic resin is also used to make custom trays for impressions. These trays produce high-quality impressions because they are accurate replications of individual oral tissues. Temporary crowns are fabricated from acrylic resin; permanent crowns are often faced with acrylic veneers.

Abrasion and Polishing

Dental restorations are usually rough and irregular after construction. In order to improve their appearance and comfort and to increase their resistance to tarnish and corrosion, they are abraded and polished. Abrasive materials capable of cutting or scratching are used to smooth the surfaces. Initially, coarse abrasives are used and sequentially followed by progressively finer materials. As a result of this process, the scratches become undetectable and the restoration's surfaces become smooth.

The polishing process may take place either intraorally or in a laboratory. If the polishing is done in the mouth, caution must be taken to prevent overheating the tooth and consequently damaging vital tissues. It is also important to choose abrasive agents which will not stain either the tooth or the restoration. Common abrasive materials used in dentistry include diamond stones, wheels, and disks; carborundum wheels and disks; aluminum oxide disks; and quartz sandpaper disks. Most of these agents are available in graduated degrees of abrasiveness.

Question Section

Directions: Each of the questions or incomplete statements below is followed by four suggested answers or completions. Select the BEST answer in each case.

1. A material that speeds up a chemical reaction without becoming involved chemically is called
   1. a solvent
   2. a base
   3. a catalyst
   4. thermoplastic

2. An excellent thermal conductor is a
   1. gold inlay
   2. zinc phosphate base
   3. composite restoration
   4. porcelain crown

3. The ability of material not to become permanently distorted under stress is called
   1. compression
   2. strain
   3. elasticity
   4. conductibility

4. Dissimilar metal restorations in the same mouth can cause pain resulting from differences in
   1. cavity preparation
   2. electrical potential
   3. thermal conductivity
   4. compressive strengths

5. Cohesion is molecular attraction between
   1. similar molecules
   2. a denture and the oral mucosa
   3. different molecules
   4. irregular surfaces

6. Flow of a material refers to
   1. continued change of the material under a given load
   2. the consistency of a material when mixing
   3. the homogeneity of gypsum products
   4. dimensional change of the material during setting

7. The stress required to fracture a material by pulling it apart is known as
   1. compressive strength
   2. ductility
   3. tensile strength
   4. pull

8. Vulcanization refers to the setting of
   1. reversible hydrocolloid
   2. mercaptan impression material
   3. zinc phosphate cement
   4. zinc oxide–eugenol

9. Which product undergoes an exothermic reaction when setting?
   1. amalgam
   2. zinc oxide–eugenol
   3. gold foil
   4. plaster

10. Study models are used
    1. as references in orthodontic cases
    2. to show shape, size, and position of teeth
    3. as an aid in treatment planning
    4. all of the above

11. Impressions are used to
    1. determine the shade of prosthetic teeth
    2. determine the best filling material
    3. fabricate cast prosthetic restorations
    4. determine the type of cement that should be used to place cast restorations

12. An impression is a
    1. negative reproduction of oral tissues
    2. flexible model
    3. metallic casting
    4. positive reproduction of a prepared tooth

13. Impression materials can be classified according to
    1. cost
    2. nature of the material as it is being removed from the mouth
    3. setting time
    4. accuracy

14. The oldest impression material is
    1. impression plaster
    2. irreversible hydrocolloid
    3. metallic oxide paste
    4. silicone impression material

15. When taking impressions of the abutments for fixed bridgework, the following materials can be used

A. plaster
B. compound
C. irreversible hydrocolloid
D. silicone
E. reversible hydrocolloid
   1. A, B, and D
   2. B, C, and D
   3. B, D, and E
   4. C, D, and E

16. Which material is thermoplastic?
   1. compound
   2. mercaptan
   3. alginate
   4. plaster

17. Which material should be tempered before using?
   1. alginate
   2. reversible hydrocolloid
   3. impression plaster
   4. metallic oxide paste

18. The impression material capable of change from gel to sol to gel is
   1. reversible hydrocolloid
   2. irreversible hydrocolloid
   3. compound
   4. silicone

19. Hydrocolloid impressions
A. are extremely accurate
B. have high tear strength
C. have low dimensional change
D. are used for final impressions to make models for partial dentures
E. must be poured immediately
   1. A, B, and C
   2. B, C, and D
   3. C, D, and E
   4. A, D, and E

20. Heavy and light body impression materials are used with
   1. mercaptan
   2. silicone
   3. reversible hydrocolloid
   4. 1 and 2

21. A perforated tray is used to carry
   1. plaster
   2. mercaptan
   3. irreversible hydrocolloid
   4. reversible hydrocolloid

22. Which material is carried in a custom tray?
   1. high fusing compound
   2. reversible hydrocolloid
   3. metallic oxide paste
   4. irreversible hydrocolloid

23. Copper bands carry which impression material?
   1. metallic oxide paste
   2. stick compound
   3. impression plaster
   4. all of the above

24. When using rubber impression material, it is necessary to coat the tray with
   1. a separating medium
   2. petroleum jelly
   3. a rubber adhesive
   4. no coating is necessary

25. Water-cooled trays are used to carry which impression material?
   1. silicone
   2. mercaptan
   3. reversible hydrocolloid
   4. impression plaster

26. A bulk of material is important when using
   1. silicone impression material
   2. reversible hydrocolloid impression material
   3. mercaptan impression material
   4. metallic oxide impression material

27. Which material undergoes hysteresis?
   1. irreversible hydrocolloid
   2. reversible hydrocolloid
   3. impression plaster
   4. metallic oxide paste

28. Syneresis is the
   1. uptake of water by hydrocolloid impressions
   2. loss of water by hydrocolloid impressions
   3. uptake of water by gypsum products
   4. expansion of elastic impression materials

29. Imbibition is the
   1. uptake of water by hydrocolloid impressions
   2. loss of water by hydrocolloid impressions
   3. increase in model size due to expansion
   4. decrease in model size due to evaporation of water

30. Undermixing irreversible hydrocolloid impression material results in
   1. a grainy mix and a model with poorer detail
   2. an increased tear strength
   3. an increased setting time
   4. finer surface detail

31. The setting time of irreversible hydrocolloid can easily be altered by
    1. using a metal spatula
    2. using a perforated tray
    3. varying the water temperature
    4. adding hard water

32. When loading a tray with irreversible hydrocolloid
    1. more material is placed posteriorly
    2. more material is placed anteriorly
    3. more material is placed in the palatal area
    4. the material is placed evenly in the entire tray

33. The setting of reversible hydrocolloid occurs
    1. only in the presence of water
    2. from the tray to the oral tissues
    3. from the oral tissues to the tray
    4. only in the presence of saliva

34. The removal of hydrocolloid impressions from the mouth is accomplished with
    1. a rocking motion
    2. a jiggling motion
    3. lateral pressure
    4. one firm movement

35. After removing a hydrocolloid impression from the mouth, the operator should
    1. immerse the impression in a warm bath
    2. tap the impression to remove saliva
    3. wash the impression to remove saliva, blood, and debris
    4. let the impression stand in the air for 1 hour

36. Placing a reversible hydrocolloid impression in 2% potassium sulfate solution for several minutes results in
    1. a hard smooth model surface
    2. an increase in the gypsum setting time
    3. a decrease in tear strength
    4. dies with finer detail

37. The addition of extra catalyst to silicone impression material
    1. lengthens the setting time
    2. decreases the setting time
    3. does not change the setting time
    4. incapacitates the material

38. When extruding mercaptan impression material, the
    1. base and the accelerator are of equal volume
    2. base and the accelerator are of equal length
    3. amount of each material is not important
    4. base and the accelerator are of equal weight

39. When mixing mercaptan and silicone impression materials
    A. they should be tempered before use
    B. they must be homogeneous
    C. use wiping, pressing motions
    D. use a flexible stainless steel spatula
    E. mix on a cool glass slab
    F. the mix should be completed in about a minute
    1. A, C, D, and F
    2. B, C, D, and F
    3. C, D, E, and F
    4. D, E, and F

40. The setting time for mercaptan impression material is affected by
    1. the shape of the impression tray
    2. the bulk of material used
    3. the amount of accelerator used
    4. an exothermic reaction

41. It is best to clean excess silicone from a patient's face
    1. after the patient arrives home
    2. as soon as it contacts the patient's face
    3. after the material has fully set
    4. with formocresol

42. What is an advantage of using rubber impression material over reversible hydrocolloid?
    1. hydrocolloid is inaccurate
    2. the hydrocolloid has a higher melting point
    3. the rubber impression material has dimensional stability
    4. all of the above

43. Compound is used
    1. to make impressions
    2. interchangeably with irreversible hydrocolloid
    3. as a final impression material in edentulous patients
    4. none of the above

44. Low fusing stick compound is used
    1. for the bulk of preliminary edentulous impressions
    2. as a substitute for inlay wax
    3. to muscle trim an edentulous impression
    4. for spruing

45. What is a disadvantage of using compound

for making impressions of teeth for prepared crowns?

1. it is inaccurate
2. the resulting dies lack sufficient detail
3. there is the probability that irreversible pulpal damage exists
4. the compound will not spring undercuts

46. Metallic oxide impression paste is used to make
   1. final edentulous impressions
   2. impressions of inlay preparations
   3. impressions of crown preparations
   4. impressions for study models

47. Metallic oxide paste is mixed on
   1. a glass slab
   2. a paper mixing pad
   3. either of the above
   4. neither of the above

48. Adding a few drops of water when mixing metallic oxide paste will
   1. slow the setting time
   2. speed up the setting time
   3. not affect the setting time
   4. destroy the paste

49. Quick-setting plaster is used
   1. in transfer registrations when constructing crowns
   2. as a wash in edentulous impressions
   3. to record jaw registrations in full denture work
   4. all of the above

50. Which material is the most difficult to remove from the patient's face?
   1. metallic oxide paste
   2. silicone impression material
   3. reversible hydrocolloid
   4. impression plaster \

51. Dies of crown preparations can be made of
   A. porcelain
   B. amalgam
   C. copper
   D. acrylic
   E. improved stone
      1. A, C, and D
      2. A, B, and E
      3. B, C, and D
      4. B, C, and E

52. Which is a gypsum product?
   1. stone
   2. plaster
   3. investment
   4. all of the above

53. Calcination of gypsum determines

1. debubblizing techniques
2. how impressions are poured
3. the physical characteristics of the resulting gypsum products
4. the type of impression material that should be used

54. When mixing gypsum products
   1. add the powder and water to the mixing bowl at the same time
   2. add the powder to water in the mixing bowl
   3. add water to the powder in the mixing bowl
   4. none of the above

55. To make a gypsum product set faster
   A. increase the water-powder ratio
   B. increase spatulation
   C. lower the water-powder ratio
   D. add an accelerator
   E. use hygroscopic materials
      1. A, B, and D
      2. B, C, and D
      3. B, C, and E
      4. C, D, and E

56. To prevent air bubbles in the final model use
   1. high water-powder ratio
   2. boxing techniques
   3. a mechanical vibrator
   4. additional catalysts

57. Hygroscopic setting expansion occurs in
   1. noble metals
   2. waxes
   3. acrylics after exothermic reactions
   4. all gypsum products immersed in water after the initial setting

58. When pouring a model from a full upper impression, add stone
   1. to the anterior teeth first
   2. to the same place on the palate
   3. to the posterior teeth first
   4. any place desired

59. When pouring a model from a full lower impression, add stone
   1. when the exothermic reaction begins
   2. to either heel and continue to add to the same place
   3. of a watery consistency
   4. anywhere in the impression

60. A reason for boxing impressions is
   1. to decrease the time necessary to finish the base of the model
   2. easy storage
   3. identification
   4. to increase the hardness of the model

61. Dowel pins are used to
    1. articulate impressions
    2. reinforce stone models
    3. reinsert individual dies in a model
    4. calcine gypsum products

62. Plaster is used
    A. to construct study models
    B. to construct dies
    C. to attach models to articulators
    D. to make models for partial denture construction
    E. to make models for fabricating full dentures
       1. A and E
       2. A and C
       3. B and D
       4. C and D

63. Plaster models
    1. contract on setting
    2. expand on setting
    3. have no dimensional change on setting
    4. have greater crushing strength than do stone models

64. The amount of water needed to mix various gypsum products is related to the
    1. water temperature
    2. irregularity of the gypsum particles
    3. impression material used
    4. capillary action

65. Dental stone is used
    1. to pour all irreversible hydrocolloid impressions
    2. for occlusal registration
    3. to construct casts used in denture construction
    4. for all of the above

66. Increasing the water–powder ratio of stone will result in
    1. a less porous model
    2. dies that can be used in constructing crowns
    3. a weaker model
    4. a thermoplastic model

67. The working time of a mix of dental stone ends when the
    1. exothermic reaction is complete
    2. stone no longer flows
    3. model can be separated from the impression
    4. material is the consistency of sour cream

68. Improved stone is used
    1. to make dies
    2. to make study models

3. for bite registrations
4. to invest wax crowns

69. Investment material is used to
    A. pour final fixed bridge impressions
    B. prepare molds in which crowns will be cast
    C. make bite registrations
    D. help solder fixed bridge units
    E. work hardened gold
       1. A, B, and C
       2. B, C, and D
       3. C, D, and E
       4. B and D

70. It is desirable to have expansion of the investment mold to compensate for the
    1. expansion of wax
    2. warping of the impression material
    3. expansion of gold
    4. shrinkage of gold

71. The function of a sprue is to
    1. form an opening for molten metal to enter the mold
    2. help polish cast restorations
    3. eliminate air bubbles on the wax patterns
    4. reproduce fine detail

72. Cracking of an investment mold before casting takes place can result from
    1. heating, cooling, and reheating the mold
    2. quenching the heated investment in cold water
    3. permitting the investment material to set
    4. all of the above

73. To remove a stone model from a metallic oxide paste impression
    1. heat the impression over an open flame
    2. cool the impression in an ice water bath
    3. soak the impression in a warm water bath
    4. tap the impression lightly with a hammer

74. Waxes are used in dentistry for
    A. forming patterns from which castings will be made
    B. taking impressions for bite registrations
    C. accurate final impressions for partial dentures
    D. boxing impressions
    E. picking up castings for soldering
       1. A, B, and C
       2. B, C, and D
       3. C, D, and E
       4. A, B, and D

75. Three general classifications of waxes are
    A. inlay wax

B. processing wax
C. paraffin wax
D. impression wax
E. beeswax
F. pattern wax
   1. A, B, and F
   2. A, C, and D
   3. B, D, and E
   4. B, D, and F

76. Desired physical characteristics of waxes may be obtained by
   1. mixing waxes with water
   2. mixing different waxes and additives
   3. passing an electric current through the wax
   4. permitting them to age

77. Which wax is not used intraorally?
   1. baseplate wax
   2. sticky wax
   3. utility wax
   4. none of the above

78. Inlay wax is used to
   1. temporarily cement inlays
   2. make inlay wax patterns
   3. invest inlay patterns
   4. box models

79. The main ingredient of inlay wax is
   1. carnauba wax
   2. paraffin wax
   3. beeswax
   4. spermaceti wax

80. At mouth temperature, inlay wax should
   1. produce galvanic stimulation
   2. constantly flow
   3. inbibe slightly
   4. have no flow

81. To prevent distortion of an inlay wax pattern
   A. avoid temperature changes
   B. store it in a dark area
   C. keep it moist
   D. manipulate it as little as possible
      1. A and C
      2. A and D
      3. B and C
      4. D and E

82. The best way to heat inlay wax is
   1. to rub it in the palms of your hands
   2. over a flame
   3. in warm water
   4. on a hot plate

83. Instruments used to carve inlay wax in the mouth should be

   1. made of plastic
   2. warm
   3. cold
   4. 1 and 3

84. It is best to invest the inlay wax pattern
   1. as soon as possible
   2. after one hour
   3. after one day
   4. any time

85. If it is necessary to store an inlay wax pattern
   1. wrap it in gauze
   2. keep it at room temperature
   3. refrigerate the pattern
   4. suspend it in air with a piece of dental floss

86. A wax pattern must be
   A. an accurate reproduction of missing tooth structures
   B. made on the tooth itself
   C. well adapted
   D. softened at room temperature
   E. properly carved
      1. A, B, and C
      2. B, C, and D
      3. A, C, and E
      4. C, D, and E

87. An important property of inlay wax is
   1. it is brittle at mouth temperature
   2. it contracts when it is being invested
   3. its complete burnout
   4. it is interchangeable with utility wax

88. Baseplate wax is used to
   1. construct wax patterns for crowns
   2. hold broken parts of dentures together
   3. contour the edges of impression trays
   4. determine occlusal relationships in full dentures

89. When attaching a baseplate rim to a shellac tray, care must be taken
   1. to avoid burning the patient
   2. not to wrap the shellac tray when heating the wax
   3. to coat the ridge area with sticky wax
   4. all of the above

90. The wax used to make a rim around an impression to contain the poured gypsum material is called
   1. boxing wax
   2. utility wax
   3. periphery wax
   4. blue wax

91. Casting wax is used

1. to replace inlay wax
2. to retain asbestos in the casting ring
3. as a pattern for metal partial frameworks
4. to hold gold casting together

92. Sticky wax is used to
    1. rebuild cusps on models
    2. take single tooth impressions
    3. take bite registrations
    4. hold fractured denture parts in a fixed position temporarily

93. Utility wax is used
    1. to wax inlays on models
    2. as a tray to hold compound
    3. as periphery wax around trays
    4. to construct bite rims

94. Impression waxes are used
    1. for bite registrations
    2. for study models
    3. to cast restorations
    4. to hold dies in position

95. Dental cements are used
    A. to hold copper dies together
    B. as temporary restorations
    C. to hold dentures
    D. as thermal insulators
    E. as a substitute for sticky wax
    F. as a luting agent
    1. A, B, and D
    2. B, C, and F
    3. B, D, and F
    4. D, E, and F

96. Which cement is irritating to the pulp?
    1. carboxylate cement
    2. zinc oxide–eugenol cement
    3. zinc phosphate
    4. ethoxybenzoic acid

97. Which cement has the highest crushing strength?
    1. zinc oxide–eugenol
    2. zinc phosphate
    3. calcium hydroxide
    4. all cements have the same crushing strength

98. Dew point is the
    1. melting point of thermoplastic materials
    2. creamy consistency of cements
    3. setting temperature of zinc oxide–eugenol cement
    4. temperature at which water vapor condenses

99. The effect of zinc oxide–eugenol on the pulp
    1. is irritating
    2. encourages pulpal fibrosis
    3. is sedating
    4. has no effect

100. Which component of zinc oxide–eugenol cement gives it strength?
    1. rosin
    2. zinc oxide
    3. zinc acetate
    4. oil of cloves

101. Why is the zinc oxide–eugenol cement mixed on a paper pad?
    1. to prevent the material from setting
    2. to make the material antimicrobial
    3. to make cleaning easier
    4. to increase the temperature

102. Which chemical accelerates the setting time of zinc oxide–eugenol cement?
    1. rosin
    2. zinc oxide
    3. zinc acetate
    4. oil of cloves

103. Which factors will accelerate the setting time of zinc oxide–eugenol cement?
    A. increased powder–liquid ratio
    B. decreased powder–liquid ratio
    C. increased rate at which the powder is added
    D. water
    E. increased temperature
    1. A, C, and D
    2. A, D, and E
    3. B, C, and D
    4. C, D, and E

104. What is the consistency of zinc oxide–eugenol cement, used as a temporary restoration?
    1. fluid
    2. firm and brittle
    3. puttylike
    4. none of the above

105. Which of the following are advantages of zinc oxide–eugenol cement?
    A. ability to use it for a sedative
    B. high compressive strength
    C. insoluble in oral fluids
    D. easily manipulated
    E. ability to control setting time
    1. A, B, and C
    2. B, C, and D
    3. C, D, and E
    4. A, D, and E

106. Zinc phosphate cement is used as a

1. permanent restoration
2. sedative
3. pulp-capping agent
4. thermal insulator under metallic restorations

107. Excess zinc phosphate cement powder left on the mixing slab is
    1. discarded
    2. returned to the bottle
    3. placed under the cement base in the cavity preparation
    4. placed over the cement base in the cavity preparation

108. If water evaporates from the liquid portion of zinc phosphate cement, the setting time is
    1. shortened
    2. not affected
    3. lengthened
    4. indefinite

109. Increasing the powder–liquid ratio of zinc phosphate cement will result in
    1. an increase in pulpal irritation
    2. decreased solubility
    3. decreased crushing strength
    4. a heterogeneous mix

110. Advantages of zinc phosphate cement include
    A. high compressive strength
    B. ease of manipulation
    C. low acidity
    D. ability to control setting time
    E. lack of irritation to the pulp
       1. A, B, and C
       2. B, C, and D
       3. A, B, and D
       4. C, D, and E

111. Which factors retard the setting time of zinc phosphate?
    A. adding small portions of powder
    B. using a disposable spatula
    C. mixing on a paper pad
    D. mixing on a glass slab
    E. decreasing initial acidity
    F. adding a drop of water
       1. A, D, and E
       2. B, C, and E
       3. B, D, and F
       4. D, E, and F

112. What is an advantage of using zinc polyacrylate cement over zinc phosphate cement?
    1. increased tensile strength
    2. decreased irritation
    3. increased crushing strength
    4. none of the above

113. What is the main component of zinc polyacrylate cement powder?
    1. zinc acetate
    2. zinc oxide
    3. methyl methacrylate
    4. polyacrylic acid

114. What is the working time of zinc polyacrylate cement?
    1. 1 minute
    2. 2 minutes
    3. 3 minutes
    4. 4 minutes

115. An advantage of using a silicate restoration is its
    1. sedative effect on the pulp
    2. anticariogenic properties
    3. high crushing strength
    4. thermal conductivity

116. Some disadvantages of using silicate restorations are
    A. its solubility in oral fluids
    B. its ability to discolor easily
    C. its lack of crushing strength
    D. its galvanic shock
    E. its ability to expand on setting
       1. A, B, and C
       2. B, C, and E
       3. B, D, and E
       4. C, D, and E

117. What is the effect of silicate restorations on the pulp tissues?
    1. sedative
    2. irritating
    3. neutral
    4. none of the above

118. Shade selection for a silicate restoration is made
    1. after the rubber dam is placed
    2. before the rubber dam is placed
    3. at the time of insertion
    4. after the placement of a cement base

119. Which factors will accelerate the setting time of silicate cement?
    A. increasing the powder–liquid ratio
    B. adding a drop of water
    C. increasing the spatulation time
    D. increasing the temperature of the mixing slab
    E. adding the powder slowly
       1. A, B, and C
       2. A, B, and D
       3. B, D, and E
       4. C, D, and E

120. Spatulating silicate cement should result in

1. wetting the powder
2. crushing the powder
3. allowing water evaporation
4. increasing the crushing strength

121. What is the mixing time of silicate cement?
   1. 1 minute
   2. 2 minutes
   3. 3 minutes
   4. 4 minutes

122. Which material is primarily used to stop noxious chemicals from reaching the pulp?
   1. calcium hydroxide
   2. zinc oxide–eugenol
   3. varnish
   4. zinc phosphate cement

123. Calcium hydroxide is used as a base primarily to
   1. protect the pulp from bacterial invasion
   2. insulate the pulp thermally
   3. insulate the pulp chemically
   4. promote secondary dentin formation

124. Advantages of calcium hydroxide are
   A. ease of manipulation
   B. low solubility in oral fluids
   C. the ability to stimulate the production of secondary dentin
   D. high compressive strength
   E. the ability to form a barrier against irritants from filling materials used
      1. A, B, and C
      2. B, C, and D
      3. A, C, and E
      4. B, D, and E

125. What is the most frequently used restorative material?
   1. silicate
   2. amalgam
   3. composite
   4. gold

126. Which is the least frequently used restoration?
   1. full crown
   2. composite
   3. porcelain jacket
   4. gold foil

127. Why is it a disadvantage if filling materials are radiolucent?
   1. they are always good thermal conductors
   2. they irritate the pulp
   3. they always cause galvanic shock
   4. it is difficult to differentiate between the restoration and recurrent decay on the radiograph

128. Pins are used in restorative dentistry to
   1. increase the crushing strength of the restorative material
   2. hold a tooth together
   3. fracture the enamel
   4. increase retention

129. Which material is least soluble?
   1. acrylic
   2. silicate
   3. composite
   4. all of the above are of equal solubility

130. Which material most closely approximates the compressive strength of amalgam?
   1. acrylic
   2. silicate
   3. composite
   4. all of the above are of equal strength

131. Which material has the roughest finished restoration?
   1. acrylic
   2. silicate
   3. composite
   4. cast gold

132. The material used in its pure form in dentistry is
   1. composite
   2. silver
   3. amalgam
   4. gold

133. Noble metals
   1. will not conduct an electrical current
   2. will not tarnish or corrode in oral fluids
   3. must be used in all oral restorations
   4. are all very soft

134. Which material has the least amount of flow?
   1. acrylic
   2. amalgam
   3. cast gold
   4. composite

135. Which would be the restoration of choice for a small cavity preparation on the mesial surface of the maxillary right central incisor?
   1. amalgam
   2. gold inlay
   3. composite
   4. porcelain jacket

136. Which would be the restoration of choice, in most cases, to restore a conservative distal occlusal cavity preparation on a maxillary right second premolar?
   1. amalgam
   2. gold inlay

3. composite
4. porcelain jacket

137. Which is the restoration of choice for a right maxillary lateral incisor fractured a third up the crown?
    1. amalgam
    2. gold inlay
    3. composite
    4. porcelain jacket

138. Which is the restoration of choice for a mandibular second molar with the distal buccal cusp missing due to decay?
    1. amalgam
    2. gold onlay
    3. composite
    4. all of the above are of equal quality

139. What is the most esthetic material that can be used in fabricating an anterior bridge?
    1. acrylic
    2. gold
    3. cobalt–chrome
    4. porcelain fused to metal

140. Acrylic resins are used for
    1. anterior restorations
    2. temporary bridges
    3. denture bases
    4. all of the above

141. Advantages of acrylic restorations are
    A. high crushing strength
    B. adhesive properties with dentin
    C. completion in one sitting
    D. insolubility in oral fluid
    E. ability to add to the existing restoration
        1. A, C, and D
        2. B, C, and E
        3. B, D, and E
        4. C, D, and E

142. Disadvantages of acrylic restorations are
    A. they are good thermal conductors
    B. they flow under stress
    C. they wear easily
    D. they have a large coefficient of expansion
    E. the excess can attach to the acrylic of adjacent teeth
        1. A, B, and C
        2. A, C, and E
        3. B, C, and D
        4. C, D, and E

143. The process of chemically combining monomer and polymer is called
    1. plating
    2. mesmerizing
    3. bonding
    4. polymerization

144. Percolation is the
    1. movement of fluids between the tooth and restoration
    2. burrowing effect of bacteria
    3. progressive degeneration of the pulpal tissues
    4. shearing effect of a hoe

145. The main component of acrylic monomer is
    1. methyl methacrylate
    2. hydroquinone
    3. sulfuric acid
    4. quartz filler

146. Acrylic restorations are retained in cavity preparations by means of
    1. base retention
    2. chemical retention
    3. physical retention
    4. both chemical and physical retention

147. Acrylic is applied to the cavity preparation
    1. in small increments
    2. in bulk amounts
    3. with an amalgam carrier
    4. both 1 and 2

148. To process denture base acrylic, it is necessary to
    1. use only acrylic teeth
    2. shake the material for 5 minutes
    3. add extra accelerator
    4. heat the material

149. When constructing a custom acrylic tray, placing it in warm water will
    1. increase its strength
    2. delay the setting
    3. speed polymerization
    4. spring the material past any undercuts on the model

150. When constructing a custom acrylic tray, it is best to remove most of the excess material with
    1. a lathe after the acrylic has set
    2. a knife before the acrylic has set
    3. high-speed burs after the material sets
    4. high-speed burs before the material sets

151. When polishing acrylic on a lathe
    A. use low speed to avoid heat buildup
    B. use copious amounts of water with the pumice
    C. keep moving the prosthesis
    D. add other abrasives to the pumice
    E. use a wire brush

1. A, B, and C
2. B, C, and D
3. B, D, and E
4. C, D, and E

152. If dentures are cleaned in boiling water, they
    1. become sticky
    2. warp
    3. melt
    4. galvanize

153. If dentures are allowed to dry
    1. they contract
    2. they crack
    3. the teeth will discolor if they are porcelain
    4. all of the above

154. To repair a fractured temporary fixed bridge
    1. the bridge is seated in the patient's mouth, and small additions of acrylic are brushed on the fractured area
    2. the bridge is seated in the patient's mouth, and a large amount of acrylic is mixed and adapted around the entire bridge
    3. the bridge is removed from the patient's mouth, sticky wax is added to hold fractured pieces together, and small amounts of acrylic are then added
    4. the bridge is removed from the patient's mouth, the fractured pieces are embedded in fast-setting plaster, and small amounts of acrylic are added

155. To repair a fractured maxillary denture
    1. the fractured denture is placed in the patient's mouth, and small amounts of acrylic are added to the fracture site
    2. the fractured denture is placed in the patient's mouth, the edges are luted together with sticky wax, and then small amounts of acrylic are added to the fractured site
    3. the fractured denture is luted together with sticky wax out of patient's mouth, then the fractured denture is embedded, and acrylic is added to the fracture site
    4. none of the above

156. To replace an intact tooth broken from a denture
    1. the site on the denture is roughened, some quick-cure acrylic is added, and the tooth is reset
    2. the tooth is luted to the denture with sticky wax; the area is then embedded in quick-setting plaster and boiled for 10 minutes

3. the lingual portion of the tooth is cut off, and the tooth is held in position while a loose mix of acrylic is vibrated into the area
4. none of the above

157. Amalgam restorations
    A. are easily inserted
    B. are relatively inexpensive
    C. have low thermal conductivity
    D. are the restoration most frequently used in dentistry
    E. resist tarnish and corrosion
       1. A, B, and C
       2. B, C, and D
       3. B, D, and E
       4. A, B, and D

158. What is the main component of composite restorative materials?
    1. methyl methacrylate
    2. zinc oxide
    3. calcium hydroxide
    4. inorganic filler

159. The type of spatula used to mix composite is
    1. plastic
    2. stainless steel
    3. iron
    4. none of the above

160. What type of base cannot be used with acrylic or composite restorations?
    1. calcium hydroxide
    2. zinc oxide–eugenol
    3. zinc phosphate
    4. all of the above materials could be used as bases with acrylic or composite restorations

161. Preventive sealant resins are placed on the
    1. occlusal surface of the tooth
    2. proximal surface of the tooth
    3. gingival third of the tooth
    4. cusp tips

162. The chemical used to etch enamel is
    1. zinc oxide
    2. methyl methacrylate
    3. phosphoric acid
    4. eugenol

163. Some uses of amalgam are
    A. for posterior restorations
    B. to rebuild teeth on which crowns will be placed
    C. as a post in endodontically treated teeth
    D. to repair fractures in porcelain jackets
    E. to make dies
       1. A, B, and D

2. A, B, and E
3. B, C, and D
4. C, D, and E

164. The largest component of amalgam alloy is
    1. silver
    2. tin
    3. zinc
    4. copper

165. A possible shape of the amalgam alloy particles is
    1. cubic
    2. spiral
    3. spherical
    4. sheetlike

166. Why is zinc sometimes not incorporated in the amalgam alloy?
    1. zinc only acts as a filler
    2. zinc weakens class II restorations
    3. zinc causes the amalgam to pit if the restoration is polished
    4. zinc causes delayed expansion of the amalgam restoration if any water is present while the amalgam is setting

167. How are surface contaminants removed from mercury?
    1. a few drops of water are added to the mercury and the bottle is shaken
    2. the mercury is filtered through a chamois filter
    3. a small magnet is used
    4. if the surface of the mercury is contaminated, the entire bottle must be discarded

168. Which factors would decrease the dental team's exposure to mercury vapors?
    A. use of premeasured capsules
    B. smooth tile floors
    C. careful handling of amalgam scraps
    D. use of an automatic plugger
    E. use of fine grit polishing agents
        1. A, B, and C
        2. B, C, and D
        3. B, D, and E
        4. C, D, and E

169. The best way to control the mercury content of an amalgam restoration is by
    1. mulling the amalgam
    2. undertriturating the amalgam
    3. adding the desired amount of mercury before mixing
    4. firmly condensing the amalgam

170. Which technique of combining mercury with amalgam alloy ensures consistent excellent results?

    1. amalgam fillings
    2. amalgam pellets
    3. premeasured capsules
    4. none of the above

171. Insufficient mercury in an amalgam mix results in
    1. an increase in thermal conductivity
    2. a grainy texture
    3. a gray staining of the gingiva
    4. excessive percolation

172. The crushing strength of amalgam is
    1. 15,000 psi
    2. 30,000 psi
    3. 45,000 psi
    4. 60,000 psi

173. The most common cause of amalgam failure is
    1. poor condensation
    2. incorrect mixing
    3. incorrect preparation
    4. not polishing the restoration

174. Amalgamation is the process of
    1. combining mercury with amalgam alloy
    2. plugging amalgam into the preparation
    3. dispensing the amalgam
    4. burnishing the amalgam against the matrix band

175. The purpose of trituration is to
    1. cause a final expansion in amalgam restorations
    2. decrease the thermal conductivity of amalgam restorations
    3. expose each amalgam particle to mercury
    4. increase galvanization

176. Undertrituration of amalgam will result in
    1. excessive expansion
    2. excessive contraction
    3. slight contraction
    4. no effect

177. Mulling the triturated amalgam results in
    1. moisture contamination
    2. increased expansion
    3. a homogeneous mix
    4. a decrease in thermal conductivity

178. A squeeze cloth is used to
    1. polish amalgam
    2. proportion the amalgam alloy
    3. filter the mercury
    4. remove the excess mercury from the amalgam mix

179. What is the working time of amalgam?

1. 1-2 minutes
2. 3-4 minutes
3. 5-6 minutes
4. 7-8 minutes

180. As amalgam is condensed, excess mercury
    1. is brought to the surface
    2. will dissolve the matrix band
    3. decreases the setting time
    4. liquefies the alloy particles

181. If amalgam is carved after it has started to set, what will occur?
    1. excessive flow
    2. chipping
    3. expansion
    4. discoloration

182. Excess mercury in the final amalgam restoration results in
    A. decreased crushing strength
    B. excessive expansion
    C. pitting when polishing
    D. increased adhesion to the preparation walls
    E. less matrix material to hold the amalgam alloy together
        1. A, B, and C
        2. A, C, and D
        3. B, D, and E
        4. C, D, and E

183. The most frequent complaint of patients shortly after amalgam restorations are placed is
    1. pain on percussion
    2. an open contact point
    3. cold sensitivity
    4. numbness around the gingiva

184. Tarnishing and corrosion of amalgam can be reduced by
    1. polishing the amalgam
    2. using a zinc oxide base
    3. increasing the tin content of amalgam alloy
    4. decreasing the size of the amalgam fillings

185. Which of the following materials are used to polish amalgam restorations in the mouth?
    A. emery
    B. garnet
    C. rouge
    D. tin oxide
    E. tripoli
        1. A, B, and C
        2. B, C, and D
        3. A, D, and E
        4. A, B, and D

186. Overheating amalgam restorations during polishing can result in
    1. creating a restoration high in occlusion
    2. shrinkage in the restoration
    3. pulpal damage
    4. an apthous ulcer

187. An advantage of using a gold restoration over an amalgam restoration is
    1. the ease of tooth preparation
    2. better adaptation to the walls of the preparation
    3. the greater edge strength of cast gold
    4. it is less expensive

188. A disadvantage of using a gold restoration is
    1. the occlusal surface is always flat
    2. the restoration must be replaced in 3 years
    3. full coverage is always necessary
    4. the expense

189. What forms of gold can be worked directly in the mouth?
    A. type I
    B. gold foil
    C. type III
    D. mat gold
    E. powdered gold
        1. A, B, and C
        2. B, C, and D
        3. B, D, and E
        4. C, D, and E

190. The composition of casting gold alloy usually contains
    A. gold
    B. tin
    C. copper
    D. stainless steel
    E. palladium
        1. A, B, and C
        2. B, C, and D
        3. A, C, and E
        4. B, D, and E

191. Gold foil is annealed
    1. to form gold oxides
    2. to remove volatile surface impurities
    3. to soften the gold
    4. to harden the gold

192. The compacting of gold foil is accomplished by the use of
    1. an explorer
    2. condensers
    3. the back of a mirror
    4. burnishers

193. Synthetic resins are used for
    A. relining dentures

B. fabricating custom trays
C. fabricating artificial teeth
D. sedative fillings
E. fabricating onlays
   1. A, B, and C
   2. B, C, and D
   3. B, D, and E
   4. A, D, and E

194. Burnishing the gold foil restoration
   1. hardens the gold
   2. increases its cohesiveness
   3. makes it an alloy
   4. increases the fineness

195. Twelve-carat gold contains what percentage of gold?
   1. 12%
   2. 25%
   3. 50%
   4. 75%

196. Casting gold is used for
   1. wrought wire
   2. soldering
   3. inlays
   4. all of the above

197. The hardness of casting gold is dependent on the
   1. amount and type of metal with which gold is alloyed
   2. shape of the final restoration
   3. type of die used
   4. investment

198. The fusion temperature of gold solder must be
   1. higher than the fusion point of the parts it is joining
   2. the same as the fusion point of the parts it is joining
   3. lower than the fusion point of the parts it is joining
   4. the fusion temperature is not considered a factor

199. Flux is used during casting to
   1. remove the oxides formed on the gold alloy
   2. lower the melting point
   3. replace casting wax
   4. speed the burnout process

200. Pickling
   1. is accomplished by soaking the casting in baking soda
   2. causes porosity in gold
   3. removes surface oxides from gold castings
   4. removes investment from gold castings

201. The primary reason for using an individual porcelain jacket is
   1. the amount of overjet
   2. esthetics
   3. crushing strength
   4. edge strength

202. A problem with a porcelain jacket is that it
   1. is not color stable
   2. is very brittle
   3. has a very high compression strength
   4. is irritating to the gingiva

203. The main component of dental porcelain is
   1. clay
   2. silica
   3. feldspar
   4. borax

204. Gutta percha is used
   1. as a dental wax
   2. as a root canal filling material
   3. as an impression material for gold posts
   4. only in occlusal restorations of molars

205. Chromium–cobalt alloys are used most in dentistry as
   1. posts to reinforce teeth
   2. intercoronal restorations
   3. orthodontic appliances
   4. frameworks for partial dentures

206. Stainless steel is used most in dentistry
   1. to strengthen amalgam
   2. in orthodontic wires
   3. to construct clasps for partial dentures
   4. to replace internal gold restorations

Answers and Explanations

1. **3** A catalyst is a material that either initiates or speeds up a chemical reaction but that does not chemically change itself. An example of a catalyst is benzoyl peroxide, which initiates polymerization in the formation of acrylics.

2. **1** Metals are excellent thermal conductors, that is, they are capable of transmitting changes in temperature. Large metallic restorations must be thermally insulated; otherwise, they will produce thermal sensitivity indefinitely in the teeth in which they are placed.

3. **3** Elasticity is the ability of a material to return to its original shape after stress has been released.

4. **2** Dissimilar metal restorations have differences in electrical potential, setting up a battery effect or galvanic current in the mouth. This can cause pain or a metallic taste in the patient's mouth.

5. **1** Cohesion is the molecular attraction between similar molecules. An example of the property of cohesion is condensation of gold foil. Adhesion is the molecular attraction between different molecules. An example of adhesion is the retention of a denture due to attractive forces of molecules between the denture, saliva, and oral mucosa.

6. **1** Flow is the dimensional change of a material under a given load. Flow is an important property to consider in evaluating filling materials and waxes.

7. **3** Tensile strength is a measure of the stress required to fracture a material by pulling it apart. The opposite of tensile strength is compressive strength, the force necessary to fracture a material by pushing it together.

8. **2** The setting or curing of mercaptan impression materials is known as vulcanization.

9. **4** Exothermic reactions are those that release energy in the form of heat. All gypsum products, including plaster, acrylic, and zinc phosphate cement, undergo exothermic reaction on setting.

10. **4** Study models are used as references to show progress in orthodontic cases; to help in treatment planning in all phases of dentistry; to show arch shape and arch relationship; to help fabricate restorations such as temporary bridges and mouth guards; to show occlusal relationships; and to help construct custom trays for final impressions.

11. **3** Impressions are used to fabricate restorations outside the mouth. If a restoration is to fit a tooth (e.g., a crown) and oral tissues (e.g., a denture), the impression must be accurate.

12. **1** An impression is a detailed, accurate negative reproduction of oral tissues. A positive reproduction, or model, which is an exact duplication of the impressed tissues, is obtained by allowing a gypsum product to set in the impression.

13. **2** The classification of impression materials is made on the basis of the nature of the material when it is being removed from the mouth. Rigid materials are impression plaster, metallic oxide paste, and impression compound; elastic materials are reversible and irreversible hydrocolloids, mercaptan or polysulfide, silicone, and polyether impression material.

14. **1** Impression plaster is the oldest impression material.

15. **3** The materials used to take impressions of abutments for fixed bridgework are impression compound, silicone impression material, reversible hydrocolloid impression material, mercaptan or polysulfide impression material, and polyether impression material.

16. **1** Compound is a thermoplastic material. A material is thermoplastic if it becomes softer when heated and harder when cooled.

17. **2** To avoid burning the oral tissues, reversible hydrocolloid should be tempered in a water bath at 110°–115°F for 5–10 minutes before using.

18. **1** Reversible hydrocolloid can change from gel to sol and back to gel by heating and cooling. This material can be reused up to four times.

19. **4** Hydrocolloid impressions are very accurate impression materials that must be poured up immediately because of their fragility and susceptibility to dimensional change.

20. **4** Mercaptan and silicone impression materials use heavy and light body materials to make fine detailed impressions. The light body, or syringe material, has low viscosity and is placed around the prepared teeth. The heavy body or tray material has high viscosity and is placed in the impression tray.

21. **3** A perforated tray is used to carry irreversible hydrocolloid.

22. **3** Materials carried in a custom tray are metallic oxide paste, impression plaster, and rubber impression materials. The custom tray can be constructed of acrylic, shellac, or compound.

23. **2** Copper bands carry low fusing compound used to make impressions of crowns or inlays. The copper band is closely adapted to the prepared tooth before the compound is placed in it.

24. **3** When rubber impression materials are used, the tray is coated with a rubber adhesive. Failure to coat the tray can result in the impression separating from the tray.

25. **3** Reversible hydrocolloid is carried to the mouth in water-cooled trays. After the tray is properly positioned in the patient's mouth, cool water is circulated through the tray.

26. **2** The strength of hydrocolloid, both reversible and irreversible, is poor. A bulk of material is therefore necessary to give strength and body to the impression. The ideal amount of rubber impression materials is 2 mm between the surface of the tray and the tooth.

27. **2** Hysteresis is the temperature lag between the gelation temperature and the liquification temperature of the gel of reversible hydrocolloid.

28. **2** Syneresis is the exuding of water from hydrocolloid impressions. This loss of water causes shrinkage of the impression, which results in an inaccurate model.

29. **1** Imbibition, the uptake of water by hydrocolloid impressions, causes an expansion of the impression; the resulting model will be inaccurate.

30. **1** Undermixing irreversible hydrocolloid impression material will yield a grainy mix that will result in an impression—and subsequently a model—with poor detail. The proper consistency of the material should be smooth and creamy within the mixing time of 1 minute.

31. **3** The most effective way to adjust the setting time of hydrocolloid is to vary the water temperature. Warmer water will accelerate the set; cooler water will retard the set. Changing the water-powder ratio will also affect the setting time, but it is a poor method because it will weaken the material physically and can alter some of its properties.

32. **2** Irreversible hydrocolloid is loaded in a perforated tray with most of the material placed anteriorly. This reduces the amount of material flowing posteriorly and thereby decreases the possibility of the patient gagging.

33. **2** Reversible hydrocolloid sets from the water-cooled tray to the oral tissues. The opposite is true with irreversible hydrocolloid, which sets on the oral tissues first.

34. **4** Hydrocolloid impressions are removed from the mouth with one firm movement. Rocking or slow removal causes increased deformation of the impression.

35. **3** After removing a hydrocolloid impression from the mouth, the impression should be washed to remove debris. After washing the impression, excess water must be removed from the impression before pouring a gypsum model.

36. **1** Reversible hydrocolloid impressions immediately upon removal from the mouth are placed in a 2% potassium sulfate solution for several minutes. The purpose is to accelerate the setting of the stone model and to give it a hard smooth surface.

37. **2** The setting time for silicone impression material is shortened by using extra catalyst, increasing the temperature, and/or increasing the humidity.

38. **2** When extruding mercaptan base and accelerator, they are proportioned in equal lengths. The volume of the base is more than that of the accelerator.

39. **2** In order to mix mercaptan and silicone impression materials, the materials should be proportioned on a paper pad, and mixed with a flexible stainless steel spatula using a wiping and pressing motion. The resultant mix should be homogeneous and should be completed in about 1 minute.

40. **3** The setting time for a mercaptan impression material is dependent on the amount of accelerator, temperature, and humidity.

41. **3** The best time to clean excess silicone impression material from a patient's face is after the material has fully set. After the material has set, it can easily be peeled off the patient's face.

42. **3** Reversible hydrocolloid impression material lacks dimensional stability because its composition is mainly water. The material gains and loses water rapidly; therefore, the reversible hydrocolloid impression should be poured immediately after removal from the patient's mouth. Rubber impression materials are more dimensionally stable as well as stronger than reversible hydrocolloids. They can also be electroplated to fabricate metal dies.

43. **1** Impression compound is used to prepare custom-made trays for edentulous mouths, to make impressions of crown preparations, to border mold custom trays, and to check occlusion for mounting casts.

44. **3** Low fusing stick compound is used to muscle trim edentulous impressions and to take impressions of teeth for crowns or inlays.

45. **4** The disadvantages of using compound for im-

pressions of teeth prepared for crowns are that it will not spring undercuts, has low thermal conductivity, and can burn the operator, assistant or patient.

46. **1** Metallic oxide impression material is used to make final impressions of edentulous areas and bite registrations.

47. **2** Metallic oxide paste is mixed on an oil-resistant paper pad, to avoid the cleaning problem of using a glass slab.

48. **2** The setting time of metallic oxide paste is decreased by adding a few drops of water and increasing the temperature, the mixing time, and/or amount of accelerator.

49. **4** Impression plaster, also known as quick-setting plaster, is used to make final impressions of edentulous mouths, to make bite registrations, and to transfer registrations so that dies of crown preparations can be properly positioned.

50. **1** Metallic oxide paste is the most difficult material listed to remove from a patient's face. Oil of orange is used for this purpose.

51. **4** Dies of crown preparations can be made of amalgam, electroplated copper, electroplated silver, or improved stone.

52. **4** Gypsum products include plaster, dental stone, improved stone, and investment.

53. **3** The calcination of gypsum is the process of heating gypsum to drive off water. This process determines the physical characteristics of the resulting powder, and subsequently the physical characteristics of gypsum products.

54. **2** When mixing gypsum products, the powder should be added to the water in the mixing bowl. This technique minimizes the amount of air trapped in the mix.

55. **2** To accelerate the setting time of gypsum products, lower the water–powder ratio, increase spatulation, add an accelerator, and use warm water or terra alba.

56. **3** To prevent bubbles from forming in the final model, a mechanical vibrator and/or vacuum mixer is used. The mix is pressed against the side of the mixing bowl; it is then firmly trapped against the laboratory bench. The debubblizer is placed in the impression to reduce the surface tension.

57. **4** Hygroscopic setting expansion occurs in all gypsum products immersed in water after the initial set. This increase in volume of the gypsum product will decrease the strength of the model. Hygroscopic expansion is part of the controlled expansion of dental investment.

58. **2** When pouring a model from a full upper im-

pression continuously add stone to the same place on the palate. This will allow the stone to slowly flow into the areas where the teeth have been impressed and will move the air out of these areas.

59. **2** When pouring a model from a full lower impression, continuously add stone to either heel of the impression. The rationale for this process is the same as that for question 58.

60. **1** Impressions are boxed to confine the model material and thereby decrease the time necessary to finish the base of the model.

61. **3** Dowel pins are used in the construction of individual dies. They permit the accurate replacement of individual dies back in a model. The pin acts as a male attachment and is inserted in a female attachment, which is produced when the model is poured.

62. **2** Plaster is used to construct study models, to attach models to articulators, and for miscellaneous uses where strength is not an important factor.

63. **2** All gypsum products expand on setting. Plaster expands more than stone, which expands more than improved stone. Increased expansion may be caused by increased spatulation, increased water–powder ratio, hygroscopic expansion, and/or the addition of certain chemicals.

64. **2** The more porous, rough, and irregular the gypsum particles, the higher the water–powder ratio needed to mix the material. With plaster, it is 1–2; with stone, 3–10.

65. **3** Dental stone is used to construct models used in constructing dentures, bite plates, and bite guards. It is also used to make orthodontic study cases.

66. **3** Increasing the water–powder ratio of any gypsum product will result in a porous, and therefore weaker, model.

67. **2** The working time, also known as the initial setting time, begins with the mixing of the gypsum powder and water. It ends when the stone no longer flows, due to the increasing crystallization and viscosity. The final setting time ends when the model can be separated from the impression.

68. **1** Improved stone is the densest gypsum product and is used to make dies from which crowns, inlays, and onlays can be constructed.

69. **4** Dental investment is used to prepare molds for cast restorations, such as crowns, inlays, onlays, and partial frameworks, and to hold fixed bridge units in place when soldering.

70. **4** It is desirable to have a controlled expansion of the investment mold to compensate for the shrinkage of gold and wax. The controlled expan-

sion of the investment is caused by setting expansion, which includes hygroscopic setting and thermal expansion. The asbestos liner of the investment ring permits expansion of the material.

71. **1** The function of a sprue is to form an opening for the entrance of the molten metal into the mold left by the wax pattern.

72. **1** Cracking of an investment mold can result from heating, cooling, and reheating the mold, too-rapid heating, and/or heating the investment before it has had time to set.

73. **3** To remove a stone model from a metallic oxide paste impression or a compound impression, soak the model and impression in warm water for several minutes.

74. **4** Waxes are used as patterns for cast restorations, bite registrations, and boxing impressions among a multitude of other impressions for partial dentures.

75. **4** Waxes can be classified as pattern waxes, including inlay wax, base plate wax, and casting wax; processing waxes, including boxing wax, sticky wax, and utility wax; and impression waxes, including corrective wax and bite wax.

76. **2** Physical characteristics of waxes can be altered by varying the components. An example is the addition of carnauba wax to inlay wax to make it harder.

77. **2** Sticky wax is not used intraorally because its high melting range will severely burn any oral tissue it contacts.

78. **2** Inlay wax is primarily used to make wax patterns for inlays, individual crowns, and fixed bridges.

79. **2** The main ingredient of inlay wax is paraffin wax (40–60%). Other constituents are added to improve the physical characteristics of the wax.

80. **4** At mouth temperature, inlay wax should have no flow, or the pattern will distort before it is removed from the mouth. The flow of inlay wax should take place at temperatures slightly above mouth temperature. If the flow temperature is much higher than the mouth temperature, oral tissues might be injured when using the wax intraorally.

81. **2** To avoid distortion of a wax pattern, it should be invested as soon as possible, manipulated as little as possible, and protected from temperature changes.

82. **2** The best way to heat inlay wax is to hold it above a flame and manipulate it until it is uniformly soft. Some components will be lost or destroyed if the wax is overheated in a flame or softened in warm water.

83. **2** When carving inlay wax in the mouth, the use of warm instruments will avoid chipping the wax.

84. **1** It is best to invest the wax pattern as soon as possible. Stresses introduced into the pattern during fabrication are released after the pattern is removed from the tooth or die. The relaxation of these stresses causes the wax pattern to distort. The longer the wax pattern is stored before investment the greater the possibility of distortion of the pattern.

85. **3** If it is necessary to store a wax pattern, it should be refrigerated to decrease possible distortion.

86. **3** A wax pattern must be an accurate reproduction of tooth structure, well adapted and properly carved. The pattern can be made on the tooth itself or on a die.

87. **3** Some important properties of inlay wax are complete burnout, close adaptation to the prepared tooth, minimal distortion, carvability, maintenance of detail, and flow just above mouth temperature.

88. **4** Baseplate wax is used to construct bite rims to record occlusal relationships, to set up artificial teeth, and to record bite registrations.

89. **2** Care must be taken when attaching wax rims to a shellac tray to avoid warping the tray. Shellac trays, as waxes, are thermoplastic materials and are easily altered by heat.

90. **1** Strips of boxing wax are used to form a rim around an impression. This will contain the poured gypsum material and facilitate finishing the model.

91. **3** Casting wax is used as a pattern for the metal framework (gold or chrome cobalt) of partial dentures.

92. **4** Sticky wax is used to hold metallic, acrylic, or gypsum parts in a fixed position temporarily. This wax is sticky only when melted: it is brittle when hard.

93. **3** Utility wax is a soft tacky wax that is often placed around the periphery of perforated metal trays to improve the contour of the tray.

94. **1** Impression waxes are used to record bite registrations and as impression material for non-undercut areas.

95. **3** Some uses of dental cements are as temporary restoration, thermal insulator, luting material, sedative base, root canal sealer, and pulp capping material.

96. **3** Zinc phosphate cement remains acidic several hours after it is set and irritating to the pulp. To avoid its irritating effects cavity varnish is often used to seal the dental tubules before this cement is applied.

97. **2** Zinc phosphate cement has the highest crushing strength of dental cements. Zinc phosphate has a crushing strength of 14,500 psi, zinc oxide-eugenol 200 psi, and calcium hydroxide 150 psi.

98. **4** Dew point is the temperature at which water vapor condenses. If a glass slab is cooled below the dew point, moisture will collect on the slab and will speed the setting time of zinc phosphate and silicate cements.

99. **3** Zinc oxide-eugenol cement sedates pulpal tissue and is therefore used when cavity preparations are near the pulp. Zinc oxide-eugenol cement is also used as a temporary restoration, as a luting medium for cast gold restorations, as a root canal sealant, as a pulp capping agent, and as a periodontal dressing.

100. **1** Rosin is added to zinc oxide-eugenol cement to increase strength and adhesion.

101. **3** A paper pad is used to mix zinc oxide-eugenol cement because of the time consuming cleanup necessary if a glass slab is used.

102. **3** Zinc acetate is added to zinc oxide-eugenol cement to accelerate the setting time.

103. **2** The setting time of zinc oxide-eugenol is accelerated by increasing the powder-liquid ratio or increasing temperature, water, and/or zinc acetate.

104. **3** The desired consistency of zinc oxide-eugenol cement when used as a temporary restoration is puttylike. This can be easily manipulated and can stand in a covered container for many hours without setting.

105. **4** ZOE is a sedative and is easily manipulated. In addition, setting time can be controlled. Its compressive strength is low, and it is highly soluble in oral fluids.

106. **4** Zinc phosphate cement can be used as a thermal insulator under metallic restorations, as a luting agent for cast gold restorations and orthodontic bands, as a temporary filling material, and to rebuild cavity and crown preparations to an ideal form.

107. **1** Excess zinc phosphate cement powder left on the mixing pad should be discarded because it may be contaminated. Placing contaminated powder with uncontaminated powder will contaminate all the powder and can change the cement's characteristics.

108. **3** The liquid portion of zinc phosphate cement consists of phosphoric acid, water, and dissolved salts. The acid-water ratio is critical and alterations will affect the setting time of the cement. Evaporation causes a lengthened (slower) setting time, and the addition of water will cause a shorter (faster) setting time.

109. **2** Increasing the powder-liquid ratio will decrease the solubility of zinc phosphate cement. Decreased solubility is desirable and therefore as much powder as possible should be mixed into the available liquid until the optimum consistency is reached.

110. **3** Advantages of zinc phosphate cement include its high compressive strength, ease of manipulation, and ability to control the setting time by changing the powder to liquid ratio. ZOP is acidic and consequently irritating to the pulp.

111. **1** The setting time of zinc phosphate cement can be retarded by using a cool glass slab, decreasing initial acidity by mixing a very small portion of powder with the liquid, adding small portions of the powder to the liquid, mixing cement over a large area to dissipate the heat, and lengthening spatulation time.

112. **2** Zinc polyacrylate cement, also known as carboxylate or polycarboxylate cement, can be used for the same purposes as the zinc phosphate cement. Advantages of zinc polyacrylate cement are that it is less irritating to pulpal tissues than is zinc phosphate cement and that it has adhesive properties.

113. **2** The main component of zinc polyacrylate cement powder is zinc oxide. The liquid is a 40% solution of polyacrylic acid in water.

114. **3** The working time for zinc polyacrylate cement is 3 minutes. This short working time is a disadvantage when cementing multiple units of bridgework.

115. **2** An advantage of using a silicate restoration is its anticariogenic effect resulting from fluoride in the powder. There is usually a lack of recurrent decay around the restored area.

116. **1** Silicate cements have the following disadvantages: they are acidic, which irritates pulpal tissues; are soluble in oral fluids; porous and therefore discolor easily; shrink on setting; lack crushing and edge strength; and are subject to dehydration, which will lead to disintegration. The life expectancy of a silicate cement restoration is 2-4 years.

117. **2** Silicate cement is acidic and therefore acts as an irritant on the pulp. The liquid is phosphoric acid (42%), the same type of liquid used in zinc phosphate cement (40%). To prevent pulpal injury, a base such as varnish, zinc oxide-eugenol, or calcium hydroxide should be used under silicate restorations.

118. **2** Shade selection for silicate cements should be accomplished before the rubber dam is placed. The dam creates an artificial background and keeps the teeth dry, making them appear lighter.

119. **2** Factors that accelerate the setting time of silicate cement are adding some water (this factor

works in the same way as when utilizing zinc phosphate cement); increasing the powder–liquid ratio (this factor will also result in a stronger, less soluble cement); spatulating for too short a period of time; and adding the powder quickly.

120. **1** Silicate cement is spatulated to wet each powder particle as completely and quickly as possible within a small area.

121. **1** The mixing time for silicate cement is about one minute. The material should be folded into the liquid as quickly as possible.

122. **3** To prevent irritating chemicals from reaching the pulp the dentinal tubules are sealed with varnish. Varnish is placed under zinc phosphate cements, amalgam restorations, silicate cements, and other materials that would have deleterious effects on the pulp. Varnish is not placed under materials which have a beneficial effect on the pulp, such as zinc oxide–eugenol and calcium hydroxide.

123. **4** Calcium hydroxide is a base placed beneath deep restorations to promote irritation of the pulp and thereby promote the formation of secondary dentin. Calcium hydroxide is also used beneath silicate restorations to neutralize the acidity of silicate cement.

124. **3** Calcium hydroxide is easy to manipulate, stimulates the production of secondary dentin, and protects the pulp from irritation from caustic filling materials. It is, however, soluble in oral fluids and does not have a high compressive strength when compared with other restorative materials.

125. **2** The material used in approximately 75% of all restorations is amalgam.

126. **4** Gold foil is the least frequently used restoration material because of esthetics, difficulty in manipulation, and cost.

127. **4** When viewing radiographs of teeth with radiolucent filling materials, it is difficult to distinguish between the restoration and recurrent decay. If the materials used are radiopaque, they are easily distinguished from decay.

128. **4** Pins are used in restorative dentistry to increase retention of filling materials. Pins are placed in the dentin and are retained by threads, cement, or friction.

129. **3** Composite is about one-tenth as soluble as acrylic. Silicate is more soluble than either composite or acrylic.

130. **3** Composites have compressive strength of 30,000 psi, which approaches the compressive strength of amalgam (45,000 psi).

131. **3** Composite restorations have a rougher finish than that of most other restorative materials. The organic matrix that holds the very hard inorganic material is worn away, and a rough finish results.

132. **4** Pure gold is used in dentistry to fabricate gold restorations directly in the mouth. Gold alloys are used for cast gold restorations.

133. **2** Noble metals are metals that will not tarnish or corrode in the oral cavity. Gold and platinum are examples of such metals.

134. **3** Cast gold has the least amount of flow. Flow is the deformation of a material under a constant load.

135. **3** The filling material of choice for a small cavity preparation on the mesial surface of the maxillary right central is composite. This material offers both conservation of tooth structure and esthetics.

136. **1** The filling material of choice for restoring a conservative distal occlusal cavity preparation on a maxillary right second premolar is amalgam. This material offers strength and reasonable cost; esthetics is usually not a factor in this area.

137. **4** The restoration of choice for an extensive fracture of central or lateral incisors is usually a porcelain jacket. This restoration offers the finest esthetic result possible.

138. **2** The restoration of choice for a molar that is missing a cusp, of the choices offered, is a gold onlay. This restoration offers the strength necessary to replace a large stress-bearing area.

139. **4** The most esthetic material for anterior bridgework is porcelain fused to metal.

140. **4** Some uses of acrylic resins are anterior restorations, bases of full or partial dentures, temporary crowns and bridges, facings on crowns, prosthetic plastic teeth, bite plates, retainers, custom-made trays, and splints.

141. **4** Advantages of acrylic restorations are that they are insoluble in oral fluids, can be finished in one sitting, are easy to repair and add to the existing restoration, act as a thermal insulator, and are easily manipulated.

142. **3** Disadvantages of acrylic restorations are that they readily wear, flow under stress, irritate pulp tissue, have a high coefficient of expansion, and shrink during setting.

143. **4** Polymerization is the formation of large molecules (polymers) from smaller units. When acrylics polymerize, they give off heat and shrink.

144. **1** Percolation is the movement of fluids between the tooth and acrylic restoration. It is caused by opening and closing of the margin because of the difference in the coefficient of expansion of the acrylic and tooth.

145. **1** The main component of the acrylic monomer

is methyl methacrylate. The powder is mostly composed of polymethyl methacrylate.

146. **3** Acrylic restorations, as well as silicate, amalgam, and so on, are physically retained in cavity preparations; therefore, mechanical retention must be built into the cavity preparation.

147. **4** Acrylic may be added to a cavity preparation by small increments, brush or Nealon technique, or by bulk amounts. In the brush technique, two dappen dishes are used, one with monomer and one with polymer. A sable hair brush is wet in the monomer and then placed in the polymer to pick up some powder. The wet powder is then placed in the cavity preparation and allowed to polymerize. This process is repeated until the preparation is overfilled. In the bulk technique, monomer and polymer are mixed on a glass slab or in a dappen dish to a puttylike consistency. The acrylic is then placed in the cavity preparation in bulk until the preparation is overfilled.

148. **4** Denture base acrylic needs heat for polymerization. Acrylics used for anterior restorations, temporary crowns, and bridges are self-curing and polymerize by the chemical reaction of their components.

149. **3** Placing self-curing acrylics in warm water will speed up polymerization by driving off excess monomer.

150. **2** When constructing a custom acrylic tray excess acrylic is best removed with a knife after adapting the acrylic to the model. The excess can be then used to make a handle for the tray.

151. **1** Polishing acrylic on a lathe requires the use of low speed, copious amounts of water with the pumice, and continuous movement of the acrylic. These factors will prevent the buildup of heat and deterioration of the acrylic.

152. **2** Cleaning dentures in excessively hot water will cause the denture base to warp and distort because processing stresses will be released.

153. **1** If dentures are left to dry, they contract. This process is reversible and if the denture is placed in water it will return to its original dimension.

154. **1** To repair a fractured temporary bridge, the bridge is seated in the patient's mouth and dried, small amounts of acrylic are added to the fractured ends of the bridge, the acrylic is allowed to set, and the bridge is then removed from the patient's mouth and polished.

155. **3** To repair a fractured denture, the denture is removed from the patient's mouth; the pieces of the denture are luted together with sticky wax on the polished surface; plaster is poured into the denture to obtain a model of the patient's mouth; after the plaster has set the sticky wax is removed from the fractured ends; the pieces of the denture are placed back on the model; denture repair

acrylic is added to the fractured ends; the acrylic is allowed to set; and the repaired denture is polished and returned to the patient.

156. **1** To replace an intact tooth in a denture, the area on the denture where the tooth has popped out is roughened; denture repair acrylic is placed on the area; the tooth is reset; and the acrylic is allowed to set.

157. **4** Amalgam is the most frequently used dental restorative material because of its ease of insertion and ability to resist tarnish and corrosion, especially when polished.

158. **4** The main component of composite (sometimes known as filled acrylic resin) is the inorganic filler. The inorganic filler consists of glass particles, fused silica, and quartz crystals. The organic portion of composites is composed of polymers.

159. **1** A plastic spatula is used to mix composites. The filler is so abrasive that abraded metal particles will be incorporated into the material if a metal spatula is used.

160. **2** Zinc oxide–eugenol bases will interfere with polymerization of acrylic and composite restorations; therefore, they should not be used as bases under these materials.

161. **1** Preventive sealant resins are usually placed in pits and fissures on the occlusal surface of the tooth. Pits and fissures are inaccessible for cleaning; therefore, they are susceptible to decay. The use of sealants has shown a reduction of decay in these areas.

162. **3** Fifty percent solution of phosphoric acid is used to etch enamel. Enamel treated in this manner has increased mechanical retention for resin materials.

163. **2** Amalgam can be used to make dies for gold and porcelain restorations, to rebuild badly broken down vital teeth so cast restorations can be placed on them, and for posterior restorations.

164. **1** The components of amalgam alloy are, as stated by the ADA, silver (65% minimum), tin (29% maximum), copper (6% maximum), and zinc (2% maximum).

165. **3** The shape of amalgam alloy particles is spherical or random filings. Spherical alloy contains less mercury in the final restoration than the filings and is therefore stronger.

166. **4** Zinc causes water to break down into hydrogen and oxygen gases. This will result in delayed expansion if moisture is present while the amalgam is setting and will weaken the restoration.

167. **2** Surface contaminants are removed from mercury by wiping a cotton ball over the surface or by filtering the mercury through a chamois filter.

168. **1** The toxic effects of mercury can occur through the skin or by inhalation of mercury vapors. Prevention by limited and careful handling and quick efficient cleanup if any spills occur is the best way to avoid mercury-related health problems.

169. **3** The best way to control the amount of mercury in the final restoration is by initially dispensing the desired amount. If too much mercury is dispensed initially, some can be removed by the use of a squeeze cloth and proper condensation, but the final restoration will probably still contain too much mercury.

170. **3** Premeasured amalgam capsules ensure correct proportioning of mercury and alloy and excellent results. The disadvantage of using this technique is that the cost of preproportioned capsules is considerably more than the office-addition techniques.

171. **2** Insufficient mercury will not wet each alloy particle and will result in an amalgam that is weak, granular, and crumbly and that might have some voids.

172. **3** The crushing or compressive strength of amalgam is at least 45,000 psi when it is fully hardened (about 24 hours).

173. **3** The most common cause of amalgam failure is incorrect cavity preparation. The next most common cause of amalgam failure is incorrect manipulation of the alloy.

174. **1** Amalgamation is the combining, chemically and physically, of mercury with amalgam alloy.

175. **3** The purpose of trituration is to remove the protective oxide coat of the amalgam alloy particles. This will allow mercury to react with the individual particles so that they can bond together.

176. **1** Undertrituration of amalgam results in expansion of the restoration, reduction in strength of the final restoration, rapid setting of the restoration, and excessive mercury in the final restoration. Overtrituration causes the alloy particles to be crushed; this increases the mercury content of the restoration and results in a weakened restoration. Overtrituration also produces a soft, soupy material that is difficult to manipulate.

177. **3** Mulling is the gathering together and homogenizing of the amalgam mix. It is accomplished by placing the fresh amalgam mix in a squeeze cloth or rubber dam and rubbing the mass between the thumb and forefinger.

178. **4** Squeeze cloths are used to remove excess mercury after trituration. The excess mercury should be carefully placed in a receptacle to prevent mercury contamination in the operatory.

179. **2** The working time of amalgam is 3–4 minutes. After this time, a new mix should be used.

180. **1** As a result of condensation, amalgam is placed in intimate contact with the cavity preparation and a dense restoration is achieved by bringing excess mercury to the surface of the restoration. This excess is then removed when carving.

181. **2** If amalgam is carved after it has begun to set it will chip, flake, and possibly fracture.

182. **1** Excess mercury in the final amalgam restoration results in fracture due to decreased crushing strength, pitting due to vaporization of excess mercury when polishing, and excessive expansion.

183. **3** The most frequent patient complaint after an amalgam restoration is placed is cold sensitivity in the newly restored tooth. Cement bases, such as zinc phosphate, at least 0.5 mm thick, act as a thermal insulator when placed under amalgam restorations.

184. **1** Tarnishing, a surface phenomenon, and corrosion, a chemical deterioration of amalgam restorations, can be substantially reduced by polishing the restorations. Polishing should not take place until 24 hours after placement.

185. **4** Pumice, emery disks, quartz disks, garnet disks, and tin oxide are included in the materials used to polish amalgam restorations intraorally. Rouge and tripoli are polishing agents but cannot be used in the mouth.

186. **3** Overheating the amalgam restoration when polishing may result in damaging the pulp or vaporization of surface mercury.

187. **3** An advantage of using a gold restoration, rather than an amalgam restoration, is the greater edge strength of cast gold. This implies greater occlusal stresses can be sustained by gold restorations.

188. **4** A disadvantage of using gold restorations is the high cost in comparison to using other filling materials.

189. **3** The forms of gold that can be worked directly intraorally are gold foil (extremely thin gold sheets), mat gold (sheets of compressed gold powder), and gold powder (powder wrapped in gold foil).

190. **3** Casting gold alloy usually contains gold, copper, palladium, silver, and zinc. Tin in a component of amalgam and stainless steel is sometimes used for temporary crowns.

191. **2** Annealing gold foil removes gaseous impurities from the surface of the gold and makes the gold cohesive. It is accomplished by heating the gold. Underannealing will not remove all the impurities and will result in gold that is not as cohesive as it should be. Overannealing will make the gold brittle and unworkable.

192. **2** Compacting of gold foil is accomplished by

the use of condensers. Each piece of gold foil is welded to the existing gold to form a solid piece of gold. The resulting restoration is as hard as a cast gold inlay. There are three types of condensers: the automatic plugger (spring activated), the pneumatic plugger (motor driven), and the hand plugger (condenser and mallet).

193. **1** Synthetic resins are used to reline dentures and to fabricate custom trays and artificial teeth. The material is not used for sedative fillings because of its caustic properties, and it is inappropriate for fabricating inlays because it is not an acceptable permanent restorative material.

194. **1** Burnishing the gold foil restoration hardens the gold and better adapts the margins of the restoration to the tooth. Burnished gold becomes noncohesive, and the surface must be roughened before additional gold can be added.

195. **3** Pure gold, 100% gold, is 24 carat. Twelve-carat gold is half pure gold, or 50% gold. Casting gold is 75-85% gold.

196. **4** Casting gold is used for cast restorations (e.g., crowns, inlays, posts) wrought wire clasps (for partial dentures), and solder (to join metals together by fusion).

197. **1** The hardness of gold depends on the amount and type of metal with which it is alloyed. The hardness of gold is ranked as follows:

Type	Uses
I (soft)	Class I and V inlays
II (medium)	Inlays
III (hard)	Crowns
IV (extra hard)	Partial denture frameworks

198. **3** Gold solder must have a lower fusion (melting) temperature than that of the parts it is connecting or the parts will melt before the solder can join them.

199. **1** Flux is used when heating the gold for casting. It removes oxides that form on the gold.

200. **3** Pickling removes surface oxides from gold castings. This process is accomplished by placing the gold casting in a strong acid solution.

201. **2** The primary reason for a porcelain jacket restoration is the excellent esthetic result. Other favorable features of porcelain restorations are that they do not irritate tissues and resist wear.

202. **2** Porcelain jacket restorations are very brittle and will not deform, but will fracture.

203. **3** The main component of dental porcelain is feldspar. Silica, also known as quartz, is the second most abundant component of porcelain.

204. **2** Gutta percha is used to seal root canals, as a temporary filling material, and to test teeth for vitality by their sensitivity to heat.

205. **4** Chromium–cobalt alloys are used as frameworks for partial dentures, dental implants, and some fixed bridgework.

206. **2** Stainless steel is used for orthodontic wires and bands and preformed crowns.

Bibliography

Benson, H.J. and Kipp, K.E. *Dental Science Laboratory Guide,* 4th ed. Dubuque, Iowa: William Brown Co., 1968.

Buonocore, M.G. *The Use Of Adhesives in Dentistry,* Springfield, Ill.: Charles C Thomas Publishers, 1975.

Craig, R.G.; O'Brien, W.J.; and Powers, J.M. *Dental Materials: Properties and Manipulation,* 2nd ed. St. Louis: The C. V. Mosby Co., 1979.

Gilmore, H.W., et al. *Operative Dentistry,* 4th ed. St. Louis: The C. V. Mosby Co., 1982.

Philips, R.N. *Elements of Dental Materials for Dental Hygienists and Assistants,* 8th ed. Philadelphia: W. B. Saunders Co., 1982.

Skinner, E.W. and Phillips, R.W. *Skinners Science of Dental Materials,* Philadelphia: W. B. Saunders Co., 1981.

Williams, D.F. and Cunningham, J. *Materials in Clinical Dentistry,* New York: Oxford University Press, 1979.

5

Chairside Assisting

Course Synopsis

Principles of Dental Auxiliary Utilization

As the demand for dentistry has increased, it has been recognized that dentists must increase their effectiveness and efficiency without increasing psychological and physical stresses. As a result, dentists have begun to apply industrial principles of work and time mangement, including delegation of duties and the increased use of four-handed dentistry. Research has shown that a dentist using one full-time auxiliary can increase production by 33%, and by using two trained auxiliaries, he or she can increase productivity by 90%.

The increased demand for dentistry is a natural outgrowth of increased public awareness, higher standards of living, increased third-party payments, and a change in attitude that access to quality health care is a right, not a privilege. An attempt to achieve equilibrium and to decrease the need for dental care has caused an increase in water fluoridation, research directed toward anticariogenic agents, and an increase in the number of dentists. The four-handed techniques discussed in this chapter have helped decrease fatigue and increase productivity in dentistry.

Work Simplification

The concepts and principles behind work simplification were borrowed from industry and applied to the dental office. Objectives were to increase worker production and decrease stress and fatigue. One of the most important concepts offered by industry was increased production through elimination or reduction of delaying factors. Analysis of physical steps through time and motion studies generated work simplification principles. These principles are as follows:

Elimination

All tasks that can be eliminated produce the highest return (100%). For example, it has been demonstrated that every time a patient rinses his or her mouth, approximately 18% of useful chair time is wasted. If this process can be eliminated through the use of high-speed suction, approximately 11 minutes per working hour can be gained.

Combination

Tasks or instruments that cannot be eliminated can be combined. Production increases range from 50% to 75%. For example, double-ended instruments decrease the number of hand transfers by as much as 50%.

Rearrangement

If elimination and combination are not inappropriate, tasks and instruments can be rearranged to facilitate utility. For example, if the three-way syringe is used more often than any other instrument, it should be located in the most accessible position.

Simplification

When any of the previous three principles are not applicable, tasks should be simplified. An example of simplification is the use of disposable prepared materials.

Standardization

If elimination, combination, rearrangement, or simplification cannot be applied, procedures should be standardized to reduce the number of variables. For instance, each time an amalgam procedure is done, it should be done in the same manner, with the same instruments.

Minimization of Motion

Stress and fatigue are decreased if movement is minimized and controlled. Industrial time and motion studies have identified five classifications of motion.

Class I motions involve only the fingers, for example, transfer of most instruments. Class II motions involve the fingers and wrists, for example, transfer of a double-handled instrument, such as scissors. Class III motions involve the use of fingers, wrist, and elbows, for instance, placement of the rubber dam clamp.

The next two classifications of motion are the most physically taxing and should be eliminated if possible. Class IV motions involve the entire arm and shoulder, such as when reaching to adjust an overhead light. Class V motions involve the entire arm and torso, as in turning to reach for an instrument. Class V motions are most fatiguing because they involve refocusing the eyes (accommodation) to different light intensities and distances.

Positioning

A basic principle of four-handed, sit-down dentistry is proper positioning of the operator, assistant, patient, and equipment. The benefits of proper positioning include minimizing physical stress of the members of the operating team while maximizing visibility and patient comfort (Fig. 22).

To help visualize the positioning relationship in the operatory, the face of the clock can be superimposed on the properly positioned dental team. The patient's mouth is located at the center of the clock, and 12 o'clock is located above the patient's head.

The following zones of activity can be identified for a right-handed operator (a mirror image is used for a left-handed operator). The operator's zone is 8 to 12 o'clock, depending on the quadrant and tooth surface being treated. The assistant's position remains constant at 3 o'clock regardless of the quadrant and tooth surface being treated; the static zone is located from 12 to 2 o'clock (this zone contains equipment that is infrequently used, such as the nitrous oxide unit and electrosurgery equipment. The transfer zone is at 5 to 8 o'clock, in which instrument transfers are made either at the patient's mouth or below the chin.

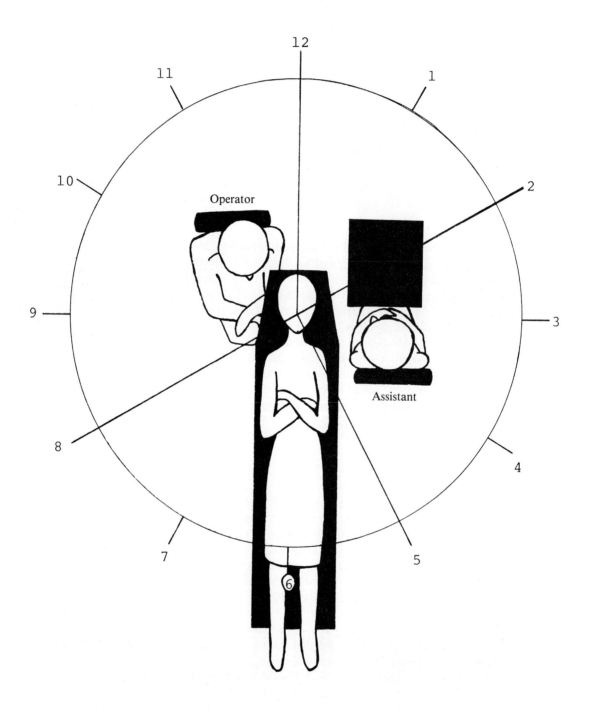

Fig. 22. Zones of operating activity. 12 to 2 o'clock, static zone; 2 to 4 o'clock, assisting zone; 4 to 8 o'clock, transfer zone; 8 to 12 o'clock, operating zone.

Seating the Patient

The manner in which an assistant introduces a patient to an operatory affects the entire procedure. The assistant should lead the patient to the operatory and, with hand motions, indicate where the patient should sit. The patient's chair should be preset at a comfortable height for a sitting position, and the chair arm should be raised, if possible. After the patient is seated the patient's napkin is secured. The assistant should then slowly tilt the chair backward until the patient's calves are parallel to the floor. If the procedure to be accomplished is located in the maxilla, the patient should be supine. If the area being treated is in the mandible, the patient's back should be between a 25- and 45-degree angle to the floor. The patient's head should be as close to the top of the dental chair and the operator as possible. The light is positioned approximately 30 inches from the operating field, and the chair is elevated to a comfortable working height for the operator. Patients who might have difficulty in a supine position include the elderly and those with respiratory or circulatory problems, or both. These patients should be treated in an upright position.

After a procedure is completed, the assistant should slowly return the patient to an upright position. The patient should remain seated until equilibrium is regained; the assistant can then dismiss the patient.

Assistant's Position

The assistant should be seated in a position as close to the patient's head as possible with eye level 6 inches above that of the operator. The thigh nearest the patient should be resting against the patient's chair; the wraparound arm of the stool, if there is one, should be placed beneath the rib cage. The assistant's feet rest on the base of the stool. Once the patient is positioned, the assistant should remain with him or her until the operator enters.

Operator Position

The operator should be positioned such that his or her back touches the back rest, thighs are parallel to the floor, and feet are resting flat on the floor.

Transferring of Instruments

It is the dental assistant's responsibility to prepare and position all instruments used for a procedure. The instruments should be placed in a manner that affords accessibility and efficiency. Once placed in the appropriate position, the instruments are transferred between the assistant and the operator in a prescribed manner.

The assistant transfers instruments from the left hand (for a right-handed operator) to the operator's right hand. During transfers, it is necessary for the operator only to use Class I motions. The stages of instrument transfer are as follows:

Signal stage. The operator makes a Class I motion, moving the instrument out of the working field while maintaining the finger rest.

Pretransfer stage. The assistant positions the instrument to be transferred parallel to the working instrument.

Midtransfer stage. The assistant holds the instrument to be transferred between the index finger and thumb and removes the instrument previously used from the operator's hand with the fourth finger of his or her left hand.

Transfer stage. The instrument to be transferred is placed in the proper position into the operator's hand.

Transfer completion stage. The assistant releases the transferred instrument, and the operator returns to the operating field. If the instrument is to be reused, it is repositioned into the pretransfer stage.

The transfer process is slightly altered when transferring a syringe or any double-handled instrument. The stages remain the same, but the operator must make a Class II motion in releasing the finger rest. With the palm facing up, the operator positions his or her hand under the patient's chin to receive the new instrument. The other steps in the transfer process remain the same.

To properly complete a transfer, both the operator and assistant must know the appropriate way in which to grasp instruments. Different instruments are held in different grasps. For example, explorers and spoon excavators are held in a pen grasp, while chisels and hatchets are held in a palm–thumb grasp. Double-handled instruments such as forceps and syringes are held in palm grasps.

Efficient transfer is an integral part in increasing productivity by using the principles of motion economy and work simplification.

Suction and Retraction

In addition to proper patient positioning and efficient instrument transfers, high-speed evacuation and proper retraction are important in increasing accessibility and decreasing stress.

The primary function of high-speed suction is to provide a working field free of saliva and debris and eliminate the use of the cuspidor during a procedure. A properly positioned suction tip will decrease the size of the area of bacterial aerosol created close to the high-speed handpiece. Concurrently, the tip can be used for retraction purposes, permitting increased visibility and protection of the patient's tissues.

A number of principles are used for suction tip placement. The assistant holds the tip in his or her right hand (when working with a right-handed operator) with a reverse palm or thumb to nose grasp. When working on a posterior tooth the tip should be positioned as close to the tooth as possible without injuring the soft tissue. The beveled tip should be held parallel with either the buccal or lingual surface of the tooth, and the edge of the tip should be even with the occlusal surface of the tooth. While working on an anterior tooth, the tip should be placed opposite the surface of the tooth being treated, with the beveled tip parallel to and bisecting the incisal edges of the teeth. The tip should not be placed on the back of the tongue or soft palate to avoid gagging. If it is placed too close to the water coolant of the handpiece, the water will be evacuated before it reaches the tooth. The tip should be positioned before the operator places the handpiece and mirror.

A mirror or suction tip, or both, can be used to retract the cheeks and tongue. The operator using the mirror and the assistant using the suction tip retract the tissue closest to each. For example, a right-handed operator working in the lower right quadrant retracts the cheek and the assistant retracts the tongue.

Tray Setups

The use of preprepared tray setups also decreases delaying factors. This system involves having trays easily accessible and containing instruments and materials needed to perform given procedures in optimum positions.

Benefits accrued by use of these tray setups include adaptability to any procedure, ease of storage, minimization of interruptions to retrieve a forgotten instrument or material, and decrease in time needed for preparing and cleaning operatories.

Trays are either plastic or metal. Plastic trays are lighter in weight and less expensive than metal trays. Moreover, they come in different colors and can be color coded for different procedures. Disadvantages of using plastic trays include inability to be sterilized and decreased durability. Because metal trays can be autoclaved, they can be opened at the time of use to insure asepsis. Disadvantages of their use include their cost and inability to be sterilized in small autoclaves.

The instruments and materials that are routinely placed on the trays are those that are used 90% of the time. This determination can be made by recording on an index card the instruments and materials used for the same procedure 10 times and analyzing the cards. The arrangement of instruments and materials on the tray is dependent on frequency of use. The more frequently an instrument or material is picked up and placed down, the more convenient and accessible it must be. For example, a tray setup used by an assistant working with a right-handed operator would have the hand instruments located on the left side of the trays. This placement is closest to where they will be used and in the most accessible part of the tray.

Hand instruments are placed vertically on an elevated mat to allow the assistant to easily see and grasp them. The tray must be kept orderly, and instruments are replaced in the same position from which they are taken.

Charting

Charting is the process of recording the present condition of the hard and soft tissues in the oral cavity. Symbols and abbreviations are used to minimize time and space on the chart. Reasons for accurate charting include facilitating treatment planning and permitting future comparisons. Dental charts are also used to identify persons involved in accidents and in other aspects of forensic dentistry. Diagnostic tools used by the dental team to chart a patient's oral condition include radiographs, study models, health history, and clinical examination.

Several tooth identification systems can be used, the most popular of which are as follows:

The Universal System

The universal system identifies the adult dentition by numbers 1–32. Number 1 is the maxillary right third molar; the numbering procedes around the maxillary arch to number 16, which is the maxillary left third molar. The mandibular left third molar is number 17, and the numbering again procedes around the mandibular arch to the mandibular right third molar designated number 32. The deciduous dentition is identified by letters A–T, beginning with the maxillary right second molar and finishing with the mandibular right second molar.

Diagrammatically, the adult dentition is identified as follows:

$$\text{RIGHT} \quad \frac{1 \quad 2 \quad 3 \quad 4 \quad 5 \quad 6 \quad 7 \quad 8 \; | \; 9 \; 10 \; 11 \; 12 \; 13 \; 14 \; 15 \; 16}{32 \; 31 \; 30 \; 29 \; 28 \; 27 \; 26 \; 25 \; | \; 24 \; 23 \; 22 \; 21 \; 20 \; 19 \; 18 \; 17} \quad \text{LEFT}$$

The Palmer System

The Palmer system divides the mouth into quadrants. Each quadrant in the adult dentition consists of the central incisor, numbered 1, to the third molar, numbered 8. For example, the maxillary right 6, is the maxillary right first molar, etc. The deciduous dentition is also divided into quadrants with the teeth identified by letters A through F. For example, the maxillary right B is the maxillary right lateral incisor.

Diagrammatically, the adult dentition appears as follows:

$$\text{RIGHT } \frac{8\ 7\ 6\ 5\ 4\ 3\ 2\ 1\ \big|\ 1\ 2\ 3\ 4\ 5\ 6\ 7\ 8}{8\ 7\ 6\ 5\ 4\ 3\ 2\ 1\ \big|\ 1\ 2\ 3\ 4\ 5\ 6\ 7\ 8} \text{ LEFT}$$

The International System

The international system, like the Palmer system, divides the adult and deciduous teeth into quadrants. The adult teeth in each quadrant are numbered 1–8 and the deciduous dentition is numbered 1–5. Another number placed before the tooth number indicates the quadrant in which the tooth is located. If the first number is 1, it represents the adult maxillary right quadrant; 2, the adult maxillary left quadrant; 3, the adult mandibular left quadrant; 4, the adult mandibular right quadrant; 5, the deciduous maxillary right quadrant; 6, the deciduous maxillary left quadrant; 7, the deciduous mandibular left quadrant; and 8, the deciduous mandibular right quadrant. In this system, number 32 represents the adult mandibular left lateral incisor and number 25 the maxillary left first molar.

An adult dentition is represented as follows:

$$\text{RIGHT } \frac{18\ 17\ 16\ 15\ 14\ 13\ 12\ 11\ \big|\ 21\ 22\ 23\ 24\ 25\ 26\ 27\ 28}{48\ 47\ 46\ 45\ 44\ 43\ 42\ 41\ \big|\ 31\ 32\ 33\ 34\ 35\ 36\ 37\ 38} \text{ LEFT}$$

The dentist using the diagnostic tools dictates the findings to the dental assistant, who records them on the patient's chart.

In addition to the tooth-identification system, symbols and abbreviations are used to transcribe the existing condition of the oral cavity. Table I presents a key to such a system.

Table I

Transcription of Existing Condition of Oral Cavity

Existing Condition	Symbol or Abbreviation
Amalgam restoration	Darkened area on the charted tooth indicating the affected surfaces
Tooth-colored restoration	Spotted area on charted tooth indicating the affected surfaces
Gold restoration	Striped area on the charted tooth indicating the affected surfaces
Crown	Striped area on the charted tooth with the initials of the type of material used: FC = Full metallic crown FCV = Full metallic crown with a veneer PJ = Porcelain jacket PM = Porcelain fused to metal crown
Restoration required	Surfaces requiring preparation are outlined on the charted tooth and left blank
Replacement of existing restoration usually due to recurrent decay or a material breakdown	Charted existing restoration is outlined

Fractured tooth structure	Two vertical lines on the charted tooth
Tooth missing	X drawn through the missing charted tooth
Impacted tooth	Entire tooth is outlined, with an arrow indicating the tooth's orientation
Root canal therapy has been performed	Darkened area on the root of the charted tooth
Root canal therapy is required	An outlined area on the root of the charted tooth
Fixed bridge	Continuous striped area on the charted teeth with the initials of the type of material used
Removable partial denture	Continuous striped area on the charted teeth that are replaced and a dark bar connecting the replaced missing teeth

The location of each existing restoration and area of the oral cavity to be treated is identified in a standard manner. All tooth surfaces facing the midline are called mesial; those away from the midline are termed distal. Surfaces of anterior teeth facing the lips are called labial and those of posterior teeth facing the cheeks are termed buccal. All surfaces that face the tongue are called lingual. The biting edges of anterior teeth are called incisal, and the chewing surfaces of posterior teeth are called occlusal.

Dental Specialties

Dental specialties recognized by the profession include operative dentistry, prosthodontics, periodontics, endodontics, oral surgery, pedodontics, orthodontics, and public health. Following is a brief description of the role of each specialty.

Operative Dentistry

Caries is a disease that affects the hard tissues (teeth) of the oral cavity. It is thought to be the result of an imbalance among a triad of factors including: the patient (host), bacteria of the oral cavity, and diet (substrate). The actual process by which caries is thought to occur is called the acid decalcification theory. This theory states that bacteria in the mouth will break down carbohydrates in uncleaned areas, leading to the production of an acid. This acid dissolves the enamel, beginning a carious lesion. The combination of oral debris, bacteria, and salivary proteins is known as plaque. Plaque adheres to teeth unless its sticky matrix is mechanically removed by brushing.

Some areas of the mouth are more susceptible to caries than are others. The susceptibility of an area is based on its ability to be either naturally or mechanically cleaned and on natural immunity. The natural immunity is a result of tooth formation and forming of lobes. Inadequate fusing can result in the formation of pits and fissures, which can later lead to carious lesions.

Caries can be diagnosed through a clinical examination in conjunction with radiographs. Radiographs are used to identify radiolucent areas in teeth that might be carious lesions, particularly in proximal areas in which clinical examination is difficult. Radiographs, however, are an adjunct to, not a substitute for, a clinical examination. Each exposed surface of a tooth must be examined to ensure that decalcification is not present.

Caries are classified by their clinical tooth locations. Pit and fissure cavities that occur on occlusal surfaces of molars and bicuspids and on lingual surfaces of upper anterior teeth are Class I caries. This class also includes cavities on the occlusal or incisal surfaces of all teeth. Class II caries involve the proximal surfaces of bicuspids and molars. Class III caries occur on proximal surfaces of incisors and cuspids, with the exceptions of lesions appearing on the incisal angles. Class IV caries are also found on the proximal surface of incisors and cuspids, but involve the incisal angle. Class V caries occur on the gingival third portion of the labial, buccal, and lingual surfaces of all teeth.

Tooth Preparation and Restoration

Preparations include both removing decay and cutting tooth structure appropriately for insertion of a restoration. The first step requires the generation of outline form, which determines the perimeters of the preparation. It includes extending the margins of the preparation into areas that will be least susceptible to caries while concurrently removing minimal healthy tooth structures. At this time gross removal of caries is accomplished. Steps are taken to ensure resistance and retention. Resistance includes those preparation features that permit the final restoration to withstand the forces of mastication. Retention includes those preparation features that permit the tooth to retain the final restoration. After these steps are taken, convenience form is achieved, permitting access to instrumentation and placement of the final restoration. At this point, the preparation is cleaned of debris and dried.

The decision to use a base and the amount and type of base depends upon the amount of dentin destroyed. Preparations cut to ideal depths require only varnishes or cavity liners. Cavity liners are used to protect the pulp from caustic restorative materials and varnishes help certain restorations resist the fluids of the oral cavity. Those preparations cut beyond ideal depth require bases that, in effect, replace lost dentin. If during the preparation significant amounts of dentin have been removed, the integrity of the pulp may be threatened. In these cases, additional cavity liners are used to promote development of secondary dentin before placement of bases.

The choice of restorative material depends on many factors, including esthetic requirements, size of preparation, and cost. The four basic restorative materials are amalgam, composite, gold, and porcelain. The properties, uses, and manipulation of these materials are addressed in Chapter 4.

Prosthodontics

The replacement of missing teeth in partially or fully edentulous mouths falls under the specialty area of prosthodontics. The task of replacement is accomplished with either fixed or removable prostheses.

Removable Prosthetic Appliances

The number of missing teeth helps determine the size and complexity of the removable prosthetic appliance. If the mouth is completely edentulous, full dentures are required. If the remaining teeth can support the forces of mastication, a partial denture can be fabricated. Fabrication of full and partial prosthetic appliances have some procedures in common, such as preliminary and final impressions and occlusal records. The impressions must be accurate representations of both hard and soft tissue structures. Alginate or compound can be used to take preliminary impressions. From these impressions, accurate trays for border molding and final impressions are fabricated. Border molding is accomplished using thermoplastic materials (compound) to accurately obtain a representation of those movable tissue areas. The final impression then represents both fixed and movable tissues.

Partial dentures rely on remaining teeth for retention and support. These teeth must be prepared to hold the components of a partial denture. Components of partial dentures include saddles, which lie on the edentulous ridges; clasps, which provide direct retention to the remaining teeth; and connectors, which connect saddles and clasps into a functioning partial denture. The success of a partial denture is a function of the design and interaction of the components (framework). By direct and indirect retention, the final prosthesis should be strong enough to resist the forces of occlusion. Once the framework is completed, bite registrations must be taken. Teeth can then be added to the framework to complete the partial denture.

Full dentures require accurate impressions for retention and comfort. An improperly fitting full denture can cause difficulty in speech, mastication, and retention. Retention depends on the surface area covered, peripheral seal, adhesion, and cohesion.

After final impressions are taken, the dentist takes accurate records of the bite (centric relation), face height (vertical dimension), face form, and tooth size in order to approximate normal structure.

Materials used in making full dentures are acrylic and porcelain. Acrylics are used for both base construction and teeth, but porcelain is used only for teeth.

Fixed Prosthetic Appliances

Fixed prosthetic appliances are used to replace missing teeth in the mouth when remaining teeth are sufficiently strong to support such appliances. A fixed prosthetic appliance, when put in place, cannot be removed. This appliance is used to restore normal mastication to keep remaining teeth from moving, as well as for esthetic purposes. Often this kind of appliance is a more satisfactory solution than a removable appliance.

In fabricating a fixed appliance, strong remaining teeth are used as abutments. The cemented bridge is attached to the abutments, which can be shaped to accept different types of retainers. Retainers can be full crowns, three-quarter crowns, onlays, or inlays. The retainers are connected to pontics, which are used to span the edentulous area. In the preferred construction, bridges have two fixed ends. Under very limited circumstances, however, bridges can have single fixed ends or cantilevers.

Frameworks are sets of retainers and pontics that are usually fabricated from precious or semiprecious metals. The esthetic replacement teeth are then fabricated and attached to the framework. These replacement teeth can be made from porcelain fused to the gold or acrylic veneers.

A bridge is designed to rely on satisfactory abutments identified by radiographs and study models. The teeth selected are prepared to accept the retainer. A temporary bridge is then fabricated to judge occlusion, esthetics, and the parallelism of abutments.

Final impressions are taken to make an accurate determination of abutment shape and the relationship of one abutment to another. Materials used for this impression include compound, rubber, and polyether impression materials.

Final impressions are sent to the laboratory, where cast frameworks are fabricated. These frameworks are then returned to the practitioner to determine whether the fit is correct. An esthetic cover of acrylic or porcelain is usually applied, and the restoration is temporarily and subsequently permanently cemented in place.

In general, a fixed bridge provides the most realistic restoration of missing teeth. However, the cost in time and money can be prohibitive.

Periodontics

Periodontics is the specialty concerned with the hard and soft tissues that support functioning teeth. These tissues are the gingiva (free and attached), the attachment apparatus, and alveolar bone.

The primary cause of periodontal disease is dental plaque. If plaque is not removed at least once every 24 hours, it begins to calcify and will eventually form calculus. Once the deposit reaches the calculus stage, it can no longer be removed by simple brushing.

Periodontal disease can be recognized with the help of radiographs and clinical examination. A full mouth series of radiographs shows the amount and type of alveolar bone loss. The depth of each sulcus can be determined by use of a periodontal probe. Sulci depths in excess of three millimeters are considered indications of periodontal disease. The most important diagnostic tool, however, is visual inspection of the color, texture, and shape of the gingiva.

Periodontal Diseases

Failure to remove bacteria and the end product of bacteria can cause an inflammatory reaction in the gingiva, called gingivitis. As the inflammation spreads, it can affect the underlying alveolar process. Once the bony support of a tooth is affected, the disease is no longer considered gingivitis. It becomes periodontitis.

A common acute disease that occurs in many young adults is called acute necrotizing ulceratous gingivitis (ANUG). Although there is no definitve etiology for this disease, an important factor seems to be stress. The characteristics of ANUG are pain, acute inflammation, sloughing of tissue between teeth, and bleeding.

Treatment of periodontal disease depends on the disease state. The most common treatment begins with scaling and prophylaxis to remove calculus and plaque. Suggested treatment for disease that has progressed somewhat can include curettage, a gingivectomy or gingivoplasty, flapping periodontal tissue, or an ostectomy or osteoplasty.

Curettaging removes the necrotic gingival tissue. This procedure is accomplished with a curette, under local anesthesia. As necrotic tissue is removed, remaining tissue can heal properly and return to its normal shape and color.

If after curettage, residual periodontal pockets or poorly formed gingiva remain with an absence of underlying bony defects, but with a sufficient amount of attached gingiva, a gingivectomy or gingivoplasty is performed. Gingivectomy refers to removal of tissue, while gingivoplasty indicates reshaping. These procedures are performed only if sufficient healthy gingival tissue remains after these surgeries.

If alveolar bone is involved, a periodontal flap is made in order to gain access to underlying osseous tissue. An ostectomy or osteoplasty—removal or reshaping of bone—can then be performed in order to return the oral cavity to an acceptable level of health.

Endodontics

Endodontics is the specialty concerned with the treatment of pulpal and periapical diseases of teeth. Some of the treatments involve pulp capping, pulpotomy, pulpectomy, instrumentation and obduration of infected root canals, and removal of diseased periapical tissues.

All diagnostic tests and aids are designed to help the practitioner make a correct diagnosis. Some of the important tests used by endodontists are as follows. Percussion is checked by striking the crown of the tooth with the handle of an instrument to determine whether a tooth is sensitive. This is done in conjunction with the percussion of adjacent teeth in order to obtain subjective separation of symptoms by the patient. Palpation, the touching of suspected areas, can help determine whether swelling is present. The mobility test, to determine the buccolingual range of movement, in conjunction with a radiograph, helps determine whether the remaining alveolar bone is sufficient to consider restoring the tooth. A radiograph is the most common diagnostic tool because it can help determine what is happening in the periapical areas of suspected teeth. Pulp testing by the use of heat and cold or small amounts of electric current determines the vitality of a tooth.

Pulpal Injury

The pulp can become diseased or irreversibly damaged from many causes. These pathologies fall into one of three categories: bacterial, chemical, or physical. Bacteria enter the pulp chamber through a carious lesion. Caustic agents contained in dental materials may also cause chemical damage. Physical damage can occur mechanically, through trauma; thermally, as a result of overheating cavity preparations; or electrically, as a result of the interaction of dissimilar metals in restored teeth.

Endodontic Treatment

Pulp capping is the process by which a minimally exposed pulp is protected by antiseptic and sedative agents. This procedure is usually indicated for permanent teeth in which good pulpal circulation is present.

A pulpotomy is the removal of that portion of the pulp contained in the crown of the tooth. This procedure is performed to maintain the vitality of the portion of the pulp that remains in the root; it is especially useful when the apices of permanent teeth have not closed.

A pulpectomy is the total removal of all pulpal tissue (pulp extirpation) and is performed when the pulp is irreversibly damaged. Techniques of asepsis, debridement, and obduration of the canal are accomplished to complete root canal treatment. Aseptic techniques include the use of rubber dam and sterile instruments and are required to prohibit harmful organisms from entering the open canal area. Access to a canal is individualized; the number of canals is dependent on the tooth being treated.

Instrumenting the canal removes the infected pulp and prepares the canal for obduration, or filling. The instrumentation is accomplished by using reamers, broaches, and files. Reamers enlarge the canal slightly and are used to measure the length of the canal. Broaches are used to remove the affected nerve and any debris from the canal. Files are used to increase the diameter of the root canal so that it can be filled. All instrumentation is done using an irrigant, which serves to break down the soft tissue in the canal and lubricate the area. The preferred irrigant is sodium hyperchlorite.

After the canal is properly instrumented, it is filled with gutta percha, a material that is compressible and that can be laterally condensed into the canal, sealing the apex. The tooth is then ready to be fully restored to function.

Oral Surgery

Oral surgery treatment ranges from simple exodontia to the most complicated maxillofacial surgery.

All patients who are scheduled to undergo treatment must undergo assessment of general physical condition, that is, knowledge of a patient's vital signs (pulse, blood pressure, respiration rate, and body temperature), past medical history, allergies, and current medication. This information is necessary to determine whether a patient can physically sustain the rigors of surgery. More complicated procedures require additional testing.

Preparation for oral surgery also includes treatment of pain and anxiety through premedication. Administration of anesthesia is either local or general, including conscious or unconscious sedation.

During oral surgery it is mandatory that aseptic techniques be followed to prohibit contamination of the operating field. The assistant must be aware of the proper procedures for handling instruments. This applies to the sterilization of instruments, as well as to their transfer.

The most common oral surgery procedure is the simple extraction. Teeth are removed with specifically designed forceps and elevators. Extractions of impacted teeth, retained roots, or alveolar bone are more complicated procedures.

Even more complicated procedures involve the treatment of fractures of the mandible or maxilla and maxillofacial surgery which may include sectioning portions of the facial area to compensate for abnormalities resulting from genetic or traumatic causes. In addition, treatment of oral cancer falls under the purview of the oral surgeon.

After treatment, a patient might suffer from pain, postoperative bleeding, and swelling. The patient must also be protected against the possibility of infection, which requires specific postoperative instructions or appropriate medication, or both.

Pedodontics

The area of dentistry concerned with the prevention, diagnosis, and treatment of children's dental problems is called pedodontics. This specialty recognizes that children present special problems to the dentist because of growth and behavioral factors. In addition, prevention and treatment of disease in the child permit identification of future problems in the adult.

Children must be given proper strategies to cope with subjective or objective fears of dental treatment. This area is addressed in detail in Chapter 7; its importance should not be underestimated.

The child's mouth contains 20 primary teeth; each quadrant contains a central incisor, a lateral incisor, a cuspid, and a first and second molar. One function of primary teeth is mastication and assimilation. Additional functions include the maintenance of space for the permanent teeth, the stimulation of growth of the jaws, and the development of speech. Primary teeth are different in size and in external and internal design from permanent teeth.

Care of the pedodontic patient requires recognition that the purpose of treatment is not simply care of the primary dentition, but management of the eruption and health of the permanent dentition as well. This involves treatment in all phases of dentistry. Particular attention is paid to prevention in an attempt to prevent caries through fluoride treatments and prophylactic operative procedures.

Thumbsucking is certainly the most common oral habit exhibited by children. It is generally agreed that if this habit is not discontinued by the time the permanent teeth erupt, deleterious effects can occur. The severity of these effects is determined by the position of the finger in the mouth and the amount of force exerted. Other detrimental habits include lip sucking or biting, tongue thrusting, and mouth breathing.

The principles of general dentistry apply to the pedodontic patient, except that the situation is dynamic, since two sets of teeth are involved. It is therefore necessary to intercept and prevent the progress of dental disease by early and consistent treatment.

Orthodontics

Orthodontics is the study of the growth and development of the jaws and face. Also included are the position of teeth, influences on development, and prevention and correction of malocclusions.

Malocclusions develop as a result of many factors. Face form, jaw relation, and the final position of teeth depend greatly on heredity. Anomalies must be corrected to provide proper functioning in the mouth. Additional factors affecting growth of structure are diet, metabolism, and poor habits, such as thumbsucking, mouth breathing, and poor swallowing habits. In addition, the number and size of teeth are important and can determine the ability of a person to have a properly functioning mouth.

Three basic classifications of occlusion were developed by Dr. Edward Angle. Class I occlusion refers to maxillary and mandibular molars in correct relationship to one another.

In Class II occlusion, the lower molars are in a distal relationship to the maxillary molars and the lower jaw is retruded. Class II occlusion is further subdivided into two categories. Division I is characterized by V-shaped arches instead of U-shaped arches and by protrusion of the maxillary incisors. Division II of the classification is characterized by maxillary arches that are wider than normal and by maxillary incisors that show a marked lingual inclination with an excessive overbite.

Class III occlusion is characterized by the mandible anterior to its normal position. Mandibular incisors might be in total crossbite in relationship to upper anterior teeth and maxillary arches might be restricted in growth.

Diagnostic tools for classifying occlusion include clinical examination, health history, tooth relationships, and soft tissue appraisal. In addition, plaster study models, bite records, and cephalometric radiographs are necessary.

Resolution of occlusal problems is usually accomplished by tooth movement through application of measured forces in the desired direction. Teeth are either tipped or moved until they reach their new positions. Some teeth are more resistant than others. For example, molars are often more resistant than are anterior teeth.

Orthodontic treatment can be either preventive or interceptive. Careful diagnosis and early treatment for relatively minor problems can minimize future patient discomfort and expense.

Public Health

Within the purview of public health dentistry fall the areas of community, municipal, state, and national dental health programs. The duties and responsibilities of dentists and auxiliaries depend on the scope of individual programs.

Many public health programs offer public education and prevention-oriented components, whereas others concentrate on research and direct patient care. The assistant's role in public health dentistry can vary greatly. In the direct provision of services, the assistant may perform tasks similar to those of an assistant in any private practice, whereas in public education, prevention, and research areas, he or she might assume complex roles involving the application of a variety of skills.

Some auxiliaries in public health dentistry are required to hold advanced degrees to meet the responsibilities of their positions. For example, an assistant involved in research concerned with effects of a fluoridation program might be called to analyze statistical information to determine incidence and prevalence rates of dental disease.

All clinical functions are regulated by state law, but auxiliaries in certain federal programs may be exempt from state restrictions. Since state laws regarding performance of functions vary from state to state, so too do the assistant's responsibilities. Some states permit assistants to perform expanded functions, tasks traditionally performed by dentists. These expanded functions include reversible tasks, such as placing rubber dams, placing and removing temporary restorations, and applying topical anesthesia.

Question Section

Directions: Each of the questions or incomplete statements below is followed by four suggested answers or completions. Select the BEST answer in each case.

1. Knowledge of the patient's medical and dental history can affect
   1. the treatment plan
   2. the drugs prescribed
   3. the frequency of appointments
   4. all of the above

2. When treating a patient with a history of rheumatic fever, the patient should
   1. be prophylactically given antibiotics
   2. be treated with the operator wearing gloves
   3. be treated without any special precautions
   4. never be placed in a supine position

3. Short appointments are given to patients with
   1. allergies
   2. heart problems
   3. aphthous ulcers
   4. rampant caries

4. Chronic respiratory problems affect the
   1. type of prosthesis a patient can wear
   2. prognosis of root canal therapy
   3. positioning of the patient
   4. design of cavity preparation

5. Which diagnostic test is an indicator of oral bacterial action?
   1. urinalysis
   2. complete blood count
   3. modified Snyder test
   4. scratch

6. When a patient appears in the office with pain, the immediate objective is to
   1. discuss future treatment plans
   2. relieve the pain
   3. discuss any outstanding bills
   4. look for any other work in the same quadrant

7. A complete oral examination should occur
   1. every visit
   2. each time the patient is recalled
   3. once every other year
   4. only in dentulous patients

8. A thorough dental examination
   1. will prevent viral infections
   2. should be standardized so that nothing is overlooked
   3. is unnecessary in edentulous patients
   4. will decrease the rate of caries formation

9. Some reasons for an anticipated increase in the demand for dental services are
   A. increase in third-party payments
   B. increase in public education
   C. increase in water fluoridation
   D. increase in plaque-control programs
   E. increase in advertising
      1. A, B, and C
      2. A, B, and D
      3. A, B, and E
      4. B, C, and E

10. Possible solutions for future workforce demands are
    A. dentists increasing the rate of work
    B. higher prices
    C. increased use of preventive measures
    D. increased use of assistants, or paraprofessionals
    E. research in anticariogenic drugs
       1. A, B, and D
       2. B, D, and E
       3. B, C, and D
       4. C, D, and E

11. The maximum amount of time can be saved by
    1. eliminating a procedure
    2. combining two procedures
    3. standardizing procedures
    4. rearranging procedures

12. A benefit of using premeasured and prepackaged materials is the
    1. lower cost
    2. assurance of correct proportioning
    3. lack of temperature regulation needed
    4. ease of storage

13. An advantage of using disposable materials is
    1. they are cheaper
    2. they save time in cleaning
    3. they can be hot-air sterilized
    4. none of the above

14. Some benefits of tray setups are
    A. they save time setting up
    B. the dentist sets them up for the assistant
    C. they eliminate delay in searching for instruments
    D. they are used only in restorative procedures
    E. they are adaptable to any procedure
       1. A, B, and C
       2. A, C, and E
       3. B, C, and D
       4. C, D, and E

15. Color coding prepared trays allows for
    1. more instruments to be placed on them
    2. easy identification of the procedure the tray is prepared for
    3. quicker autoclaving
    4. multiple use of each tray

16. Hand instruments on prepared tray setups are placed in
    1. order of use
    2. the order the assistant prefers
    3. size order
    4. random sequence

17. What problem does a randomly prepared tray setup present?
    1. instruments may be missing
    2. instruments must be located
    3. they appear disorderly
    4. all of the above

18. The best position for the instrument tray is
    1. over the patient
    2. over the operator's lap
    3. over the assistant's lap
    4. in back of the assistant

19. The most anxiety-producing procedure in dentistry is the
    1. removal of the matrix band
    2. placement of the rubber dam
    3. use of the high-speed evacuation
    4. administration of local anesthesia

20. When is the anesthetic syringe prepared?
    1. when the dentist is seated
    2. when the patient is seated
    3. before the patient is seated
    4. when the patient makes an appointment

21. Preparation of the anesthetic syringe by the assistant includes
    A. engaging the stylet
    B. placement of the carpule
    C. placing the anesthetic in the carpule
    D. placement of the topical anesthetic
    E. loosening the cap covering the needle
       1. A, B, and C
       2. A, B, and E
       3. B, D, and E
       4. C, D, and E

22. The assistant adjusts the bevel of the needle so
    1. it is parallel to the mandible
    2. it is perpendicular to the mandible
    3. it is at a 45-degree angle to the mandible
    4. none of the above

23. During the administration of local anesthesia aspiration will
    1. damage the mandibular artery
    2. be extremely painful
    3. determine if the lumen of the needle is in a blood vessel
    4. ensure profound anesthesia

24. Which instrument is run by compressed air?
    1. high-speed handpiece
    2. air-driven low-speed handpiece
    3. air–water syringe
    4. all of the above

25. How fast can the high-speed handpiece revolve?
    1. 10,000 rpm
    2. 45,000 rpm
    3. 250,000 rpm
    4. 500,000 rpm

26. What is the best coolant when using the high-speed drill?
    1. air
    2. high-speed evacuation
    3. cool water
    4. no coolant is necessary

27. How often should the high-speed handpiece be cleaned and lubricated?
    1. each day
    2. every third day
    3. each week
    4. each month

28. Some reasons why patients desire to rinse their mouths are to
    A. save time for the dentist
    B. delay treatment
    C. eliminate the need for rubber dam
    D. rid themselves of pooled fluids and solids
    E. refresh their mouths after treatment
       1. A, B, and E
       2. B, C, and D
       3. B, C, and E
       4. B, D, and E

29. High-speed evacuation
    A. increases the patient's desire to rinse
    B. decreases the patient's desire to rinse
    C. is used only with a rubber dam
    D. decreases the aerosol emanating from the patient's mouth
    E. increases visibility
       1. A, C, and E
       2. A, D, and E
       3. B, C, and D
       4. B, D, and E

30. Which is a technique for holding the high-speed suction tip?
    1. palm–thumb grasp
    2. inverted modified pen grasp
    3. thumb to nose grasp
    4. any of the above

31. When working in the posterior area of the mouth, the high-speed evacuation tip is placed
    A. over the occlusal surface of the tooth being prepared
    B. at the occlusal height of the tooth being prepared
    C. parallel to the buccal or lingual surface of the tooth being prepared
    D. after operator places the mirror
    E. as close as possible to the tooth being prepared
       1. A, B, and C
       2. B, C, and D
       3. B, C, and E
       4. C, D, and E

32. When working in the anterior part of the mouth, the high-speed suction tip is held
    1. below the incisal edge of the tooth being prepared

    2. on the opposite side of the tooth being prepared
    3. in the retromolar area
    4. in the vestibule

33. Several ways an assistant can help increase the dentist's visibility are
    A. using high-speed evacuation
    B. eliminating the use of certain instruments
    C. using the air–water syringe
    D. retracting soft tissues
    E. using premixed materials
       1. A, B, and C
       2. A, C, and D
       3. B, C, and D
       4. C, D, and E

34. If a right-handed operator is preparing a mandibular right molar for a crown preparation, the assistant retracts
    1. the tongue
    2. the cheek
    3. both the tongue and cheek
    4. neither the tongue nor the cheek

35. Indirect vision refers to
    1. looking through protective glass
    2. looking through a mirror
    3. looking directly at an object
    4. using prism lighting

36. Work surfaces should be located
    1. 2 inches below the elbow
    2. 4 inches below the elbow
    3. even with the elbow
    4. 2 inches above the elbow

37. The front edge of the assistant's chair should be
    1. even with the head of the patient's chair
    2. 12 inches from the side of the patient's chair
    3. even with the patient's elbow
    4. even with the patient's mouth

38. The assistant's eye level when seated is
    1. even with that of the dentist
    2. 4–6 inches below that of the dentist
    3. 4–6 inches above the patient's shoulder
    4. 4–6 inches above that of the dentist

39. The assistant's chair should have
    1. a wraparound arm located under the rib cage
    2. a wraparound arm located on the lower part of the back
    3. a small square back
    4. only a seat

40. When seated in working position, the patient's calves should be

1. perpendicular to the floor
2. parallel to the floor
3. at an angle of 25 degrees from the floor
4. varied according to the arch being worked on

41. When seated in working position, the patient's back should be
    1. parallel to the floor
    2. perpendicular to the floor
    3. at an angle of 25 degrees from the floor
    4. varied according to the arch being worked on

42. The patient's head should be positioned
    1. in the middle of the chair
    2. as close to the assistant as possible
    3. in whatever position the patient finds most comfortable
    4. at the end of the chair and close to the operator's side of the chair

43. What happens to the saliva when the patient is positioned in the supine position and the rubber dam is in place?
    1. the patient chokes on the saliva
    2. the dentist allows the patient to rinse frequently
    3. the patient swallows the saliva
    4. the assistant must evacuate the saliva with high-speed suction

44. If a patient jumps out of the chair after being treated in the supine position
    1. he or she will feel giddy
    2. his or her mouth will feel dry
    3. he or she might feel faint
    4. nothing will happen

45. If the operator is seated at the 11 o'clock position and the patient is seated in an upright position
    1. the labial surface of anterior teeth will not be directly visible to the operator
    2. the lingual surface of lower anterior teeth will not be directly visible to the operator
    3. both are true
    4. none of the above

46. How does the operator signal for an instrument transfer?
    1. by nodding his or her head
    2. by moving his or her fingers
    3. by pointing to the next instrument needed
    4. by calling out the next instrument needed

47. Which instrument is used in the palm–thumb grasp?

1. high-speed handpiece
2. scissors
3. straight chisel
4. anesthetic syringe

48. Which instrument is used in the pen grasp?
    1. high-speed handpiece
    2. scissors
    3. straight chisel
    4. anesthetic syringe

49. When working with a right-handed dentist, which hand does the assistant use to transfer instruments?
    1. right hand
    2. left hand
    3. either hand
    4. no assistance is required

50. Hand instruments are transferred
    1. at the patient's mouth
    2. in back of the patient's head
    3. to the left of the patient's head
    4. to the right of the patient's head

51. Double-handled instruments are transferred
    1. under the patient's chin
    2. at the patient's mouth
    3. behind the patient's head
    4. over the assistant's tray

52. The assistant holds the hand instrument to be transferred between
    1. thumb and forefinger
    2. small finger and palm
    3. thumb and palm
    4. small finger and forefinger

53. The assistant retrieves the operator's hand instruments with
    1. thumb and forefinger
    2. small finger
    3. whole hand
    4. none of the above

54. Prepared materials should be held by the assistant
    1. over a waste receptacle
    2. over the prepared tray
    3. over the operator's lap
    4. as close to the area of the operation as possible

55. Some benefits of using rubber dams are that they
    A. permit controlled amounts of saliva through the dam
    B. permit optimum use of dental materials
    C. permit easier communication between patient and doctor
    D. keep debris out of the patient's mouth

E. help retract the tongue and cheek
   1. A, B, and D
   2. B, C, and E
   3. B, D, and E
   4. C, D, and E

56. During the placement of a rubber dam, an explorer can be used to
   1. secure the rubber dam
   2. invert the rubber dam
   3. punch small holes, for the anterior teeth, in the rubber dam
   4. all of the above

57. The rubber dam napkin is used to
   1. place the dam
   2. secure the dam
   3. avoid irritation around the patient's mouth
   4. help the patient swallow

58. A lubricant can be used on the rubber dam to
   1. retard the flow of saliva
   2. help clamp the last tooth
   3. repair a torn dam
   4. make it easier for the dam to be slipped between the teeth

59. When applying a rubber dam, dental floss can be used to
   1. help secure the dam
   2. force the dam between the teeth being isolated
   3. invert the dam around the teeth being operated on
   4. all of the above

60. When placing a rubber dam to prepare an anterior tooth
   1. a large hole must be made for breathing
   2. the entire arch should be isolated
   3. one large hole should expose all the anterior teeth
   4. silicate restorations should be protected from desiccation

61. What aids are used to diagnose caries?
   A. a millimeter probe
   B. broaches
   C. a sharp explorer
   D. a ball burnisher
   E. bite-wing radiographs
   1. A, C, and D
   2. B, C, and D
   3. C and E
   4. C, D, and E

62. Recurrent caries refers to
   1. decay that begins inside of the tooth
   2. root caries only
   3. caries around the margins of restorations
   4. occlusal decay only

63. If carious lesions are not restored the subsequent problem will involve the
   1. cortical bone
   2. pulpal tissues
   3. buccal mucosa
   4. periodontal membrane

64. A mesial occlusal cavity preparation is an example of a
   1. Class I cavity preparation
   2. Class II cavity preparation
   3. Class III cavity preparation
   4. Class IV cavity preparation

65. A cavity preparation in the gingival third of the lingual surface of an upper molar is an example of a
   1. Class II cavity preparation
   2. Class III cavity preparation
   3. Class IV cavity preparation
   4. Class V cavity preparation

66. A cavity preparation that includes the mesial incisal angle of a maxillary central incisor is classified as a
   1. Class I cavity preparation
   2. Class II cavity preparation
   3. Class III cavity preparation
   4. Class IV cavity preparation

67. A cavity preparation that involves the mesial surface of a mandibular central incisor is classified as a
   1. Class I cavity preparation
   2. Class II cavity preparation
   3. Class III cavity preparation
   4. Class IV cavity preparation

68. A cavity preparation that involves the buccal pit of a lower molar is an example of a
   1. Class I cavity preparation
   2. Class II cavity preparation
   3. Class III cavity preparation
   4. Class IV cavity preparation

69. The toilet of the cavity preparation refers to
   1. resisting dislodgment of filling materials
   2. retaining of filling material in the cavity preparation
   3. removal of debris from the cavity preparation
   4. removal of undermined enamel

70. A problem that can be encountered when

placing a mesial occlusal amalgam restoration in the upper first premolar is
1. esthetics
2. a naturally weak lingual cusp
3. the lack of a minor embrasure
4. difficulty in removing decay

71. What is a fulcrum?
1. the amount of amalgam flow in 24 hours
2. the maximum amount of amalgam in a cavity preparation
3. a type of matrix retainer
4. the stationary point of a lever system

72. During a Class II amalgam procedure, the rubber dam is removed
1. before checking the patient's occlusion
2. before condensing the amalgam
3. before removing the matrix band
4. after the matrix band is in position

73. Which of the following is not used to evaluate an amalgam restoration?
1. mirror
2. burnisher
3. articulating paper
4. dental floss

74. What instrument is not used in the placement of a Class III amalgam restoration?
1. amalgam carrier
2. condenser
3. spoon excavator
4. matrix band retainer

75. A wooden wedge is used to
1. prevent gingival amalgam overhang
2. plug amalgam into small preparations
3. extract teeth
4. splint loose teeth

76. In a mesial occlusal cavity preparation, at what point is the amalgam placed first?
1. on the occlusal surface
2. in the proximal box
3. in the distal portion of the preparation
4. it does not matter which part of the cavity preparation is filled first

77. Factors that determine instrument selection for restorative procedures are the
A. color shade of the tooth
B. surface of the tooth being restored
C. tooth being restored
D. number of teeth in a patient's mouth
E. health of the patient
1. A, B, and C
2. B and C
3. C and D
4. C, D, and E

78. A bevel is a
1. sharp instrument
2. jerking movement
3. puncture wound
4. sloping surface

79. When preparing which of the following cavity preparations would a miniature head on a handpiece be most useful?
1. the occlusal surface of a mandibular premolar
2. the buccal surface of the maxillary third molar
3. the incisal edge of a lower incisor
4. the proximal surface of an upper incisor

80. Which technique of drying a cavity preparation can be injurious to the pulp?
1. cotton pledgets
2. short blasts of air
3. a steady stream of air
4. none of the above

81. Hand-cutting instruments are used in restorative dentistry to
1. remove deep carious lesions
2. refine cavity preparations
3. trim excess restorative material
4. all of the above

82. The placement of which restorative materials is most likely to cause postoperative discomfort?
1. composite
2. gold foil
3. amalgam
4. silicate

83. Which is not a recognized dental specialty?
1. radiology
2. pedodontics
3. periodontics
4. endodontics

84. The function of the periodontium is to
1. prevent caries
2. support the teeth
3. prevent vertical food impaction
4. aid the tongue in cleansing the teeth

85. What is gingivitis?
1. inflammation of the soft tissue surrounding the tooth
2. inflammation of the cortical bone
3. inflammation of the teeth
4. inflammation around the apical foremen

86. What is periodontitis?
1. inflammation of the soft tissue which surrounds the teeth

2. inflammation of teeth
3. the stage of periodontal disease involving loss of bone that supports the teeth
4. the removal of soft tooth-accumulated material

87. A pocket can be differentiated from a sulcus because a pocket
    1. cannot be cleaned by the patient
    2. is a pathological condition
    3. should be eliminated if possible
    4. all of the above

88. Iatrogenic disease is
    1. pathology of the salivary glands
    2. a self-inflicted oral disease
    3. a disease caused by the operator
    4. a viral disease of the palate

89. Another name for Vincent's disease is
    1. acute necrotizing ulcerative gingivitis
    2. an acute ear infection
    3. aphthous ulcer
    4. herpetic lesions

90. A furcation in periodontics refers to
    1. a surgical procedure
    2. mobility of anterior teeth
    3. the radicular area of multirooted teeth
    4. a dry mouth

91. A splint is an appliance that
    1. holds broken teeth together
    2. connects and stabilizes mobile teeth
    3. holds soft tissue against bone
    4. keeps sutures covered after surgery

92. Which coolant is used with the ultrasonic scaler?
    1. air
    2. water
    3. alcohol
    4. no coolant is necessary

93. Osteoplasty is the
    1. recontouring of gingival tissue
    2. recontouring of bony defects
    3. implanting of bone
    4. treatment of choice in gingivitis

94. Gingivectomy is the
    1. surgical removal of the mucogingival junction
    2. surgical removal of the apex of a tooth
    3. replacement of inflamed gingival tissue
    4. surgical elimination of the gingival pocket

95. Incision and drainage are used to treat a
    1. periodontal abscess
    2. granuloma
    3. cyst
    4. furcation

96. A periodontal dressing is analogous to
    1. cleaning teeth
    2. suturing
    3. a mouth bandage
    4. protecting the periodontium from plaque

97. Exfoliation of a primary tooth occurs by
    1. resorption of the root of the primary tooth
    2. extraction of the primary tooth
    3. pushing of the primary tooth by the permanent tooth
    4. bacterial degeneration of the primary tooth

98. What pedodontic technique can be used to allay a child's fear?
    1. stopping the child from breathing
    2. separating the child from parent
    3. covering the child's eyes
    4. tell, show, and do

99. Techniques used alleviate a child's fear of dental treatment are to
    A. permit the child to participate
    B. threaten the child with physical punishment
    C. use no anesthesia
    D. give the child some controls
    E. use sedating medications
       1. A, B, and C
       2. A, D, and E
       3. B, D, and E
       4. C, D, and E

100. To aid in the management of a difficult child, the dentist may
    1. strap the child in the chair
    2. scream at the child's parent
    3. spank the child
    4. prescribe premedication

101. To maintain a calm atmosphere with children, the operator should
    1. talk softly in monotone speech
    2. move with sudden movements
    3. speak loudly in the child's ear
    4. not talk directly to the child

102. A piece of equipment used in both pedodontics and orthodontics is a(n)
    1. face bow
    2. spot welder
    3. arch wire
    4. bead sterilizer

103. When making alginate impressions on children, which arch should be taken first?
    1. mandibular
    2. maxillary
    3. there is no benefit in taking one arch before the other
    4. take both arches simultaneously

104. Removal of the coronal portion of the pulp is called
    1. pulp capping
    2. pulpotomy
    3. apical retention
    4. indirect pulp capping

105. What appliance is used to maintain the space of a prematurely lost second primary molar?
    1. a space opener
    2. a space maintainer
    3. a space saver
    4. it is not necessary to maintain this space

106. Full coverage of a deciduous molar usually indicates the use of
    1. an amalgam crown
    2. an acrylic crown
    3. a stainless steel crown
    4. any of the above

107. A mixed dentition consists of
    1. deciduous and permanent teeth existing simultaneously in a child's mouth
    2. deciduous teeth in the wrong places
    3. permanent teeth that are rotated
    4. permanent teeth in the wrong places

108. Preventive orthodontics include
    1. the proper use of space maintainers in the primary dentition
    2. sound restorative dentistry to retain primary teeth
    3. the placement of fixed bridges in the adult dentition
    4. all of the above

109. A cause of malocclusion can be
    1. placement of large amalgam restorations
    2. a coarse diet
    3. oral habits
    4. all of the above

110. A result of malocclusion can be
    1. decreased enamel solubility
    2. difficulty in plaque removal
    3. root absorption
    4. increased thermal sensitivity

111. A result of orthodontic treatment may be
    1. teeth more prone to periodontal disease
    2. improved appearance
    3. a speech impediment
    4. all of the above

112. Angle's classification of malocclusion is based on the
    1. shape of the maxilla
    2. relationship between the first molars and the orbit
    3. relationship between the maxillary and mandibular first molars
    4. number of teeth in the mandible

113. The information needed for the diagnosis and treatment planning of an orthodontic case is
    A. the medical history
    B. photographs
    C. radiographs
    D. the knowledge of amalgam restorations present
    E. study models
    F. the age of all members of the family
    1. A, B, C, and E
    2. B, C, E, and F
    3. C, D, and F
    4. D, E, and F

114. Cephalometry is
    1. compression of the skull
    2. studying soft tissues of the head
    3. a technique of maintaining orthodontic movement
    4. making measurements of the skull

115. What is ankylosis?
    1. restricted movement of muscles
    2. the fusion of root with the surrounding bone
    3. calcium deposits in the pulp
    4. sores at the corner of the mouth

116. The orthodontic condition of a tooth moving in bone is analogous to
    1. a knife cutting through meat
    2. a hammer removing a nail
    3. a wire slowly moving through a block of ice
    4. turning a screw

117. An important function of the dental assistant in an orthodontic practice is
    1. to motivate and reinforce oral home care
    2. to make a preliminary reinforcement
    3. to bend the arch wire and place it in the patient's mouth
    4. all of the above

118. An advantage of using fixed, rather than removable, orthodontic appliances is
    1. the ease of keeping the teeth clean

2. elimination of dependence upon patient cooperation
3. ease of insertion in the patient's mouth
4. that fixed appliances can only be used on children

119. A technique to attach buccal tubes to molar bands is
1. finger pressure
2. spot welding
3. cementation
4. use of rubber bands

120. What is used to tie the arch into orthodontic brackets?
1. separating wire
2. buccal tubes
3. ligature wire
4. finger springs

121. On which surface(s) is the arch wire located?
1. occlusal surface only
2. labial surface only
3. lingual surface only
4. labial or lingual surface

122. The attachment of anterior plastic brackets directly to teeth can be accomplished by
1. ZOP comentation
2. soldering
3. acid etch bonding
4. spot welding

123. Cervical anchorage (headgear) is an
1. appliance that exerts distal forces on maxillary teeth
2. intraoral appliance that constricts the mandible
3. intraoral appliance that moves teeth anteriorly
4. appliance that enlarges the palate

124. After active orthodontic treatment is finished, what appliance is used to stabilize the teeth?
1. thin rubber bands
2. a retainer
3. a night guard
4. molar bands

125. Possible causes of irreversible pulpal damage are
A. carious invasion
B. trauma
C. x-rays
D. the use of irreversible hydrocolloid
E. chemical irritation
  1. A, B, and D
  2. A, B, and E
  3. B, D, and E
  4. C, D, and E

126. The information necessary for the diagnosis and treatment planning for root canal therapy is
A. radiographs
B. vitality of the tooth
C. study models
D. clinical examination
E. centric relation
  1. A, B, and D
  2. B, C, and E
  3. B, D, and E
  4. C, D, and E

127. Rubber dam is used in endodontics
1. to prevent the patient from breathing through his or her mouth
2. for asepsis
3. to accomplish quadrant dentistry
4. to prevent the patient from seeing the instruments

128. Pulpectomy is the
1. removal of the coronal portion of the pulp
2. removal of the entire pulp
3. entrance into the pulp chamber
4. slow degeneration of the pulp

129. Obtaining a measurement of the length of the root canal ensures
1. profound anesthesia
2. not irritating the periapical tissues by extending instruments beyond the apex of the root
3. a sterile root canal
4. no future pain

130. An important principle during instrumentation of a root canal is the
1. extension of the instrument 2 mm beyond the apex of the tooth
2. forcing of the instrument to the apex of the root
3. sequential use of instruments
4. rotary motion of the instrument

131. Endodontic files are used
1. to enlarge the root canal
2. to remove the contents of the pulp chamber
3. as drains in an endodontic abscess
4. to reduce the occlusal forces on an endodontically treated tooth

132. Culturing of the root canal determines
1. whether any vital tissue is left in the canal
2. the type of filling material which will be used
3. asepsis of the canal

4. the brittleness of the endodontically treated tooth

133. Sterilization of the root canal is accomplished by
   1. mechanical means
   2. using EDTA
   3. using silver points to seal the canal
   4. culturing after instrumentation

134. Gutta percha is used to
   1. irrigate the root canal
   2. gain access to the root canal
   3. fill the root canal
   4. sterilize the root canal

135. At which steps during root canal therapy are radiographs taken?
   A. at the beginning of each visit
   B. at measurement
   C. after the pulp is extirpated
   D. at the fitting of the master point
   E. after the final fill
      1. A, B, and D
      2. B, C, and D
      3. B, D, and E
      4. C, D, and E

136. Various medicaments are used in endodontic therapy to
   A. irrigate canals
   B. strengthen the coronal portion of the tooth
   C. increase asepsis
   D. fit the master point
   E. aid instrumentation
      1. A, B, and C
      2. A, C, and E
      3. C, D, and E
      4. B, D, and E

137. Between endodontic visits, temporary filling materials are used to
   1. provide thermal insulation
   2. prevent contamination of the canals by saliva
   3. prevent purulent material from escaping from the canals
   4. prevent electrical stimulation of the periodontal membrane

138. An apicoectomy is the
   1. chemical sterilization of the root apex
   2. root canal treatment of primary teeth
   3. procedure performed before reinforcing an endodontically treated tooth
   4. surgical removal of the apex of the root

139. Hemisection refers to
   1. an irreversible pulpitis
   2. a densensitizing solution

3. the removal of a root from a multi-rooted tooth
   4. the removal of the root apex

140. A function of a fixed bridge is
   1. to help move teeth
   2. to prevent movement of teeth
   3. to make cleaning easier
   4. all of the above

141. Diagnostic aids in fixed prosthetics are
   1. radiographs
   2. study models
   3. clinical examination
   4. all of the above

142. The teeth that support a fixed bridge are called
   1. abutments
   2. pontics
   3. ridge laps
   4. partials

143. The following restorations can be used to retain a fixed bridge
   A. porcelain jackets
   B. three-quarter crowns
   C. inlays
   D. full crowns
   E. amalgam restorations
      1. A, B, and C
      2. B, C, and D
      3. B, C, and E
      4. C, D, and E

144. Individual units of a fixed bridge are held together by
   1. acrylic
   2. solder
   3. porcelain
   4. aluminum

145. What type of restoration is used to reinforce an endodontically treated tooth before a crown is fabricated?
   1. an acrylic core
   2. a copper band
   3. an aluminum shell
   4. a gold post

146. Cantilever bridges
   1. are the most common bridges made
   2. are used only to replace molars
   3. always use three abutments
   4. have abutments on only one side

147. Temporary bridges are used
   A. for esthetics
   B. for durations of 1 week or less
   C. for mastication
   D. for investing procedures

E. to decrease thermal sensitivity
1. A, B, and C
2. A, C, and E
3. B, C, and D
4. C, D, and E

148. To adapt a copper band to closely approximate a crown preparation
1. use rubber impression material
2. festoon the band
3. recut the preparation
4. cut the gingival attachment

149. The process of transforming a copper band impression into a copper plated die is called
1. electroplating
2. annealing
3. electrosurgery
4. casting

150. Electrosurgery is used to
1. cut tooth structure
2. cut bone
3. copper plate dies
4. remove gingival tissue

151. Epinephrine-impregnated cord is used to
1. stimulate a patient who has fainted
2. dry the prepared tooth
3. tie stone dies together
4. stop gingival bleeding and retract the gingiva

152. An advantage of the elastic impression technique is that
1. no tissue retraction is necessary
2. a composite model is obtained
3. the material is cheaper
4. the procedure requires no assistance

153. A plaster–alginate impression is used to
1. check the fit of individual castings
2. pour study models
3. pick up transfer copings
4. make temporary crowns

154. The purpose of temporary cementation of a fixed bridge is
1. to check the reaction of the supporting tissue to the prosthesis
2. to permit the patient to evaluate the prosthesis
3. to permit the bridge to settle on the abutments
4. all of the above

155. Shade selection is accomplished using
1. natural light
2. the dental light
3. fluorescent light
4. black light

156. A disadvantage of a fixed bridge is that it
1. loosens the abutment teeth
2. must be remade every two years
3. interferes with the tongue during swallowing
4. is difficult to clean beneath the bridge

157. The adaptation by patients to wearing full mandibular dentures is dependent on the
1. age of the patient
2. number of sore spots that appear after 2 days
3. patient's desire to wear dentures
4. length of time it takes to construct dentures

158. An immediate denture
1. is constructed in one visit
2. is made of shellac
3. replaces only the anterior teeth
4. is inserted during the same appointment the remaining teeth are extracted

159. The relationship of the maxillary and mandibular teeth when they contact is called
1. contact point
2. vertical dimension at rest
3. occlusion
4. processing

160. Mandibular dentures are not as retentive as maxillary dentures because
1. gravity works against mandibular dentures
2. mandibular teeth work harder than maxillary teeth during mastication
3. the mandibular ridge needs tissue conditioning
4. mandibular dentures cover less surface area

161. Full dentures are
1. more efficient than is natural dentition
2. less efficient than is natural dentition
3. as efficient as natural dentition
4. none of the above

162. How is the maxillary denture retained in place?
1. cohesion
2. adhesion
3. close adaptation to the tissue surface
4. all of the above

163. During mastication, full dentures
1. move all the time
2. move sometimes
3. do not move
4. click together

164. Tissue conditioning

1. is used to help final casts
2. takes place at the time the denture is inserted in the patient's mouth
3. returns unhealthy tissue under a denture to a healthy state
4. is accomplished by using wax rims

165. What part of the partial denture holds it to the abutment tooth?
    1. the saddle area
    2. the rigid connector
    3. the surveyor
    4. the clasps

166. The part of the partial denture that lies over the ridge is called the
    1. saddle
    2. rigid connector
    3. surveyor
    4. clasp

167. A surveyor is used in partial denture construction to
    1. determine the placement of clasps
    2. attach wax rims
    3. determine the placement of artificial teeth
    4. determine the placement of the palatal bar

168. The function of the preliminary impression in full denture construction is to
    1. construct wax rims
    2. help mount final casts
    3. construct a custom tray
    4. help make adjustments after insertion

169. A facebow is used to
    1. insert the denture in the patient's mouth
    2. contour the wax rims
    3. mount the upper cast on an articulator
    4. check the bite

170. Wax bite blocks are used to
    1. record vertical dimension
    2. determine sore spots
    3. construct custom trays
    4. flask dentures

171. Flasking is part of the process to
    1. make adjustments after a denture is inserted
    2. attach wax bite rims
    3. check the bite
    4. heat-cure acrylic

172. The portion of the denture that should not be polished is the
    1. part touching the tongue
    2. part contacting the denture-bearing mucosa
    3. part touching the cheeks
    4. all parts must be polished

173. After dentures are inserted sore spots are
    1. common
    2. infrequent
    3. nonexistent
    4. ignored

174. The purpose of relining a denture is to
    1. alter the occlusion
    2. readapt the denture base to the existing tissue conditions
    3. make a custom tray
    4. take bite registration

175. A biopsy is
    1. any lesion in the oral cavity
    2. the surgical removal of an abscessed tooth
    3. the removal of tissue for diagnostic purposes
    4. the radical removal of a cancerous lesion

176. The condition in which the mandible is located ahead of the maxilla is called
    1. prognathism
    2. micrognathism
    3. retrusion
    4. centric relation

177. The function of a stylet is to
    1. remove soft tissue lesions
    2. section impacted teeth
    3. engage the rubber plunger of an anesthetic carpule
    4. none of the above

178. General anesthetics are administered
    1. for nerve blocks
    2. to render the patient unconscious
    3. routinely in most dental offices
    4. without any risks

179. Common reasons for extracting teeth include
    A. periodontal disease
    B. mucoceles
    C. caries
    D. sinus infection
    E. impaction
       1. A, B, and C
       2. A, C, and E
       3. B, D, and E
       4. C, D, and E

180. An impaction is
    1. a succedaneous tooth
    2. a tooth that will not erupt fully
    3. any tooth that is ankylosed
    4. a tooth that never fully develops

181. An instrument that holds a tissue flap away from the operating field is called a
    1. pick
    2. retractor
    3. elevator
    4. hemostat

182. An abscess is
    1. a collection of serous fluid
    2. a pathway for fluid drainage
    3. a localized collection of pus
    4. always infrabony in nature

183. A drain is placed to
    1. create a pathway for fluid to leave the body
    2. hold bone fractures together
    3. treat ANUG
    4. treat dry sockets

184. A cyst is
    1. found in the pulp of primary teeth
    2. a cell-lined sac
    3. a passageway for nerves
    4. always connected to an abscess

185. After an extraction, the best technique to stop bleeding is
    1. medicating with antibiotics
    2. applying indirect pressure
    3. applying direct pressure
    4. placing a drain in the extraction socket

186. Rinsing with warm salt water
    1. causes clot formation
    2. helps relieve pain
    3. causes edema
    4. decreases the number of oral microbes

187. The suture material that can be resorbed by the body is
    1. gut
    2. nylon
    3. braid
    4. none of the above

188. The treatment of fractures is
    1. the placement of a drain
    2. immediate mobilization
    3. immobilization
    4. bony transplants

189. Trismus is
    1. a calcium deposit in the buccal mucosa
    2. a grinding habit
    3. the restricted opening of the mouth
    4. caused by sudden changes in temperature

190. A dry socket is a(n)
    1. decrease in the salivary flow

    2. lesion in the parotid duct
    3. embrasure between the lower molars
    4. breakdown of the blood clot in an extraction socket

Directions: Each question names an instrument. MATCH these instruments with the number that describes the function of the instrument.

Questions 191–195
191. Broach
192. Reamer
193. Glass bead sterilizer
194. Luer-Lok syringe
195. Paper points
    1. absorbs moisture in the root canal
    2. sterilizes instruments before use
    3. seals the apical foramen
    4. extirpates the pulpal contents
    5. determines the sterility of the root canal
    6. carries irrigating solution to the canal
    7. gains entrance and cleanses the root canal

Questions 196–200
196. Matrix band
197. Gingival marginal trimmer
198. Amalgam condenser
199. Cleoid–discoid carver
200. Amalgam carrier
    1. places amalgam in the cavity preparation
    2. compresses amalgam into the cavity preparation
    3. prevents gingival overhang
    4. limits the filling material to the confines of the tooth
    5. cleanses the cavity preparation
    6. shapes the restoration
    7. removes undermined enamel

Questions 201–205
201. Ultrasonic scaler
202. Curette
203. Scaler
204. Periodontal probe
205. Pocket marker
    1. hand instrument used to remove supragingival calculus
    2. measures the distance between the gingiva and the bone
    3. a knife used to bevel the gingiva
    4. removes the crevicular epithelium
    5. reduces the height of bone
    6. punctures the gingiva at the base of a gingival pocket
    7. its vibrating movement knocks debris off teeth

Questions 206–210
206. Heatless stone
207. Rag wheel

208. Mandrel
209. Vulcanite bur
210. Rubber wheel
    1. smooths roughness in metals
    2. finishes composite restorations
    3. grossly reduces an acrylic prosthesis
    4. prevents ditching of amalgam restorations
    5. holds unmounted stones
    6. polishes acrylic prosthesis with pumice
    7. grossly reduces a metal prosthesis

Question 211–215
211. Bone file
212. Forceps
213. Straight elevator
214. Periosteal elevator
215. Rongeurs
    1. removes broken root tips
    2. extract teeth by rotation or luxation
    3. reflects tissue flaps
    4. reduces fractured bone edges
    5. extracts teeth by elevation
    6. smooths sharp bone edges
    7. removes bone with its nipping beaks

Questions 216–220
216. Burnisher
217. Orange stick
218. Pneumatic condenser
219. Articulator
220. Spoon excavator
    1. checks the adaptation of crowns
    2. welds gold foil
    3. helps seat crowns
    4. imitates oral movements
    5. removes pressure from edentulous areas
    6. hand instrument that removes decay
    7. adapts margins of restorations

Questions 221–225
221. Plastic instrument
222. Locking college pliers
223. Leather mallet
224. Chisel
225. Rim-lock tray
    1. helps seat crowns
    2. retracts the gingiva
    3. holds medicated cotton pledgets
    4. flushes debris from cavity preparation
    5. inserts composite filling material
    6. carries alginate impression material
    7. removes unsupported enamel

Questions 226–230
226. Bur 8
227. Bur 33
228. Bur 57
229. Bur 558
230. Bur ½

1. tapered fissure bur
2. cross-cut fissure bur
3. inverted cone bur
4. pointed diamond stone
5. small round bur
6. large round bur
7. finishing stone

Directions: MATCH the lettered illustrations in *Fig. 23* **with the corresponding questions.**

231. Identify the curette, periodontal probe, and syringe
    1. b, d, and f
    2. c, j, and n
    3. i, k, and m
    4. o, h, and a

232. Identify the interproximal knife, pocket marker, and locked college pliers
    1. c, g, and i
    2. e, j, and o
    3. g, k, and m
    4. l, m, and p

233. Identify the ronguers, scalpel, and topical anesthetic applicator
    1. c, j, and e
    2. i, l, and d
    3. m, f, and b
    4. o, k, and n

234. Identify the needle holder, periosteal elevator, and the bone chisel
    1. c, o, and m
    2. e, j, and k
    3. g, d, and h
    4. l, p, and n

Directions: MATCH the lettered illustrations in *Fig. 24* **with the corresponding questions.**

235. Identify the bunsen burner, dappen dish, and gold foil annealing tray
    1. e, g, and n
    2. l, j, and b
    3. m, l, and c
    4. r, p, and o

236. Identify the gold foil spring condenser, enamel hatchet, and straight enamel chisel
    1. c, f, and g
    2. e, l, and o
    3. h, j, and n
    4. g, m, and i

237. Identify the spoon excavator, stick compound, and gold foil condenser points
    1. k, b, and r
    2. f, n, and e
    3. j, a, and q
    4. g, i, and o

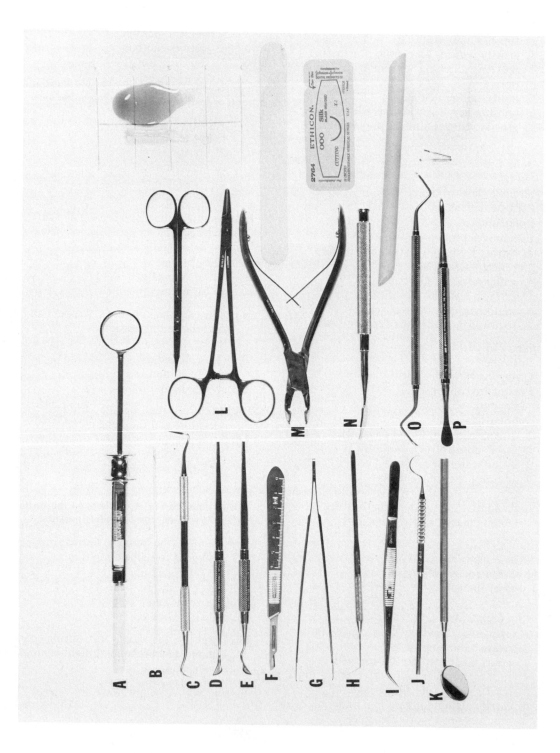

Fig. 23

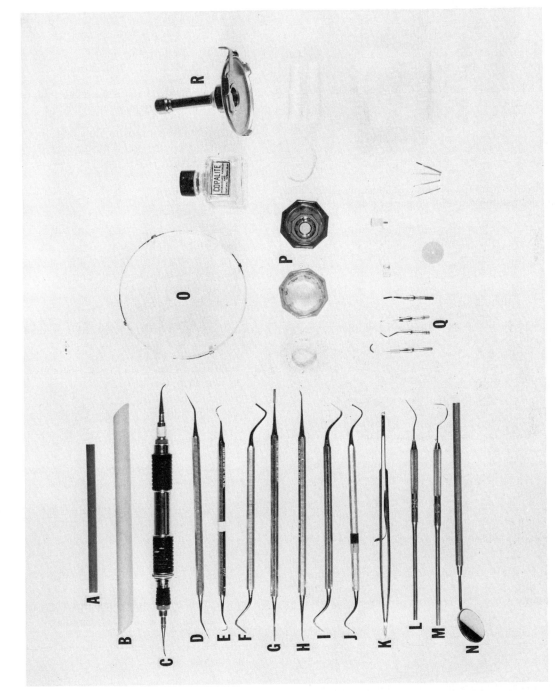

Fig. 24

Directions: MATCH the lettered illustrations in *Fig. 25* **with the corresponding questions.**

238. Identify the rubber dam clamps, endodontic explorer, and articulating paper and holder
 1. a, c, and f
 2. k, e, and b
 3. g, d, and j
 4. h, i, and c

239. Identify the culture tube, hemostat, and spoon excavator
 1. b, j, and e
 2. f, k, and c
 3. i, a, and d
 4. h, c, and f

Directions: MATCH the lettered illustrations in *Fig. 26* **with the corresponding questions.**

240. Identify the plastic instrument, stainless steel crowns, and spatula
 1. b, k, and c
 2. d, j, and g
 3. h, e, and k
 4. a, f, and b

241. Identify the base applicator, dappen dish, and locking pliers
 1. b, f, and h
 2. d, j, and g
 3. c, e, and a
 4. j, b, and e

Directions: MATCH the lettered illustrations in *Fig. 27* **with the corresponding questions.**

242. Identify the anterior rubber dam clamp, high volume evacuation tip, and rubber dam frame
 1. g, b, and f
 2. h, e, and d
 3. j, c, and a
 4. k, d, and b

243. Identify the rubber dam punch, rubber dam clamp forceps, and premolar rubber dam clamp
 1. a, f, and g
 2. b, c, and i
 3. c, d, and h
 4. e, a, and j

Directions: MATCH the lettered illustrations in *Fig. 28* **with the corresponding questions.**

244. Identify the orthodontic bands, band pusher, and ligature wire
 1. i, d, and a
 2. h, i, and f

 3. b, h, and d
 4. j, e, and h

245. Identify the band removing pliers, ligature cutters, and scaler
 1. a, d, and i
 2. b, c, and f
 3. d, h, and c
 4. e, b, and j

Directions: MATCH the lettered illustrations in *Fig. 29* **with the corresponding questions.**

246. Identify the composite finishing burs, composite matrices, and cotton pledgets
 1. i, m, and j
 2. e, d, and h
 3. c, g, and f
 4. m, b, and n

247. Identify the composite applicator, enamel hoe, and 17 explorer
 1. e, g, and j
 2. f, d, and k
 3. h, a, and i
 4. j, b, and e

Directions: MATCH the lettered illustrations in *Fig. 30* **with the corresponding questions.**

248. Identify the curette, plastic instrument, and crown shears
 1. e, d, and a
 2. f, b, and j
 3. g, f, and d
 4. h, g, and c

Directions: MATCH the lettered illustrations in *Fig. 31* **with the corresponding questions.**

249. Identify the vulcanite burs, rubber impressions syringe, and retraction cord
 1. a, b, and i
 2. d, c, and e
 3. h, g, and b
 4. i, a, and c

Directions: MATCH the lettered illustrations in *Fig. 32* **with the corresponding questions.**

250. Identify the wax spatula, copper bands, and peeso pliers
 1. d, g, and b
 2. e, d, and c
 3. g, h, and a
 4. h, b, and e

251. Identify the Baade pliers, bunsen burner, and stick compound
 1. a, g, and c

2. b, h, and i
3. c, f, and h
4. e, g, and f

Directions: MATCH the lettered illustrations in
***Fig. 33* with the corresponding question.**

252. Identify the tissue forceps, periosteal elevator, and suction tip
    1. a, b, and c
    2. a, d, and f
    3. b, e, and g
    4. c, d, and e

Directions: MATCH the lettered illustrations in
***Fig. 34* with the corresponding questions.**

253. Identify the needle holder, bone file, and syringe
    1. a, h, and l
    2. c, e, and f
    3. d, g, and k
    4. i, j, and l

254. Identify the curette, straight elevator, and tissue forceps
    1. b, c, and i
    2. k, c, and f
    3. e, h, and j
    4. g, i, and l

255. Identify the tissue tweezers, scissors, and scalpel
    1. j, i, and b
    2. d, g, and l
    3. e, h, and k
    4. f, k, and l

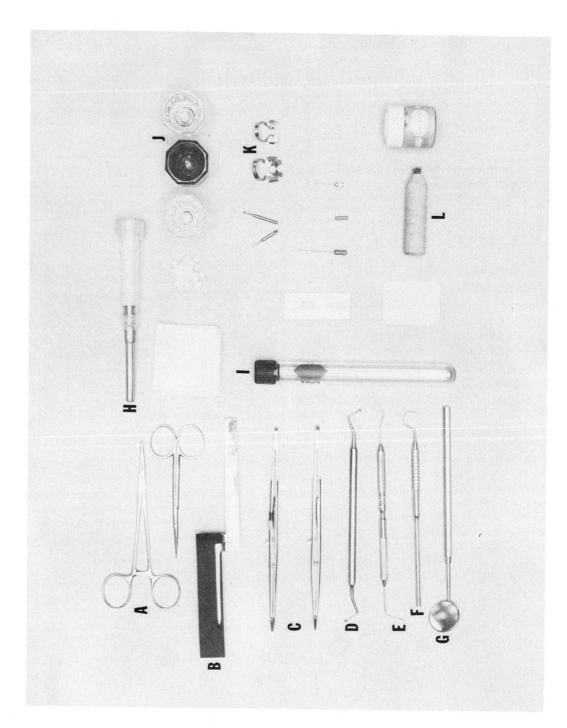

Fig. 25

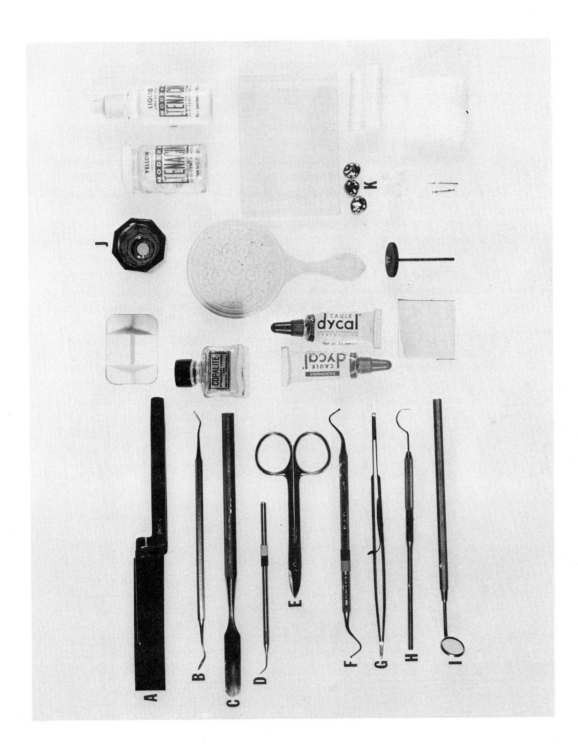

Fig. 26

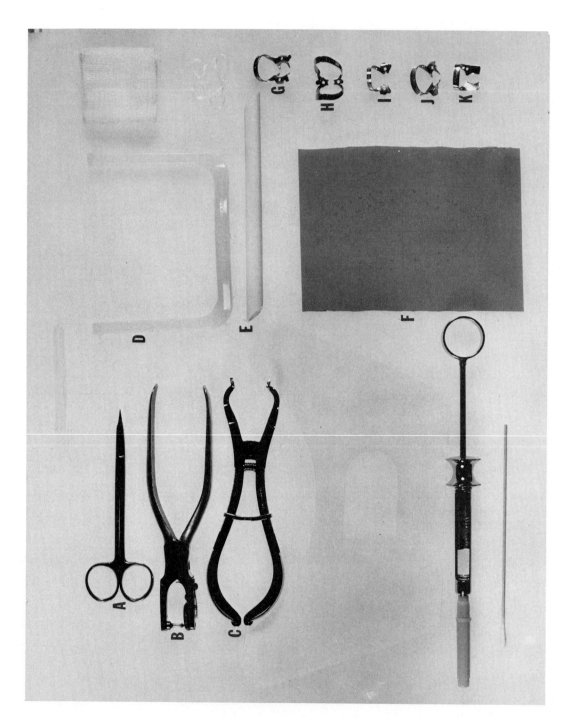

Fig. 27

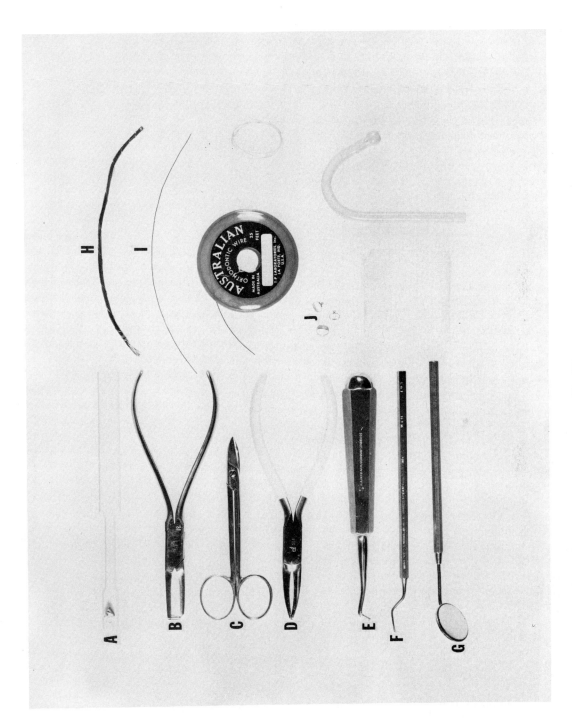

Fig. 28

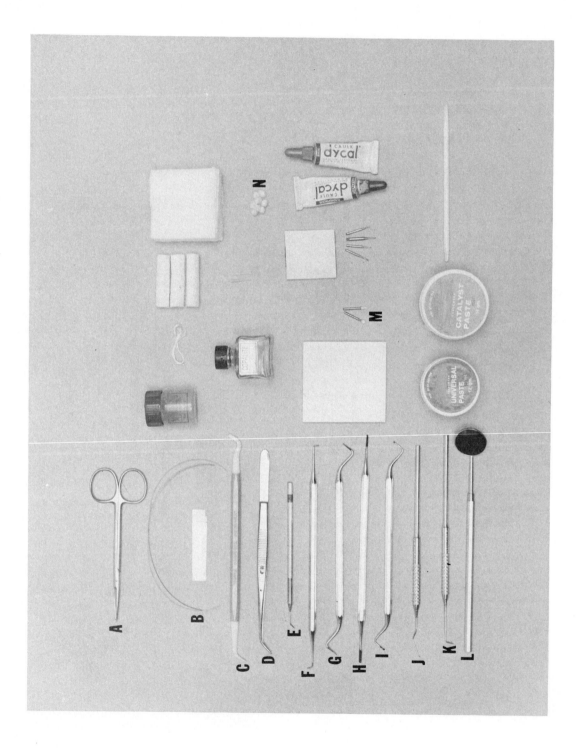

Fig. 29

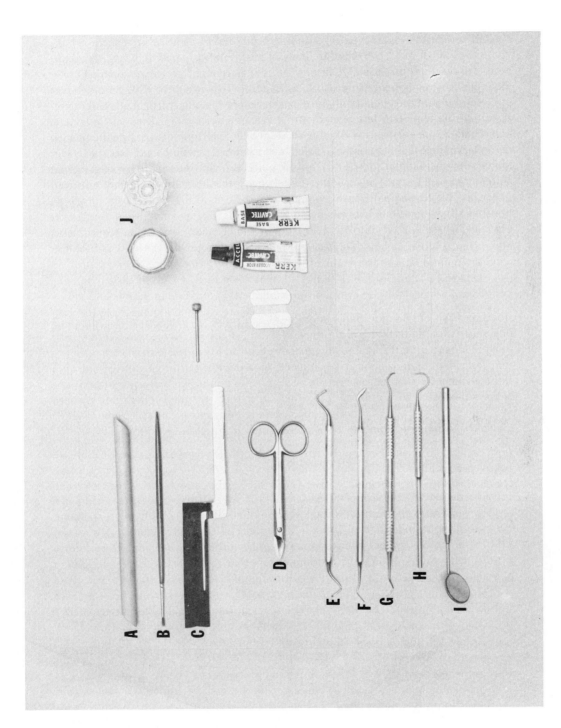

Fig. 30

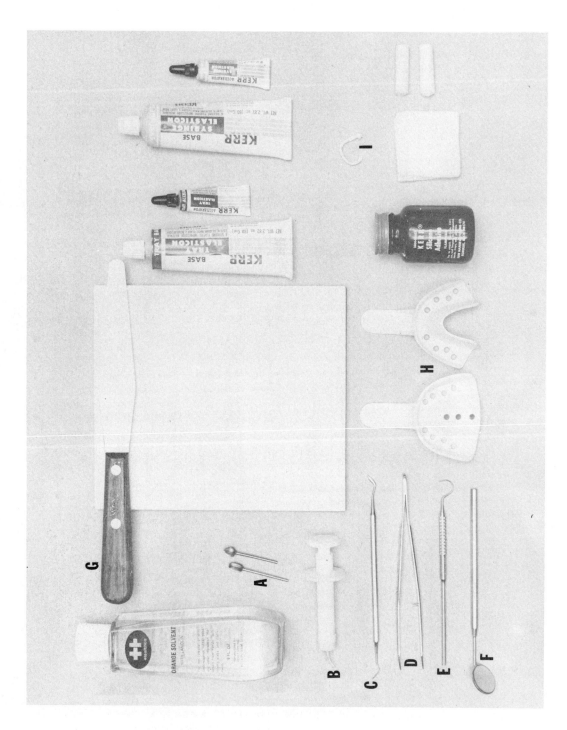

Fig. 31

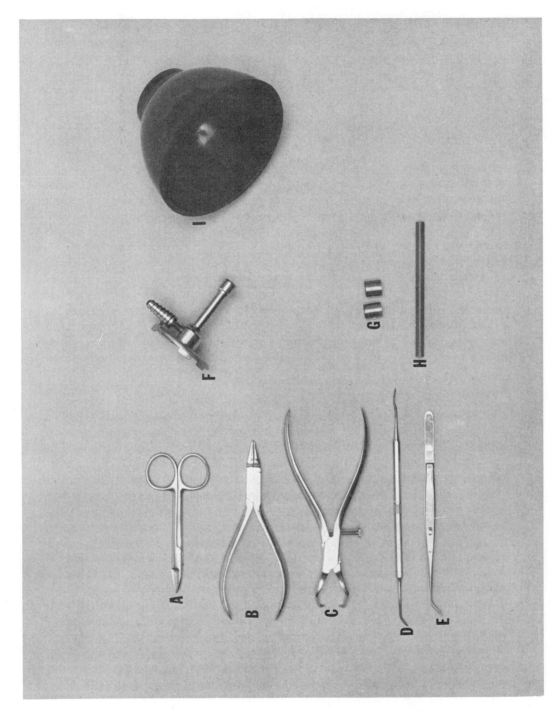

Fig. 32

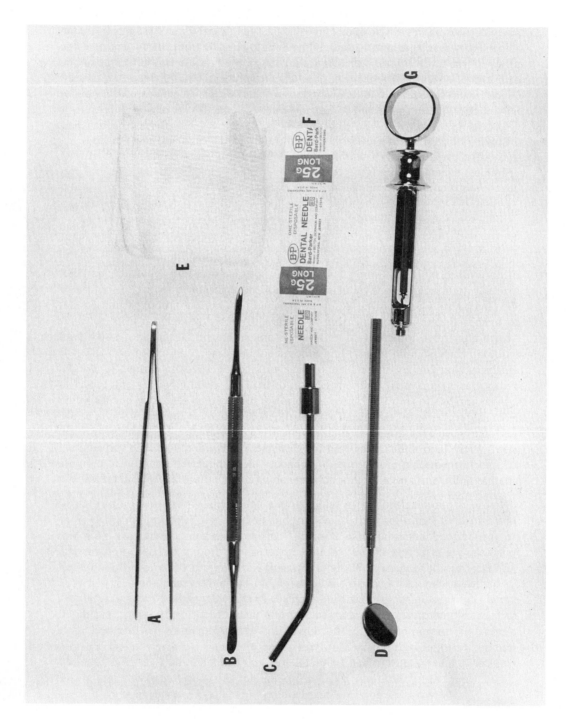

Fig. 33

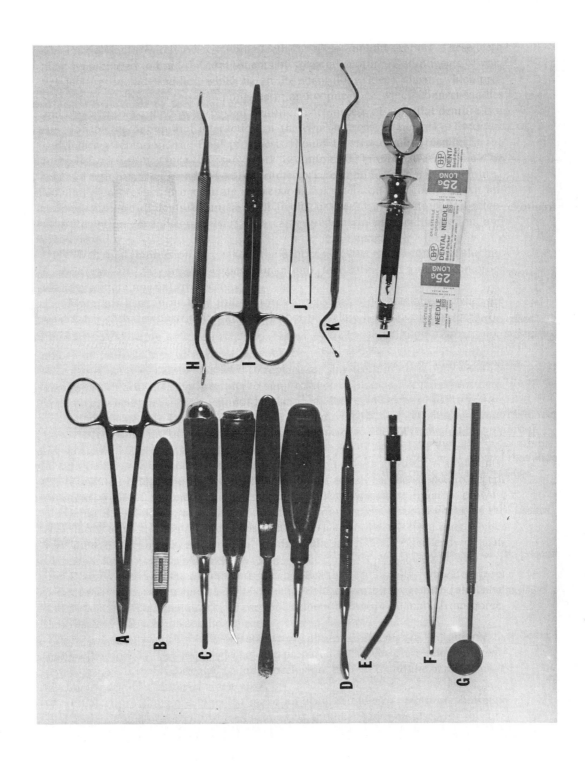

Fig. 34

Charting Exercises

Directions: To review charting, read each item in the charting exercise and record it on the given dental chart. Only refer to the dental chart you have completed when answering the charting questions. Do not write words when charting the given conditions. Use drawings and abbreviations when possible.

Charting Exercise 1

1. The maxillary right third molar is a mesioangular impaction.
2. The maxillary right first molar needs a full crown.
3. The maxillary right second premolar has a distal occlusal amalgam restoration present.
4. The maxillary right canine has a Class III mesial composite restoration present.
5. The maxillary right central incisor has a Class V buccal composite restoration present.
6. A maxillary mesiodens is exposed in the oral cavity.
7. The maxillary left central incisor has a distal incisal fracture and a periapical area.
8. The maxillary left lateral incisor has a Class III distal composite restoration that must be replaced.
9. There is a fixed bridge between the maxillary left canine and the maxillary left second premolar to replace the first premolar.
10. The maxillary left third molar is missing.
11. There is a mandibular removable partial denture replacing the right first, second, and third molars and the left first, second, and third molars.
12. The mandibular left first premolar has a mesial occlusal amalgam restoration present and must be replaced.
13. The mandibular left lateral incisor has a Class IV mesial incisal composite restoration present.
14. The mandibular right canine has a Class V buccal gold foil restoration present.
15. The mandibular right second premolar has a full crown present.

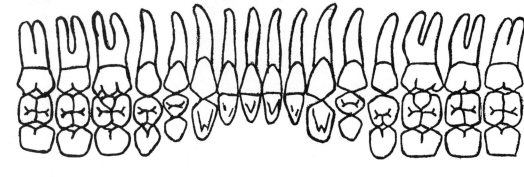

Left

Right

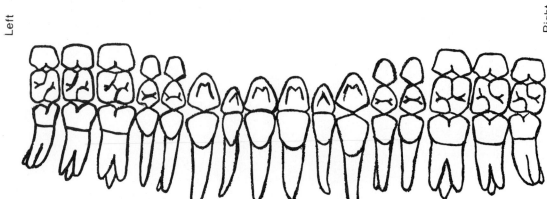

Questions 256–265 (Charting Exercise 1)

256. How many teeth are missing?
    1. 2
    2. 4
    3. 6
    4. 8

257. How many teeth need restorations?
    1. 2
    2. 4
    3. 6
    4. 8

258. How many teeth have existing restorations?
    1. 2
    2. 6
    3. 10
    4. 14

259. Which tooth is impacted?
    1. maxillary right third molar
    2. maxillary left third molar
    3. mandibular right third molar
    4. a mesiodent

260. What is the classification of the restoration in the lower left lateral incisor?
    1. Class I
    2. Class II
    3. Class III
    4. Class IV

261. What condition exists on the upper right second premolar?
    1. a crown is needed
    2. a distal occlusal amalgam is present
    3. a gold foil is present
    4. the tooth is missing

262. A supernumerary tooth is present between the
    1. maxillary left canine and left second premolar
    2. maxillary central incisors
    3. mandibular central incisors
    4. maxillary right lateral incisor and right central incisor

263. How many restorations must be replaced?
    1. 2
    2. 4
    3. 6
    4. 8

264. Which tooth has a periapical area?
    1. maxillary right canine
    2. maxillary left central incisor
    3. mandibular left canine
    4. mandibular right second premolar

265. Which tooth is fractured?
    1. maxillary right canine
    2. maxillary left central incisor
    3. mandibular left canine
    4. mandibular right second premolar

Charting Exercise 2

1. The maxillary right third molar has distal occlusal decay.
2. The maxillary right second molar has a mesial amalgam restoration present.
3. The maxillary right first premolar has a Class V buccal composite restoration present.
4. The maxillary right canine has a Class III mesial composite restoration which must be replaced.
5. The maxillary left central incisor has a full crown present.
6. There is a fixed bridge between the maxillary left canine and the maxillary left first molar replacing the maxillary left first and second premolars.
7. The maxillary left third molar is vertically impacted.
8. The mandibular left second molar is missing.
9. The mandibular left first molar has a mesial occlusal distal amalgam restoration present.
10. The mandibular left first premolar has a Class V buccal gold foil restoration present and distal occlusal decay.
11. The mandibular left lateral incisor has a Class IV mesial incisal composite restoration present.
12. The mandibular left central incisor has Class IV mesial decay.
13. The mandibular right central incisor is fractured midway down the crown.
14. The mandibular right second premolar has a mesial occlusal distal amalgam restoration present.
15. The mandibular right second molar has a mesial occlusal amalgam restoration present with recurrent decay around the margins.
16. The mandibular right third molar is to be extracted.

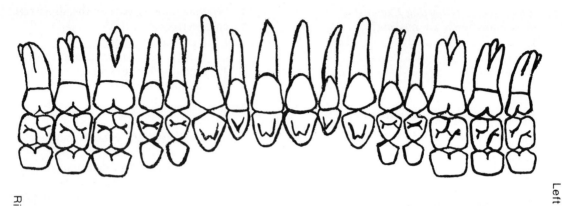

Right

Left

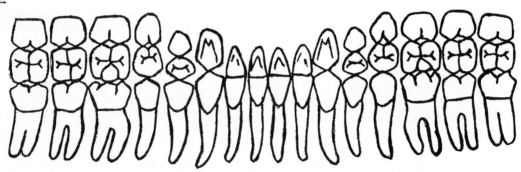

Questions 266–276 (Charting Exercise 2)

266. How many teeth are missing?
    1. 1
    2. 3
    3. 5
    4. 7

267. How many teeth need restorations?
    1. 2
    2. 4
    3. 6
    4. 8

268. How many teeth have existing restorations?
    1. 2
    2. 6
    3. 10
    4. 14

269. Which tooth is to be extracted?
    1. maxillary left third molar
    2. mandibular left second molar
    3. mandibular left central incisor
    4. mandibular right third molar

270. How many teeth are replaced with a fixed bridge?
    1. 1
    2. 2

    3. 3
    4. 4

271. What restoration exists on the mandibular left first premolar?
    1. a composite restoration
    2. an amalgam restoration
    3. a gold foil restoration
    4. a full crown

272. How many amalgam restorations are present?
    1. 2
    2. 4
    3. 6
    4. 8

273. What classification of restoration is needed on the maxillary right canine?
    1. Class I
    2. Class II
    3. Class III
    4. Class IV

274. How many teeth need distal occlusal restorations?
    1. 1
    2. 2
    3. 3
    4. 4

275. Which tooth is fractured?
    1. maxillary right central incisor
    2. maxillary left third molar
    3. mandibular left lateral incisor
    4. mandibular right central incisor

276. How many composite restorations exist?
    1. 1
    2. 2
    3. 3
    4. 4

Charting Exercise 3

1. The maxillary right third molar has mesial occlusal decay.
2. The maxillary right second molar has a distal occlusal amalgam restoration present.
3. There is a maxillary removable partial denture replacing the right and left first and second premolars.
4. The maxillary right lateral incisor is restored with a porcelain jacket.
5. The maxillary right central incisor has Class I lingual decay.
6. The maxillary left canine has a Class III mesial composite restoration present.
7. The maxillary left first molar has Class V buccal decay.
8. The maxillary left second molar is not present.
9. The mandibular left third molar is a distoangular impaction.
10. There is a fixed bridge between the mandibular left second molar and the mandibular left first premolar replacing the second premolar and the first molar.
11. The mandibular left central incisor has a Class III mesial composite restoration which must be replaced.
12. The mandibular right lateral incisor has a fractured mesial incisal angle.
13. The mandibular right second premolar has a distal occlusal inlay restoration present.
14. The mandibular right second molar has a Class V lingual amalgam restoration present.

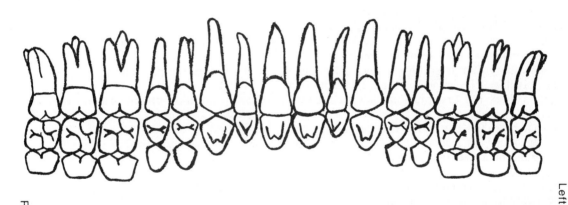

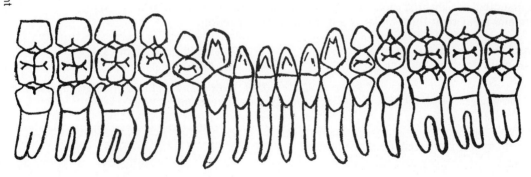

Right

Left

Questions 277–285 (Charting Exercise 3)
277. How many teeth are missing?
    1. 1
    2. 3
    3. 5
    4. 7

278. How many teeth need restorations?
    1. 1
    2. 3
    3. 5
    4. 7

279. How many teeth have existing restorations?
    1. 2
    2. 4
    3. 6
    4. 8

280. The mandibular right second premolar has a(n)
    1. amalgam restoration
    2. gold inlay
    3. carious lesion
    4. defective restoration

281. How many teeth are replaced by the removable partial denture?
    1. 2
    2. 4
    3. 6
    4. 8

282. How many Class V carious lesions are present?
    1. 1

    2. 2
    3. 3
    4. 4

283. How many teeth are replaced by fixed bridgework?
    1. 1
    2. 2
    3. 3
    4. 4

284. Which tooth has a restoration that must be replaced?
    1. maxillary right third molar
    2. mandibular left third molar
    3. mandibular left central incisor
    4. mandibular right lateral incisor

285. What exists on the maxillary left canine?
    1. mesial Class III composite restoration
    2. lingual Class I carious lesion
    3. buccal Class V carious lesion
    4. mesial incisal composite restoration

Charting Exercise 4

1. The maxillary right third molar has Class V buccal decay.
2. The maxillary right second molar has distal occlusal decay.
3. There is a cantilever bridge to replace the maxillary right first premolar. The maxillary right first molar and the maxillary right second premolar are the abutments.
4. The maxillary right lateral has a Class III mesial composite restoration present.
5. The maxillary left canine has Class III distal decay.
6. The maxillary left first premolar has an occlusal amalgam restoration present which has recurrent decay.
7. The maxillary left first molar needs a full crown.
8. The maxillary left second molar has a mesial occlusal inlay restoration present.
9. The mandibular left first premolar is missing.
10. The mandibular left canine has a periapical area.
11. A lower removable partial denture replaces the four mandibular incisors. .
12. The mandibular right canine has a periapical area.
13. The mandibular right second premolar has mesial occlusal decay.
14. The mandibular right first molar has a distal occlusal amalgam restoration present.
15. The mandibular right third molar is a mesioangular impaction.

Questions 286–295 (Charting Exercise 4)

286. How many teeth are missing?
    1. 2
    2. 4
    3. 6
    4. 8

287. How many maxillary teeth need restoration?
    1. 1
    2. 3
    3. 5
    4. 7

288. Which tooth needs root canal therapy?
    1. maxillary left canine
    2. mandibular left first premolar

    3. mandibular right canine
    4. mandibular right third molar

289. How many surfaces of amalgam restorations are present?
    1. 1
    2. 2
    3. 3
    4. 4

290. What condition is present on the mandibular left canine?
    1. gold inlay
    2. gold foil
    3. composite
    4. buccal Class V carious lesion

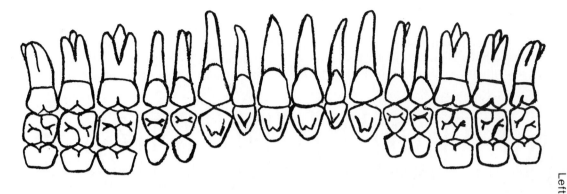

Right

Left

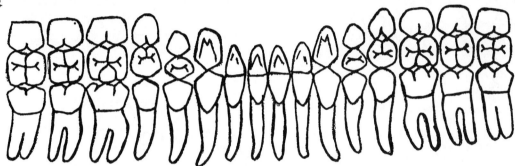

291. Which tooth is replaced by a pontic?
1. maxillary right first molar
2. maxillary right first premolar
3. maxillary right second premolar
4. maxillary left first molar

292. What is the position of the impacted tooth?
1. mesioangular
2. distoangular
3. vertical
4. inverted

293. Which tooth has a restoration that must be replaced?
1. maxillary right second molar
2. maxillary left canine

3. maxillary left first premolar
4. mandibular right first molar

294. A Class III composite exists on which tooth?
1. maxillary right lateral incisor
2. maxillary left canine
3. mandibular left canine
4. mandibular right canine

295. What condition exists on the maxillary right third molar?
1. impaction
2. distal occlusal amalgam restoration
3. mesial occlusal caries
4. Class V buccal caries

Charting Exercise 5

1. The maxillary right third molar has occlusal decay.
2. The maxillary right first molar has a mesial occlusal distal amalgam restoration present.
3. The maxillary right second premolar is missing.
4. The maxillary right canine has a Class III distal restoration present.
5. The maxillary right central incisor has Class V buccal decay.
6. The maxillary left central incisor has a Class IV mesial composite restoration present.
7. There is a fixed bridge between the left canine and the first molar replacing the first and second premolars.
8. The maxillary left second molar has a mesial occlusal amalgam restoration present which must be replaced.
9. The mandibular left third molar is a mesial angular impaction.

10. The mandibular left first molar needs a full crown.
11. The mandibular left first premolar has a full crown present.
12. The mandibular left lateral incisor has a Class V buccal gold foil restoration present.
13. The mandibular right first premolar has distal occlusal decay.
14. The mandibular right first molar has Class V lingual decay.
15. The mandibular right third molar has a mesial occlusal amalgam restoration present.

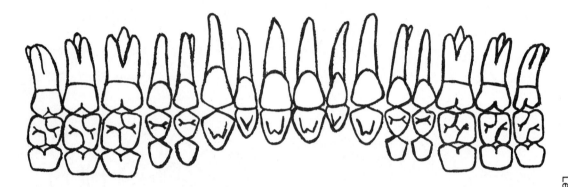

Right

Left

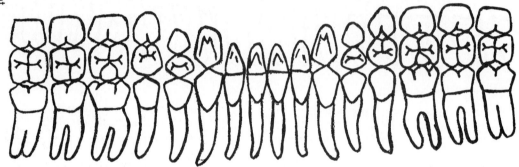

Questions 296–304 (Charting Exercise 5)

296. How many teeth are missing?
    1. 1
    2. 3
    3. 5
    4. 7

297. How many surfaces of restorations are needed in the maxillary arch?
    1. 2
    2. 4
    3. 6
    4. 8

298. What condition exists on the maxillary left central incisor?
    1. buccal Class V decay
    2. gold foil
    3. mesial incisal composite restoration
    4. mesial Class III caries

299. How many surfaces of amalgam restorations are present?
    1. 1
    2. 3
    3. 5
    4. 7

300. Which tooth needs a full crown restoration?
    1. maxillary left second molar
    2. mandibular left third molar
    3. mandibular left first molar
    4. mandibular right first molar

301. Which tooth has a restoration that must be replaced?
    1. maxillary right canine
    2. maxillary left second molar
    3. mandibular left lateral incisor
    4. mandibular right first molar

302. Which cavity classification exists on the mandibular right first molar?
    1. Class I
    2. Class II
    3. Class IV
    4. Class V

303. How many teeth are replaced by the maxillary fixed bridge?
    1. 1
    2. 2
    3. 3
    4. 4

304. How many teeth need restorations in the mandibular arch?
    1. 1
    2. 2
    3. 3
    4. 4

Charting Exercise 6

1. The maxillary right third molar has mesial occlusal distal decay.
2. The maxillary right second molar has a Class V buccal amalgam restoration present.
3. The maxillary right first premolar is missing.
4. The maxillary right canine has a Class III distal composite restoration present.
5. There is a fixed bridge between the maxillary right lateral incisor and the maxillary left canine replacing the two central incisors.
6. The maxillary left second premolar needs a full crown.
7. The maxillary left first molar has a mesial occlusal distal amalgam restoration present.
8. The maxillary left third molar should be extracted.
9. There is a mandibular removable partial denture replacing the mandibular left first, second and third molars and the right first molar.
10. The mandibular left second premolar has a full crown present.
11. The mandibular left central incisor has Class IV distal incisal decay.
12. The mandibular right central incisor has a Class V buccal composite restoration present.
13. The mandibular right second molar has a mesial occlusal amalgam restoration present which must be replaced.
14. The mandibular right third molar is vertically impacted.

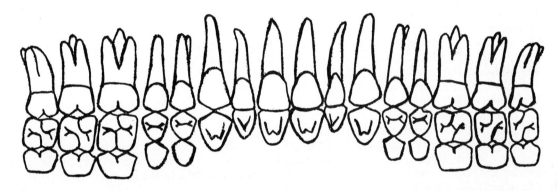

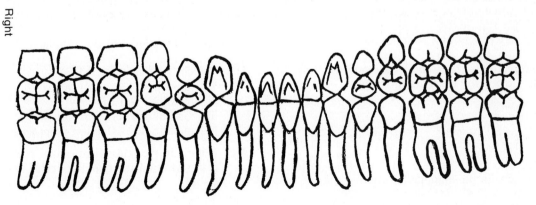

Right

Left

Questions 305–312 (Charting Exercise 6)

305. How many teeth are replaced?
    1. 2
    2. 4
    3. 6
    4. 8

306. How many surfaces of amalgam restorations are present?
    1. 2
    2. 4
    3. 6
    4. 8

307. What is the position of the impacted molar?
    1. mesioangular
    2. distoangular
    3. vertical
    4. horizontal

308. What condition exists on the mandibular left second premolar?
    1. full crown
    2. gold inlay
    3. gold foil
    4. amalgam restoration

309. How many surfaces need restorations in the mandibular arch?
    1. 2
    2. 4
    3. 6
    4. 7

310. Which tooth is to be extracted?
    1. maxillary right third molar
    2. maxillary left third molar
    3. mandibular left third molar
    4. mandibular right third molar

311. How many surfaces of composite restorations are present?
    1. 1
    2. 2
    3. 3
    4. 4

312. Which tooth needs a crown?
    1. maxillary right first premolar
    2. maxillary left second premolar
    3. mandibular left second premolar
    4. mandibular right first molar

Charting Exercise 7

1. The maxillary right third molar is missing.
2. There is a fixed bridge between the maxillary right first premolar and the maxillary right second molar. The maxillary right second premolar and first molar are missing.
3. The maxillary right lateral incisor has a Class III mesial composite restoration present.
4. The maxillary right central incisor has Class III distal decay.
5. The maxillary left canine has a porcelain jacket.
6. The maxillary left second premolar has distal occlusal decay.
7. The maxillary left second molar has a mesial occlusal distal amalgam restoration present.
8. The mandibular left third molar is vertically impacted.
9. The mandibular left first molar has mesial occlusal decay.
10. The mandibular left first premolar has Class V buccal decay.
11. There is a fixed bridge between the mandibular left canine and the mandibular right canine; the mandibular left central and lateral and the mandibular right central and lateral are missing.
12. The mandibular right first premolar is not present.
13. The mandibular right second molar has a mesial occlusal distal amalgam restoration which must be replaced.
14. There is a 14-mm periodontal pocket between the maxillary left second and third molars.

Questions 313–322 (Charting Exercise 7)

313. How many teeth are missing?
    1. 2
    2. 4
    3. 6
    4. 8

314. How many surfaces of teeth need restorations in the mandibular arch?
    1. 2
    2. 4
    3. 6
    4. 8

315. Which tooth is impacted?
    1. maxillary right third molar
    2. maxillary left canine
    3. mandibular left third molar
    4. mandibular right first premolar

316. What is the classification of the cavity restoration on the maxillary right lateral incisor?
    1. Class I
    2. Class II
    3. Class III
    4. Class V

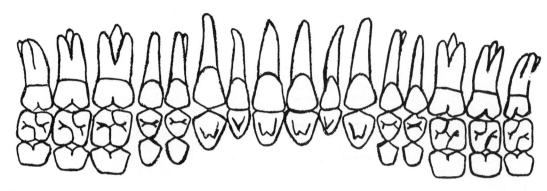

Right

Left

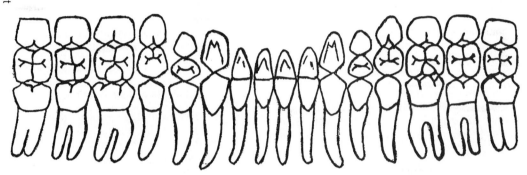

317. How many surfaces of amalgam restorations are present in the maxillary and mandibular arches?
    1. 2
    2. 4
    3. 6
    4. 8

318. Where is the periodontal pocket located?
    1. between the maxillary right second and third molars
    2. between the maxillary left second and third molars
    3. distal to the mandibular left first molar
    4. between the mandibular right canine and second premolar

319. Which teeth are abutments for a fixed bridge in the mandibular arch?
    1. mandibular right and left canines
    2. mandibular right canine and second premolar

3. mandibular left canine and first premolar
    4. mandibular lateral incisors

320. What condition exists on the maxillary left canine?
    1. full gold crown
    2. porcelain jacket
    3. three-quarter crown
    4. gold inlay

321. Which tooth has a restoration that must be replaced?
    1. maxillary left central incisor
    2. maxillary left second molar
    3. mandibular right second molar
    4. mandibular right third molar

322. What condition exists on the mandibular left first premolar
    1. Class I caries
    2. Class V buccal caries
    3. Class V buccal composite
    4. Class V lingual caries

Answers and Explanations

1. **4** Knowledge of the patient's medical and dental history can affect the treatment plan, prognosis, drugs prescribed, treatment of a medical emergency, and frequency and length of appointments.

2. **1** Patients with a history of rheumatic fever are usually prophylactically given antibiotics before dental treament. The purpose is to avoid the possibility of the patient succumbing to bacterial endocarditis as a result of bacteria being introduced into the bloodstream during the dental procedure.

3. **2** Short appointments are given to patients who, for either physical or mental reasons, should not be stressed by long dental appointments. Some of these patients have mental disorders, heart problems, and/or respiratory problems.

4. **3** Chronic respiratory problems affect the positioning of the patient. These patients find breathing easier when they are seated in an upright position.

5. **3** The modified Snyder test is a colormetric test of the amount of acid-producing bacteria in the saliva. This test is an indicator of the patient's caries susceptibility.

6. **2** The immediate objective when treating patients in pain is to relieve the pain.

7. **2** A complete oral examination should take place each time the patient is recalled. Individual patient requirements dictate the length of time between recall visits.

8. **2** A thorough dental examination should be standardized to prevent overlooking any pathology. An example of the sequence of the examination might be soft tissue, occlusal relationship, radiographs, and individual teeth.

9. **3** Some reasons for an anticipated increase in the demand for dental services are increased third-party payment by insurance companies and the federal government, increased public education due to mass media, increased advertising by dentists and companies dealing in dental health products, and the increased socioeconomic level of the population.

10. **4** Possible solutions for the anticipated increase in demand are increased use of preventive measures, increased use of assistants by dentists trained in dental auxiliary utilization, research in

anticariogentic drugs, increased number of dental schools, and increased size of the existing dental schools.

11. **1** The maximum amount of time can be saved by eliminating a procedure. If a patient spends 10 minutes an hour to rinse, high-speed evacuation can eliminate the need to rinse. The operating team would then gain 10 minutes each hour.

12. **2** Benefits of using premeasured and prepackaged materials are assurance of correct proportioning, therefore receiving the optimum properties of materials, and saving the time needed for measuring. The disadvantage is the increased cost.

13. **2** Advantages of disposable materials are saving time in cleaning, assurance of sharp needles, and scalpel blades and sterilization.

14. **2** Benefits of tray setups are that they save time when setting up, eliminate delay in searching for instruments during a procedure, adapt to any procedure, can be set up by anyone in the office, and are easily stored.

15. **2** Color coding trays allows easy identification of the procedure the tray is prepared for (e.g., blue tray for amalgam restoration, white tray for prophylaxis).

16. **1** Hand instruments are placed on the prepared tray in their order of use and on the side of the tray closest to the patient. After a hand instrument is used it is replaced in its original position.

17. **4** Randomly prepared tray setups can cause the assistant to search the tray for any instrument or supply needed, and get up to get a missing instrument in the middle of a procedure. A patient's impression of the office may be influenced by the disorderliness of the tray and the subsequent problems it causes.

18. **3** The best position of the instrument tray is over the assistant's lap.

19. **4** In the administration of local anesthesia, empathy, understanding, and a gentle technique used by the dental team are invaluable in helping to decrease the patient's anxiety.

20. **3** The anesthetic syringe should be prepared before the patient is seated in order for it to be ready for immediate use. Any instruments or materials that are prepared will save valuable patient chair time.

21. **2** The assistant prepares the syringe by placing the carpule in the syringe, placing the needle on the syringe, engaging the stylet in the rubber plunger of the carpule, loosening the needle cover and testing the syringe to be sure the anesthetic comes out.

22. **1** After the assistant has passed the syringe to the operator, he or she removes the needle cover and rotates the bevel of the needle so it will be parallel to the mandible when the anesthetic is injected. This avoids tearing the periosteum, which can cause postoperative pain.

23. **3** The purpose of aspiration is to find out if the lumen of the needle is in a blood vessel. If blood is aspirated the needle is moved to another location before the local anesthetic is deposited.

24. **4** Most handpieces and the air–water syringes are run by compressed air. Compressed air is produced in the dental office by an air compressor.

25. **3** The high-speed handpiece can revolve up to 250,000 rpm. The low-speed handpiece works at variable speeds from 1 to 30,000 rpm.

26. **3** The best coolant when using the high-speed handpiece is cool water. A coolant is used to dissipate the heat produced by the rapidly revolving bur and avoid damage to the pulpal tissues.

27. **1** As indicated in the manufacturer's directions on maintenance, the high-speed handpiece should be cleaned and lubricated daily for optimum use and long mechanical life.

28. **4** Patients might wish to rinse for the following reasons: to delay treatment (especially true of young patients), to rid themselves of pooling fluids or solids (caused by poorly positioned or inadequate suction), to refresh their mouths after treatment (often after treatment is completed patients have a foul taste and a desire to eliminate it by rinsing), to refresh their mouths before treatment (thinking they have foul-smelling breath), and to take a break during treatment.

29. **4** High-speed evacuation will decrease the patient's desire to rinse because there will be no pooling of fluids or any solid material remaining in the patient's mouth. It decreases the amount of bacteria-laden aerosol emanating from the patient's mouth and increases visibility by keeping the operating field clear of water and debris.

30. **3** The assistant, when working with a right-handed operator, holds the suction tip in the right hand with a thumb-to-nose grasp. For finer tactile sense, the assistant may hold the suction tip in a grasp in which all the fingertips are on the tip.

31. **3** The suction tip is placed posteriorly at the occlusal height, parallel to the buccal or lingual surface and as close as possible to the tooth being prepared.

32. **2** When working in the anterior area of the mouth, the suction tip is placed on the opposite side of the tooth being prepared, and parallel to the labial or lingual surface of the tooth being prepared. The lumen should bisect the incisal edge of the tooth being prepared.

33. **2** An assistant can increase the operator's visibility by using high-speed suction to keep the operating field clear, using the air–water syringe to keep the field clear and the operator's mirror clean, retracting soft tissues such as the tongue and cheek, and adjusting the operating light to better illuminate the operating field.

34. **1** When working on the lower right molars, the operator is in the 9 o'clock position, and the assistant retracts the tongue as the operator retracts the right cheek. The operator working on the lower left quadrant retracts the tongue while the assistant retracts the left cheek.

35. **2** Indirect vision refers to seeing by looking into a mirror. Often dental work must be accomplished in this manner because of the shape and location of structures in the oral cavity. Direct vision refers to seeing without the use of a mirror.

36. **1** All work surfaces should be located 2 inches below the elbow.

37. **4** The front edge of the assistant's chair should be even with the patient's mouth. The side of the assistant's chair should be in contact with the patient's chair.

38. **4** The assistant's eye level is 4–6 inches above the dentist's eye level. This permits the assistant to have maximum visibility of the operating field and not interfere with the dentist's visibility.

39. **1** The assistant's chair should have five castors for stability, a padded seat for comfort, a foot rest, an easily adjustable control, and a wraparound arm in front and to the left of the assistant. This area will be located beneath the rib cage; it offers support when the assistant leans over the operating field.

40. **2** When seated in working position the patient's calves are parallel to the floor when working on either the mandibular or maxillary arches.

41. **4** The position of the patient's back depends on the arch being treated. If the maxillary arch is being treated the back of the chair is usually parallel to the floor. If the mandibular arch is being treated the back of the chair is usually at an angle of 25 degrees from the floor.

42. **4** The patient's head should be positioned at the very end of the chair and as close to the operator's side of the chair as possible. This will allow the operator to work on the patient without leaning over the patient's chair.

43. **3** A patient in the supine positioni is capable of swallowing saliva that pools in the back of the mouth.

44. **3** If a patient jumps out of the chair after being treated in a supine position he or she will not have an opportunity to regain circulatory equilibrium. This can cause fainting due to lack of blood to the brain.

45. **3** If the operator is seated at the eleven o'clock position and the patient is seated upright, the operator will not have direct vision to see any teeth.

46. **2** The operator signals for an instrument transfer by a fingers only movement (Class I movement). The operator retains his or her finger rest and moves his or her fingers, holding the instrument being used away from the operating field. The assistant then grasps the instrument and replaces it with the next instrument to be used.

47. **3** The straight chisel is used in a palm–thumb grasp. Considerable power can be generated using this grasp and proper precautions should be taken to prevent injury to the patient.

48. **1** The high-speed handpiece is used in a pen grasp. This instrument is used with brushstroke motions.

49. **2** When working with a right-handed dentist, the assistant transfers instruments with the left hand and holds the high-speed suction tip in the right hand.

50. **1** Hand instruments and handpieces are transferred at the patient's mouth.

51. **1** Double-handled instruments (e.g., rubber dam forceps, extraction forceps, scissors) and the anesthetic syringe are transferred beneath the patient's chin.

52. **1** When transferring an instrument, the assistant holds it between the thumb and forefinger, parallel to the instrument being used, close to the operating field, and opposite the working end, which is pointed toward the surface at which it will be used.

53. **2** The assistant retrieves the operator's hand instruments with the small finger. Almost all instruments, including handpieces, can be retrieved in this manner.

54. **4** Materials should be mixed just before use and be brought as close to the area of operation as possible. This will minimize the motion necessary for the operator to obtain these materials.

55. **3** Some benefits of using a rubber dam are that it permits optimum use of dental materials due to the elimination of moisture; keeps debris out of the patient's mouth; retracts the tongue and cheek, thereby allowing better visibility and protection to these tissues; avoids the problem of rinsing; stops the patient from talking; prevents the patient from swallowing endodontic instruments; and prevents contamination of pulpal tissue by oral fluids.

56. **2** When placing a rubber dam, an explorer or plastic instrument may be used to invert the dam around the teeth being prepared. Inversion of the dam places the free edge of the dam into the gingival sulcus and thereby prevents the bur from cutting the dam during tooth preparation.

57. **3** The rubber dam napkin is used to avoid irritation around the patient's mouth by absorbing fluids and avoiding direct contact of the rubber dam with the patient's face.

58. **4** A lubricant can be placed around the holes punched in the rubber dam to facilitate the placement of the rubber dam between the teeth. A lubricant can also be used at the corners of the patient's mouth, to help avoid irritation.

59. **4** During the application of a rubber dam, dental floss may be used to help secure the dam (by tying the floss around the most anterior tooth being isolated), force the dam between the teeth being isolated, invert the dam around the teeth being prepared, and serve as a safety string on the rubber dam clamp so that it can be retrieved if swallowed or aspirated.

60. **4** When placing a rubber dam anteriorly all silicate restorations must be protected with a lubricant to avoid desiccation. Silicate restorations, when desiccated, become more opaque and unesthetic.

61. **3** The two ways to diagnose carious lesions are clinically and radiographically. Bite-wing radiographs are the radiograph of choice to diagnose caries on the proximal surfaces of teeth. A sharp explorer is used to determine caries clinically.

62. **3** Recurrent caries refers to carious lesions around the margins of existing restorations. If such caries occur, additional tooth structure is lost from the caries and subsequent restorative process.

63. **2** Carious lesions are not self-limiting and if they are not restored they will progress to involve the pulpal tissues. Pulpal tissues invaded by carious lesions are irreversibly damaged and the tooth will require root canal therapy if it is to be retained.

64. **2** Class II cavity preparations include the occlusal and one or two proximal surfaces of premolars and molars.

65. **4** Class V cavity preparations are located in the gingival third of the facial or lingual surfaces of all teeth.

66. **4** Class IV cavity preparations involve the proximal surface and the incisal angle of incisors and canines.

67. **3** A cavity preparation that involves the mesial or distal surface of an anterior tooth is classified as a Class III cavity preparation.

68. **1** A cavity preparation which involves the buccal pit of a lower molar is classified as a Class I cavity preparation.

69. **3** The toilet of the cavity preparation refers to cleaning and drying the preparation. This is accomplished by washing the preparation with water or hydrogen peroxide followed by drying the preparation with intermittent blasts of air.

70. **1** The mesial surface of the upper first premolar is often visible when a patient smiles; therefore, it can present an esthetic problem if it is restored with amalgam.

71. **4** A fulcrum is the stationary point of a lever. Examples of fulcrums in dentistry are the condyle of the mandible and the finger rests on a tooth during instrumentation.

72. **1** The rubber dam is removed after condensation of a Class II amalgam preparation in order to check the patient's occlusion.

73. **2** Burnishers are not used to evaluate amalgam restorations. They are used to adapt restorative materials, such as amalgam and gold foil, to the margins of the cavity preparation.

74. **3** The spoon excavator is a stainless steel hand cutting instrument. It is used to remove decay from teeth and not for the placement of amalgam.

75. **1** A wooden wedge is used to prevent gingival amalgam overhang by securing the gingival portion of the matrix band against the tooth, stop interproximal bleeding by applying direct pressure, and separate teeth by wedging action.

76. **2** Amalgam is first placed in the proximal box of a Class II cavity preparation. If the occlusal portion of the cavity preparation were filled first, it would be very difficult to gain access to the proximal box.

77. **2** Factors which determine instrument selection for restorative procedures are the tooth and the surface being prepared, and the type of restoration being placed.

78. **4** A bevel is a sloping surface. In dentistry, bevels are used for cavity preparation, hand cutting instruments and the ends of needles.

79. **2** When preparing a cavity preparation on the buccal surface of the maxillary third molar there is usually little room to operate and a miniature head on a handpiece is useful. The anatomic restrictions in this area include the cheek and the ramus of the mandible.

80. **3** A steady stream of warm air may desiccate the dentin and be injurious to the pulp. The correct way to dry a cavity preparation is to use cotton pledgets and/or short blasts of air.

81. **4** Hand-cutting instruments used in restorative dentistry and their uses are the spoon excavator, to remove carious lesions; the hoe, to refine cavity preparation; the hatchet, to refine cavity preparation; the chisel, to refine cavity preparation; the knife, to remove excess restorative material; the file, to remove excess restorative material; and the cleoid–discoid, to carve restorative material.

82. **2** The placement of gold foil will most likely produce some postoperative discomfort. The discomfort is usually caused by the firm condensation needed to place this restorative material and is most often transient in nature.

83. **1** Radiology is not a recognized dental specialty. Recognized dental specialties are dental public health, endodontics, oral pathology, oral surgery, orthodontics, pedodontics, periodontics, and prosthodontics.

84. **2** The function of the periodontium is to support the teeth. Periodontal disease is the destruction of this supporting mechanism, which can lead to the loss of a tooth.

85. **1** Gingivitus is inflammation of the gingival tissues surrounding the teeth. The etiology is usually poor oral hygiene, which allows plaque to remain on the teeth. If treated in its early stages by removal of the irritants, the disease process is reversible.

86. **3** Periodontitis is a stage in periodontal disease wherein there is destruction of bone supporting the teeth. This condition is often the extension of untreated gingival inflammation (gingivitis). If periodontitis is not treated it will progress until teeth are lost due to the lack of supporting bone.

87. **4** A gingival sulcus is a healthy condition of the gingiva. It is cleansable and therefore can be maintained in health by the patient. A pocket is a pathological condition that cannot be cleansed by the patient. If not eliminated, pockets usually progress and cause further destruction of the supporting apparatus of the teeth.

88. **3** Iatrogenic disease is pathology caused by the work of the operator. Some examples of iatrogenic dentistry are overhanging amalgam, improperly contoured restorations, roughened tooth surfaces, improperly placed orthodontic bands, and poorly designed and constructed prostheses.

89. **1** Another name for Vincent's disease is acute necrotizing ulcerative gingivitis (or trench mouth). It is caused by poor oral hygiene, physical stress, mental stress, and smoking. The gingival tissue is red and puffy; it bleeds easily, lacks interdental papillae, is painful, and has a fetid odor.

90. **3** A furcation refers to the radicular area of multirooted teeth. Furcations in teeth with two roots are called bifurcations. Furcations in teeth with three roots are called trifurcations.

91. **2** A splint is an appliance that connects and stabilizes mobile teeth. Splints are made of various materials including cast gold, wire, and amalgam.

92. **2** A coolant is needed to dissipate the heat produced around the tip of the ultrasonic scaler as a result of its rapid back-and-forth motion.

93. **2** Osteoplasty is the recontouring of bony defects. The procedure is performed to obtain an anatomical condition that can be maintained in health by the patient.

94. **4** Gingivectomy is the surgical elimination of a gingival pocket so the patient can completely eliminate the plaque surrounding his or her teeth.

95. **1** Incision and drainage are used to treat a periodontal abscess. A periodontal abscess, part of the body's defense mechanism, forms when a foreign body, food, calculus, or other particle becomes lodged in a periodontal pocket.

96. **3** A periodontal dressing is analogous to a mouth bandage. The dressing makes the patient more comfortable by protecting the surgical area from trauma, mouth fluids, and other irritants.

97. **1** Exfoliation (or shedding) of primary teeth occurs by the resorption of the primary root. A tooth that has been exfoliated appears to be only a crown. The first teeth normally exfoliated are the mandibular primary central incisors.

98. **4** "Tell, show, and do," is a pedodontic technique that can be used to help allay a child's fear. The operator first tells the child what is going to happen. Then, with the child holding a mirror, he or she shows the child what is going to happen and then does the procedure.

99. **2** Techniques used to alleviate a child's fear of dental treatment are allowing the patient to participate, giving the patient some control, using medication, talking in a calm voice, being honest, and giving support to the patient.

100. **4** To aid in the management of a difficult child the dentist may prescribe premedication. Premedication is usually a short-acting barbiturate used to sedate the child.

101. **1** To maintain a calm atmosphere with children, the operator should talk softly and in monotone speech, move smoothly with no surprises or jerky motion, use simple and not fear-producing vocabulary, and build trust by telling the truth.

102. **2** A spot welder is used in both pedodontic operative procedures and orthodontics. In pedodontic operative procedures custom-made ma-

trix bands are constructed by spot welding crimped band material. In orthodontics custom bands are made by spot welding, and the attachment of certain tubes and brackets to these bands is also accomplished by spot welding.

103. **1** When making alginate impressions for children it is best to take the mandibular arch first. This will avoid any possibility of gagging and will decrease the possible fear and discomfort of the procedure.

104. **2** The removal of the coronal portion of the pulp is called pulpotomy. In pedodontics there are several types of pulpal therapies possible: direct pulp capping, a small exposure of a vital pulp is medicated with calcium hydroxide; indirect pulp capping, dentin affected by the carious process is medicated with calcium hydroxide or zinc oxide-eugenol; and pulpectomy, complete removal of a necrotic pulp, and filling of the root canals with an inert material.

105. **2** If a second primary molar is prematurely lost, a space maintainer is placed in the mouth to maintain the room necessary for the normal eruption of the permanent second premolar. The use of either a removable or fixed space maintainer is dictated by the situation.

106. **3** A stainless steel crown is usually indicated for full coverage of a deciduous molar. This restoration is less expensive and easier to construct than a cast gold restoration. It protects the deciduous molar, enabling it to function and permitting normal eruption of the succedaneous tooth.

107. **1** A mixed dentition exists when there are deciduous and permanent teeth existing simultaneously in a child's mouth. This condition begins when the first permanent molars erupt, at age 6, and lasts until the second primary molars are exfoliated, at about age 12.

108. **4** Preventive orthodontics is the aspect of dental practice concerned with measures that must be taken to maintain and promote the normal relationship of teeth to each other and to the surrounding tissue. Preventive orthodontics includes replacement of missing teeth when indicated, sound restorative dentistry, patient education, judicious extractions, and habit therapy.

109. **3** Causes of malocclusion are genetic: (1) jaw and tooth size not in harmony, (2) incorrect number of teeth, (3) altered eruption patterns, (4) abnormal muscular forces of the tongue and lips; systemic: (1) altered eruption patterns, (2) Dilantin hyperplasia; and/or local: (1) loss of teeth due to caries, periodontal disease, or injury, (2) habits, (3) cysts or growths.

110. **2** Some possible effects of malocclusion are difficulty in plaque removal, compromised function,

compromised esthetics, and disruption of normal orofacial growth.

111. **2** The result of orthodontic treatment is proper alignment of teeth and jaws, which can lead to improved function and esthetics and facilitate the maintenance of teeth and supporting tissue.

112. **3** Angle's classification of malocclusion is based on relationship of the maxillary and mandibular first molars. Class I, the maxillary and mandibular first molars are in correct relationship; Class II, the maxillary first molar occludes anterior to the mandibular first molar; Class III, the maxillary first molar occludes posterior to the mandibular first molars.

113. **1** Diagnostic aids used in orthodontics are the medical and dental histories, intraoral and extraoral radiographs, study models, and photographs.

114. **4** Cephalometry is the part of orthodontic diagnosis which studies the measurement of the skull to determine skeletal pattern. The measurements are taken from tracings of extraoral radiographs (lateral plates and posterior anterior plates).

115. **2** Ankylosis is the direct fusion of the root of a tooth with the surrounding bone. The root of a primary tooth that is ankylosed might not resorb and permit the permanent tooth to erupt. The treatment for an ankylosed deciduous tooth that is preventing the eruption of the succedaneous tooth is extraction.

116. **3** The orthodontic movement of a tooth in bone is analogous to a wire slowly moving through a block of ice. As a tooth moves, bone is resorbed and deposited in the same way that ice that melts and resolidifies as a wire moves through it.

117. **1** An important function of the dental assistant in an orthodontic practice is to motivate and reinforce oral home care. When appliances are cemented in place it is much more difficult for patients to keep their teeth clean. Unless the patient exercises excellent home care, caries and periodontal problems can increase.

118. **2** An advantage of using fixed rather than removable appliances is that fixed appliances eliminate the dependence upon patient cooperation. The elimination of variables, such as the amount of time a patient wears an appliance, usually ensures a greater amount of successful treatment.

119. **2** A technique whereby buccal tubes (or metal brackets) are attached to molar bands is spot welding, sometimes followed by soldering.

120. **3** Ligature wire is used to tie the arch wire into brackets. Rubber bands can also be used to hold the arch wire in the brackets and tubes.

121. **4** The arch wire can be located on either the labial or lingual surface. When activated, an arch wire applies force to slowly move teeth.

122. **3** Acid etch bonding is currently being used to attach clear plastic brackets directly to anterior teeth. This technique is more esthetically pleasing to many patients than the metal bands and brackets.

123. **1** Cervical anchorage is an appliance that attaches intraorally to the maxillary molars and protrudes extraorally to attach to an elastic band that fits around the patient's neck. This appliance provides distal forces to move the molars.

124. **2** After active orthodontic treatment is finished, a retainer is used to stabilize the teeth in the correct position.

125. **2** Some possible causes of irreversible pulpal damage are bacterial (direct invasion or invasion via a periodontal pocket), physical (trauma or temperature), and/or chemical.

126. **1** Diagnostic aids in endodontics are medical and dental histories, radiographs, the clinical examination, and vitality tests.

127. **2** The rubber dam is used in root canal therapy to maintain asepsis and protect the patient from swallowing instruments.

128. **2** Pulpectomy is the complete removal of the pulpal tissues. This procedure is usually accomplished by using a barbed broach.

129. **2** Obtaining a measurement (or length) of the root canal will avoid the possibility of irritating periapical tissues by overextending instruments beyond the apex of the root. Measurement is obtained by placing a reamer in the canal and by taking a radiograph.

130. **3** An important principle of root canal instrumentation is the sequential use of instruments. The operator begins instrumentation with the instrument with the smallest diameter and gradually enlarges the canal using instruments with progressively larger diameters.

131. **1** Three endodontic instruments are used in the root canals; files, used to enlarge and shape the canal; broaches, used to remove pulpal tissue from the canal; and reamers, used to check the path and length of the canal.

132. **3** Culturing is a technique to check the asepsis of the root canal. If bacteria are present in the canal the operator must reinstrument the canal in an attempt to further sterilize the canal.

133. **1** Sterilization of the root canal can be accomplished by mechanical and chemical means.

134. **3** The two materials commonly used to fill root canals are gutta percha and silver points.

135. **3** In root canal therapy, radiographs are taken before treatment begins, for measurement control, for fit of master point, and after final obturation.

136. **2** Some functions of medicaments used in endodontic therapy are irrigation (sodium hypochlorite, hydrogen peroxide, Zephiran chloride), increasing asepsis (irrigants, disinfectants, antibiotics), aiding in instrumentation (EDTA, acids), and sealing the canal (ZOE, chloropercha).

137. **2** Temporary filling materials are used to seal the root canals from saliva and other contaminants between root canal therapy visits. If there is pain caused by material trying to escape from the tooth (gases, purulent material, or other fluids), no temporary sealing material is placed, thereby providing an exit for these materials.

138. **4** An apicoectomy is the surgical removal of the apex of the root. The procedure consists of flapping the gingival tissue over the designated area and removing bone to gain access to the root apex. The operator then cuts the root apex off and curettes the periapical infection. The flap is then sutured closed over the designated area.

139. **3** Hemisection is performed when the periodontal condition of one root threatens the survival of the tooth. Hemisection requires that root canal therapy be performed before surgical removal of a root.

140. **2** Fixed bridges function to prevent movement of the remaining teeth, restore function of the missing teeth, and create an esthetic appearance.

141. **4** Some diagnostic aids used in fixed prosthetics are medical and dental histories, radiographs, clinical examination, and study models.

142. **1** Teeth that support a fixed bridge are called abutments. Other parts of a fixed bridge are retainers (b), which are restorations, crowns, or inlays that are permanently cemented on abutments (a), pontics (c), which are the replacements for the missing teeth and are connected to the retainers, and connectors (d), which attach the pontics and retainers.

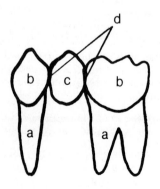

Fig. 35

143. **2** Retainers for fixed bridges include full crowns, including all gold, veneer, and porcelain fused to gold; three-quarter crowns; inlays; and onlays.

144. **2** Individual units of a fixed bridge are held together by solder. Solder is a metal that fuses two metals together.

145. **4** A gold post is used to reinforce an endodontically treated tooth before a crown preparation is made. Endodontically treated teeth are more brittle than are nonendodontically treated teeth; to prevent further fractures of these teeth, they should be reinforced before a crown is fabricated for them.

146. **4** Cantilever bridges are fixed bridges with abutments on only one side. These bridges are used for esthetics and to eliminate the need for a removable bridge.

147. **2** Temporary bridges are used for esthetics, mastication, decreased thermal sensitivity, stabilizing teeth, as a model for the permanent bridge, and for decreased contact sensitivity.

148. **2** To adapt a copper band to closely approximate a crown preparation it is necessary to select a band, anneal it, festoon it, and crimp it.

149. **1** The process of transforming a copper band impression into a copper-plated die is called electroplating. A metallic-plated die is more resistant to scratching and chipping than is a stone die.

150. **4** Electrosurgery is used in fixed prosthetics to remove gingival tissue before making final impressions with elastic materials. This procedure must be fully controlled by the operator and should allow tissue repair and regrowth after healing has taken place.

151. **4** Epinephrine-impregnated cord is used to stop gingival bleeding and to retract the gingiva before taking an impression with an elastic impression material. Epinephrine is a vasoconstrictor that stops the bleeding and the physical presence of the cord causes the gingival retraction.

152. **2** An advantage of the elastic impression technique is that a composite model is obtained. This enables the technician to see the relationship of the prepared tooth to the adjacent oral structures. The composite model may also be used to record the relationship between the abutments and pontics needed for soldering.

153. **3** A plaster–alginate impression is used to pick up transfer copings. After a model is poured from the resulting impression the exact relationship of crown preparations to each other and to surrounding tissues can be seen. A soldering index, used to assemble the bridge, can be obtained from this model.

154. **4** The purposes of temporary cementation of a fixed bridge are to check the reaction of the supporting tissues to the prosthesis, to permit the bridge to settle on the abutments, to let the patient evaluate the prosthesis, and to allow for subsequent laboratory work on the prosthesis if desired.

155. **1** Shade selection is accomplished in natural light with the aid of a shade guide. The shade of the acrylic or porcelain will depend upon several factors, some of which are the shade of adjacent teeth, the shade of patient's face, and the individual teeth involved (central incisors might be lighter than canines).

156. **4** A disadvantage of a fixed bridge is the difficulty in cleaning beneath the bridge. Plaque left under the pontics or next to the abutment teeth can cause damage to the supporting tissues or to the abutments themselves and can shorten the life of the prosthesis. Aids such as toothpicks, dental floss, or small brushes can be used by the patient on a daily basis to keep the bridge and supporting structures plaque free.

157. **3** The adaptation by patients to wearing dentures is primarily dependent on their desire to wear dentures. Wearing dentures has a variety of implications to different patients. Some implications and expectations are that the person is now old, the denture is a foreign body, and the denture will improve in function and in the patient's general health.

158. **4** An immediate denture is inserted into the patient's mouth during the same appointment in which the remaining teeth, usually anterior, are extracted. Some advantages are improved healing at the extraction sites, greater patient comfort, shorter adaptation period, improved function, and improved appearance.

159. **3** The relationship of the maxillary and mandibular teeth when they contact is known as occlusion. When constructing prosthetic appliances that replace teeth, the dentist attempts to restore the patient's occlusion.

160. **4** Maxillary dentures are more retentive than are mandibular dentures because they cover a larger surface area. Increased contact area permits more adhesive and cohesive forces to retain the denture.

161. **2** Full dentures are less efficient than is natural dentition. It is the patient's adaptability to the prosthesis that makes dentures useful appliances.

162. **4** Factors that influence denture retention are the size of contacting area and proximity of contacting surfaces. These factors permit adhesive and cohesive forces to retain the denture.

163. **1** During mastication, full dentures move all the time.

164. **3** Tissue conditioning is used to return unhealthy tissue, caused by an ill fitting denture, to a healthy condition. This procedure must be accomplished before final impressions are made to construct a new denture. The treatment entails placing a soft material in the patient's present denture that will permit the unhealthy tissue to recover.

165. **4** The clasp of the partial denture contacts the abutment teeth. It functions to stabilize and retain the denture.

166. **1** The saddle of the partial denture contacts the edentulous ridge. Replacement teeth are placed on the saddle area.

167. **1** A surveyor is used in partial denture construction to determine the path of insertion of the partial denture and the placement of clasps by determining the greatest circumference of the tooth.

168. **3** The function of the preliminary impression is to obtain a model on which a custom tray is fabricated. The custom-made tray is used to make a second and more accurate impression of the denture-bearing surface.

169. **3** A facebow is used to mount the upper cast on an articulator. This mounting should transfer the relationship of the maxilla to the temporomandibular joint accurately to the articulator.

170. **1** Wax bite blocks are used to record vertical dimension, centric relation, and facial contour, and to set up denture teeth.

171. **4** Flasking is part of the process to heat-cure acrylic. Flasking is the placement of the wax denture in metal containers known as flasks. The wax and acrylic or shellac base plate is replaced by a natural-appearing acrylic denture base.

172. **2** The portion of the denture that should not be polished is the part contacting the denture-bearing mucosa. If adjustments are made on the tissue side of the denture they can be smoothed with a small rubber wheel.

173. **1** Sore spots are common after dentures are inserted. This should be explained to patients and they should be told to return to the office for denture adjustments when this occurs. After inserting new dentures often a series of visits are necessary to alleviate sore spots and make the patient comfortable.

174. **2** A denture is relined to improve the readaptation of the denture base to the underlying tissue. This procedure is made necessary by the resorption of bone in the denture supporting area.

175. **3** A biopsy is a surgical procedure that removes tissue for diagnostic purposes. There are several types of biopsies: excisional, in which the entire lesion is removed; incisional, in which a wedge-

shaped piece of a large lesion is removed; aspiration biopsy, in which a piece of lesion is removed with a large lumen needle; and smear biopsy (exfoliative cytology), in which cells of a lesion are scraped off.

176. **1** Prognathism is the condition in which the mandible is located ahead of the maxilla. The correction of this bony defect is a combination of surgery and orthodontic treatment. The mandible is cut bilaterally and moved posteriorly to a position of desired occlusion. The mandible is then stabilized for approximately 6 weeks.

177. **3** The function of a stylet is to engage the rubber plunger of a local anesthetic carpule. After engaging the stylet the operator can aspirate to determine whether the lumen of the needle is located in a blood vessel. Upon aspirating, if blood is drawn into the carpule, the lumen of the needle is moved to a different location before depositing the local anesthetic.

178. **2** General anesthetics render patients unconscious by their effect on the central nervous system. These anesthetics can be administered by inhalation or by intravenous injection. The administration of general anesthetics requires special equipment and training and has a risk which limits its use in the dental office.

179. **2** Teeth are commonly extracted because of extensive caries, periodontal disease, orthodontic considerations, fractures, impactions, or involvement in surgical sites of fracture or neoplasms.

180. **2** An impaction is a tooth that will not erupt fully. Most impacted teeth are third molars. These teeth are surgically removed because of pain, to avoid damage to adjacent teeth, or to prevent future complications.

181. **2** An insturment that holds a tissue flap away from the operating field is called a retractor. Proper retraction offers the operator better access and visibility to the surgical site while protecting the flap and surrounding tissue from the unnecessary trauma.

182. **3** An abscess is a localized collection of pus. The specific name of the abscess is derived from its location. It can be periapical, periodontal, pericoronal, or subperiosteal.

183. **1** A drain is a piece of material, usually rubber or gauze, that creates a pathway whereby fluid can leave the body.

184. **2** A cyst is a cell-lined sac that may or may not contain fluid. Cysts are classified as either congenital or developmental.

185. **3** Application of direct pressure is the best technique to stop bleeding after extractions. Direct pressure is applied by having the patient bite on a gauze compress, which is placed directly over the extraction site for 30–45 minutes. This process leads to formation of a blood clot in the extraction site, which is the first step in healing.

186. **4** Rinsing with warm salt water decreases the number of microorganisms in the mouth and thereby promotes healing and helps prevent infection.

187. **1** A suture material that is resorbed by the body is gut. Other suture materials are silk, cotton, nylon, and wire. Sutures are used to approximate closely the edges of a wound.

188. **3** The treatment of fractures is the approximation of the parts (reduction) followed by immobilization (fixation) until the bone heals. Reduction can be accomplished by closed reduction, manipulation of the fracture without exposing the bone, or by open reduction, in which the fractured ends of the bones are exposed. Immobilization of the mandible or maxilla is accomplished by wiring the upper and lower teeth together.

189. **3** Trismus is the restricted opening of the mouth. It can be caused by infection, trauma, muscle spasm, or swelling.

190. **4** A dry socket (localized osteitis) is a breakdown of a blood clot in an extraction socket. It may be caused by infection, poor blood supply to the area, excessive trauma during extraction or improper postoperative care. Treatment of a dry socket consists of irrigation of the socket and packing it with guaze and an anodyne.

191. **4**

192. **7**

193. **2**

194. **6**

195. **1**

196. **4**

197. **7**

198. **2**

199. **6**

200. **1**

201. **7**

202. **4**

203. **1**

204. **2**

205. **6**

206. **7**

207. **6**

208. **5**

209. **3**

210. **1**

211. **6**

212. **2**

213. **5**

214. **3**

215. **7**

216. **7**

217. **3**

218. **2**

219. **4**

220. **6**

221. **5**

222. **3**

223. **1**

224. **7**

225. **6**

226. **6**

227. **3**

228. **1**

229. **2**

230. **5**

231. **4**

232. **1**

233. **3**

234. **4**

235. **4**

236. **1**

237. **3**

238. **2**

239. **3**

240. **1**

241. **2**

242. **2**

243. **2**

244. **4**

245. **2**

246. **4**

247. **1**

248. **3**

249. **1**

250. **1**

251. **3**

252. **1**

253. **1**

254. **2**

255. **1**

Charting Exercises

For answers 256–322 refer to charts 1–7 (pages 210–213).

256. **4**	273. **3**	290. **2**	307. **3**
257. **2**	274. **2**	291. **2**	308. **1**
258. **3**	275. **4**	292. **1**	309. **2**
259. **1**	276. **3**	293. **3**	310. **2**
260. **4**	277. **4**	294. **1**	311. **2**
261. **2**	278. **3**	295. **4**	312. **2**
262. **2**	279. **4**	296. **2**	313. **4**
263. **1**	280. **2**	297. **2**	314. **3**
264. **2**	281. **2**	298. **3**	315. **3**
265. **2**	282. **1**	299. **4**	316. **3**
266. **2**	283. **2**	300. **3**	317. **3**
267. **3**	284. **3**	301. **2**	318. **2**
268. **3**	285. **1**	302. **4**	319. **1**
269. **4**	286. **3**	303. **2**	320. **2**
270. **2**	287. **3**	304. **3**	321. **3**
271. **3**	288. **3**	305. **3**	322. **2**
272. **2**	289. **3**	306. **3**	

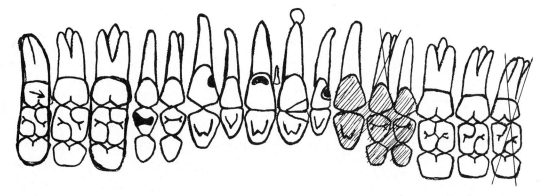

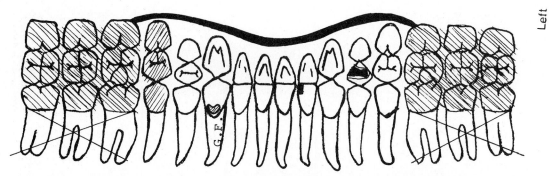

Right

Left

Chart 1

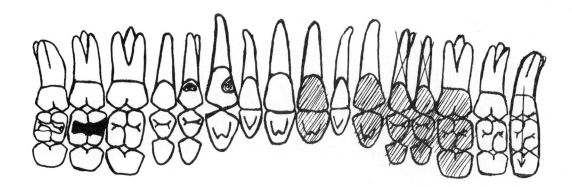

Right

Left

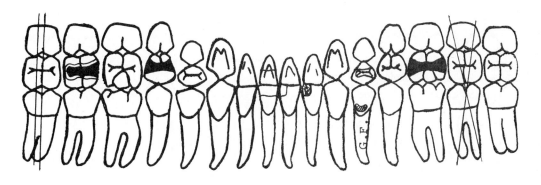

Chart 2

Right

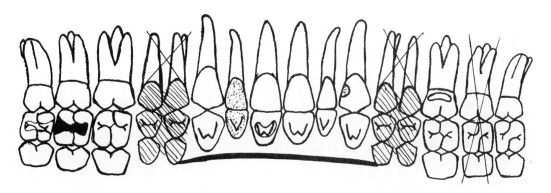

Left

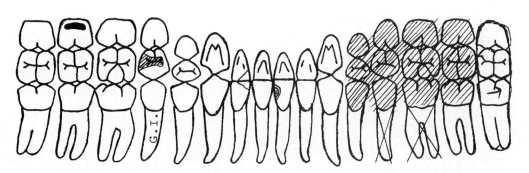

Chart 3

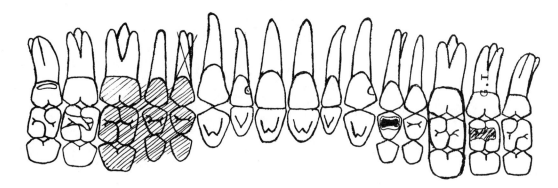

Right

Left

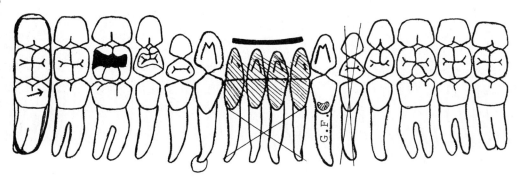

Chart 4

Right

Left

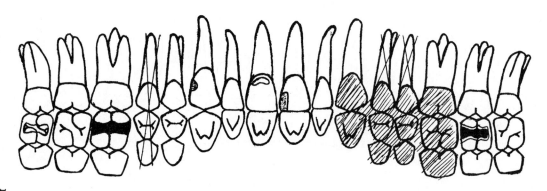

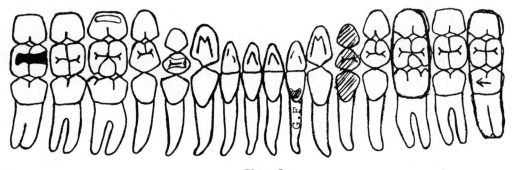

Chart 5

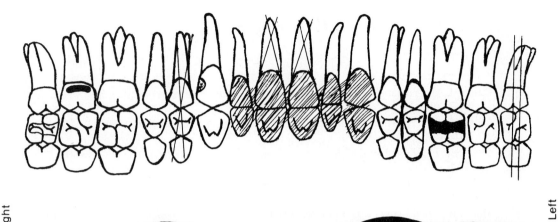

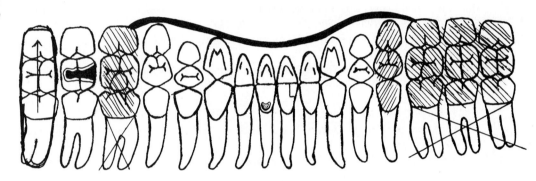

Chart 6

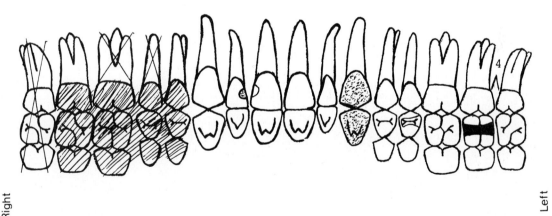

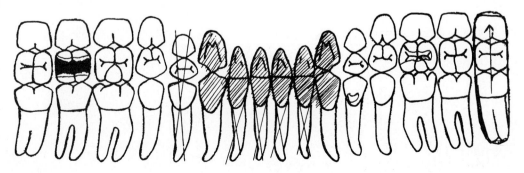

Chart 7

Bibliography

Carter, L.M.; Yaman, P.; and Ladley, B.A. (eds). *Dental Instruments,* St. Louis: The C. V. Mosby Co., 1981.

Chasteen, J.E. *Essentials of Clinical Dental Assisting,* 2nd ed. St. Louis: The C. V. Mosby Co., 1980.

Chasteen, J.E. *Four Handed Dentistry in Clinical Practice,* St. Louis: The C. V. Mosby Co., 1978.

Ladley, B.A. and Wilson, S.A. *Review of Dental Assisting,* St. Louis: The C. V. Mosby Co., 1980.

Miller, B.F. and Keane, C.B. *Encyclopedia and Dictionary of Medicine, Nursing, and Allied Health,* 2nd ed. Philadelphia: W. B. Saunders Co., 1978.

Richardson, R.E. and Barton, R.E. *The Dental Assistant,* 5th ed. New York: McGraw-Hill Inc., 1978.

Robinson, G.E., et al. *Four Handed Dentistry Manual,* 4th ed. Birmingham: University of Alabama School of Dentistry, 1978.

Spohn, E.E.; Halouski, W.A.; and Berry, T.C. *Operative Dentistry Procedures for Dental Auxiliaries,* St. Louis: The C. V. Mosby Co., 1981.

Torres, H. and Ehrlich, A. *Modern Dental Assisting,* 2nd ed. Philadelphia: W. B. Saunders Co., 1980.

Wolfson, E. *Four Handed Dentistry for Dentists and Assistants,* St. Louis: The C. V. Mosby Co., 1974.

Zwemer, T.J. *Boucher's Clinical Dental Terminology,* St. Louis: The C. V. Mosby Co., 1982.

6

Preventive Dentistry

Course Synopsis

Introduction

Current statistics demonstrate that almost the entire population of the United States experiences, at some time, either caries or periodontal disease. Knowlege of disease prevention concepts and patient education skills are becoming mandatory for dental auxiliaries. Auxiliaries must be aware of the individual patient's needs in order to avoid arousing anxiety. Properly designed prevention programs decrease patient resistance to changing poor habits by providing patients with new strategies for success. Auxiliaries work with patients to teach and motivate them to assume greater responsibility in participating in their own treatment, thereby minimizing future dental problems. As the loss of teeth caused by caries and periodontal disease decreases, a concomitant reduction in dental expenses for the patient results. This chapter addresses the basic skills and concepts for preventing diseases of the oral cavity.

Tooth Deposits

Materia alba is a white or grayish mass of oral debris that accumulates around the gingival margins. It is unesthetic and can be removed by vigorous rinsing or by a water–irrigating device.

Plaque is a dense, gelatinous layer of bacteria that adheres to the teeth and gingival tissues and can only be removed by brushing. Plaque formation is directly related to caries and gingival inflammation. If plaque is not removed, it calcifies and a mineralized mass called calculus results. Only dental instruments such as scalers and curettes are effective in the removal of calculus, which usually collects just above or below the gingival margin and occasionally on any tooth surface.

Stains appear as a result of diet or behavioral habits. They can be extrinsic, on the tooth structure, or intrinsic, within the tooth itself. Extrinsic stains often come from food, tobacco, coffee, and tea and range from yellow and green in children to dark stains in adults. Intrinsic stains can occur during tooth formation and are more often caused by medication or systemic diseases. A common form of intrinsic stain is a result of ingestion of tetracycline during the calcification stage of tooth development.

Oral Physiotherapy

Cleaning teeth is necessary to prevent the buildup of plaque and to provide the stimulation necessary to maintain a healthy gingiva. Instruments and materials that can be used by the patient to clean the teeth include the toothbrush, floss, dentifrices, disclosing tablets and solutions, perio-aids, rubber tips, wooden wedges, water–irrigating devices, interproximal brushes, and floss threaders and holders.

Toothbrushes and Brushing Techniques

The proper toothbrush should be approximately ½ inch wide and contain three or four rows of evenly spaced soft bristles. The tip of each bristle should be rounded, polished, and approximately 0.007 inches in diameter. The handle should be 5–6 inches in length to enable easy access to all areas of the mouth.

Most common methods of brushing are the roll, modified Stillman, Bass, and the Charters' techniques. The roll technique is the simplest; bristles are placed at the gingival margin of the teeth with the side of the bristles resting on the gingiva with mild pressure. The brush is then rolled to the occlusal surface, and the process is repeated approximately 10 times on each tooth surface. Occlusal surfaces are cleaned with a back-and-forth motion. A drawback of this technique is that the sulcus is not cleaned.

The modified Stillman technique is used to remove plaque from the cervical and exposed proximal areas. The bristles of the brush are placed at a 45-degree angle to the apex of the tooth. The brush, lying firmly against the gingiva, is vibrated in a rotary motion. If this technique is used, it is particularly important that the brush be soft, to prevent laceration of the gingiva. It should be noted that with this technique, the bristles do not enter the sulcus.

The Bass technique is effective for patients with gingival inflammation and deep periodontal sulci. The bristles of the toothbrush are placed at a 45-degree angle to the long axis of the tooth and are gently placed into the sulcus. The brush is gently vibrated back and forth for 10–15 seconds in each area.

The Charters' technique was designed to stimulate the gingival margin around each tooth. It is most effective when interdental spaces are open, as often occurs after periodontal surgery. The bristles are pointed toward the occlusal surfaces at a 45-degree angle to the tooth surface. The brush is moved with a small, circular motion, with the bristle ends remaining stationary; however, the ends do not enter the sulcus.

Dental Floss

The interproximal areas of the teeth are the most frequent sites of gingivitis. Brushing is generally not an effective method of cleaning these areas. An important aid for the removal of interproximal plaque is dental floss, which must be manipulated properly to avoid damaging tooth structure or gingiva. Flossing correctly can be difficult for the patient to learn; each patient must be given sufficient support to ensure that the method is learned properly. A piece of floss that is either waxed or unwaxed, approximately 18 inches long, should be wrapped around the middle finger or index finger of each hand until the fingers are about 2 inches apart. The floss is then guided interproximally with the thumb or index finger through the contact area with a see-saw motion and placed against the distal or mesial tooth surface. An up-and-down motion is then used to cleanse the surfaces.

Other Oral Physiotherapy Aids

Dentrifices, or toothpaste, serve several functions. In addition to cleaning accessible tooth areas, polishing teeth, decreasing the incidence of dental caries, and promoting gingival health, toothpaste or powder decreases mouth odors and provides a sensation of oral cleanliness. Ingredients of toothpaste include water, which acts as a solvent; abrasives, which clean and polish; detergents, which provide foaming action; humectant, which prevents dehydration; and binders, which join the solid and liquid ingredients. Often, fluoride is added to provide increased protection against caries.

Disclosing tablets and solutions are nontoxic, nonirritating, inexpensive dyes that identify plaque by coloring the deposits. Many deposits on teeth are not visible, and the tablets or solutions help the patient visualize these areas before or after brushing and flossing.

A perio-aid is a plastic handle that has a hole located at either end. Toothpicks are pressed into each hole and broken off. The instrument is used to place the toothpick end gently against the tooth surface in the sulcus to scrape away unwanted deposits.

A rubber tip is a cone-shaped piece of rubber used to stimulate the gingiva. The tip can be an independent instrument or located at the end of a toothbrush handle. The side of the tip is pressed against the gingiva with sufficient pressure to cause some blanching of the tissue and is then moved in circular motions. A rubber tip is useful in reshaping the gingiva after periodontal surgery, improving keratinization of tissue, and reducing the severity of interproximal inflammation.

Wooden wedges are triangular shaped balsawood wedges. They are used for cleaning the interproximal areas where there are exposed tooth surfaces due to gingival recession. Care must be taken to use this device properly because gingival tissue may be traumatized if the adjoining teeth are forced apart.

Water-irrigation devices remove loose food debris around teeth. They are an adjunct to toothbrushing but are not a substitute for it, since these instruments do not remove plaque. They are useful for patients with orthodontic and fixed prosthetic appliances.

Floss threaders are plastic metal devices used to thread floss under and between the pontics of fixed bridges and splinted teeth. These devices are important, since these areas are difficult to reach and are susceptible to plaque retention.

Interproximal brushes are cone-shaped nylon brushes used to remove plaque in open interproximal and bifurcated and trifurcated root areas.

Mouthwashes can be classified into two categories: cosmetic and therapeutic. Cosmetic rinses have no dental value that has been scientifically substantiated. Therapeutic rinses include sodium fluoride and phosphate acidulate fluoride solution, which have been proved effective in reducing the incidence of dental caries.

Fluorides

The most efficient and economical method of decreasing the prevalence of dental caries is the use of fluoride. Fluorides can be administered systemically through addition to the water supply and vitamin supplements or applied topically (directly onto the exposed surfaces of erupted teeth). Fluoride itself is a mineral nutrient essential in the formation of sound teeth and bones. However, if too much fluoride is absorbed during tooth developmental periods, the teeth can appear mottled.

Systemic Fluorides

Many people receive fluoride in their drinking water in the amounts of 1 part per million (ppm). If a community's central water supply is not fluoridated, individual community organizations, such as a school, can supplement their water supplies. In addition, fluoride supplements in the form of chewable tablets or liquids can be added to a child's daily diet.

Topical fluoride is applied directly to the surfaces of teeth and may be either an adjunct to fluoridated water or the sole source of fluoride for a child. Common topical fluoride agents include sodium fluoride, acidulated phosphate fluoride, and stannous fluoride.

Sodium fluoride is available in a 20% aqueous solution. This type of topical fluoride is considered less effective than are acidulated phosphate fluoride and stannous fluoride. A series of four treatments are given with intervals of several days.

Acidulated phosphate fluoride has proved more effective than sodium fluoride alone and is applied topically every 6 months.

Stannous fluoride is used in an 8% aqueous solution. Single applications are given at 4- or 6-month intervals, beginning at age 3 years. This type of fluoride is most commonly available in fluoridated toothpaste.

Occlusal sealants, also known as pit and fissure sealants, are caries reducing agents which are applied directly to caries free tooth surfaces to seal anatomical faults in the enamel of primary and permanent teeth. The most prevalent sites for caries are occlusal surfaces where lesions begin in the anatomical faults. The tooth surface being treated is etched with phosphoric acid, and a resin sealant that mechanically bonds to enamel is applied and polymerized. This process results in the formation of a physical barrier, decreasing the possibility of caries formation.

Tests for Disease Susceptibility

In some cases clinical and radiographic examinations are insufficient in demonstrating factors that indicate the reasons a patient is highly susceptible to caries or periodontal disease. Additional etiological tests are used to find these answers.

The Snyder test is used to determine the activity of acidogenic bacteria in the saliva. The patient expectorates a small amount of saliva into a test tube that contains a blue-green dextrose medium. Acid produced by the oral bacteria turns the solution medium yellow. The amount of color change indicates the amount of acid producing bacteria in the oral cavity and greater levels of acidic bacteria indicate higher susceptibility to caries.

The modified Dreizen test measures the acid-buffering capacity of saliva. The ability of saliva to buffer the acidogenic action of bacteria found in plaque is an important factor in dental caries resistance. The patient chews a small piece of parafin wax in order to collect saliva. The saliva is placed in a test tube containing pH indicator solution. Lactic acid is added a drop at a time to this mixture until a pH level of 5 is reached. This point is the critical pH value at which enamel begins to decalcify. Patients who require the addition of fewer than 10 drops of lactic acid in the salivary solution are usually caries prone.

The lingual C test determines whether a patient is deficient in vitamin C, which is a factor in periodontal health. A dye is placed on the tongue; if it does not disappear, a deficiency might exist.

Nutrition and Diet Analysis

Good nutrition is essential for the maintenance of oral hygiene. Dietary counseling is given to patients to provide them with the knowledge necessary to maintain a dietary balance. Four basic food groups provide the sources for a balanced diet.

Dairy products consisting of different types of milk, yogurt, cheese, ice cream, custards, and puddings are an excellent source of protein, riboflavin, and calcium. The recommended daily allowance (RDA) for both children and adults is three or more servings. For pregnant women, this amount is increased to four or more servings daily.

Meats, poultry, and fish provide high-quality protein, iron, and B vitamins. The RDA is two or more servings daily.

Fruits and vegetables provide vitamins that are eliminated by the body and must be replenished daily. This food group also provides minerals essential to good health and fiber, which is receiving increased attention as a part of a balanced diet. Four or more servings a day should be derived from this food group.

Breads and cereals provide B vitamins, protein, and iron. Sources include whole grains and enriched cereals. Nutrients are often lost during processing and added later to compensate for this loss.

Suggested snack foods that aid the maintenance of good oral health include fresh fruits and vegetables, protein foods (cheese, fowl, eggs, fish, plain yogurt, and meat), milk, fruit and vegetable juices, and sugar-free soft drinks.

Table I indicates the function and sources of key nutrients and problems and diseases that can arise from deficiencies.

Table I

Key Nutrients

Nutrient	Functions	Sources	Deficiency
Proteins	Build and maintain body tissues; help body carry on normal processes	Animal meat, poultry, fish, milk, cheese, eggs, plants (soybean)	Kwashiorkor, marasmus
Carbohydrates	Supply energy	Sugars, syrups, cereals, grains, bread, jam and jelly, pasta, crackers, pretzels, dried fruits	None specifically, but excessive intake can lead to dental caries
Fats	Provide insulation and support for internal body organs	Oils, butter, egg yolks, nuts, meats	None, but excessive fat intake can lead to coronary disease
Vitamins			
A	Assists in proper maintenance of epithelial cells; plays role in vision	Fish, liver, oils, vegetables, yellow fruits	Night blindness, severe drying of skin
D	Builds and maintains bones and teeth; regulates calcium and phosphorus metabolism	Milk, fish, eggs, liver, butter, sunshine	Rickets; poor tooth development
E	Essential for normal reproduction	Wheat germ, vegetable oil, green vegetables	Unknown
B_1 (thiamine)	Helps normal body function growth; assists in carbohydrate metabolism	Yeast, wheat germ, whole grains, pork, liver	Retards growth, nerve disorders, beriberi
B_2 (riboflavin)	Contributes to normal function of body cells	Fish, eggs, whole grains, liver, meat, greens	Glossitis, cheilosis, dermatitis
B_6	Contributes to normal function of body cells	Meat, liver, vegetables, whole-grain cereals	Anemia, skin lesions

Table I (continued)

Key Nutrients

Nutrient	Functions	Sources	Deficiency
B$_{12}$	Contributes to blood regeneration	Liver, milk, cheese	Pernicious anemia; neurological disturbances
K	Contributes to normal blood clotting	Green vegetables, cabbage, cauliflower, soybean oil	Defective clotting
Niacin	Helps other cells use nutrients	Yeast, eggs, milk, green vegetables	Pellagra
Pantothenic acid	Assists in proper metabolism	Yeast, liver, kidney, eggs	Lack of proper metabolism
Folacin	Contributes to normal function of cells	Plant foods, greens, liver	Unknown
Biotin	Helps body use proteins, carbohydrates, and fats	Kidney, liver	Epithelial sensitivity; muscular pains
C	Aids in resisting infections; healing and maintaining a healthy gingiva; strengthens blood vessels	Citrus fruits, broccoli, parsley, green vegetables	Scurvy

Plaque-Control Programs

Prevention and interception of dental disease occur only when patients have the knowledge and skills that enable them to participate in these processes. Educating and motivating patients to make a commitment to prevention is accomplished in a plaque-control program. Information is presented to patients to change their behavior in an effort to make them primarily responsible for maintaining good oral hygiene. A sample program follows:

Visit 1. Patients are made aware of how tooth-accumulated materials form. Basic instruction in brushing and flossing is provided, and disclosing agents are used to permit patients to see and remove deposits from teeth.

Visit 2. Techniques of brushing and flossing are reviewed and adjunct oral physiotherapy techniques are introduced based on patient need. Tests to assess oral disease susceptibility are done during this visit. Patients are provided with basic nutritional guidelines and a self-administered diet history review sheet.

Visit 3. Results and implications of caries susceptibility tests are reviewed with patients. Diet history is reviewed, and constructive behavioral strategies helpful in changing poor habits are suggested. Home care is reviewed.

Visit 4. All previous sessions are reviewed for reinforcement. During this visit patients are asked to describe or exhibit their individual strategies for prevention and to assess their own success. This visit can be repeated until success is achieved.

Question Section

1. Plaque formation begins at the
   A. gingival margin of the tooth
   B. occlusal surface of the tooth
   C. proximal surface of the tooth
      1. A and B
      2. A and C
      3. B and C
      4. all of the above

2. Which of the following factors contributes to periodontal disease?
   A. plaque
   B. materia alba
   C. food debris
   D. calculus
      1. B and E
      2. A, C, D, and E
      3. B, C, D, and E
      4. all of the above

3. An acquired pellicle
   A. forms within minutes after brushing
   B. is removed by irrigation or rinsing
   C. is the first sign of periodontal disease
   D. is very susceptible to extrinsic stain
      1. A
      2. A and C
      3. B, C, and D
      4. all of the above

4. Plaque is
   A. invisible
   B. bacterial
   C. stain on teeth
   D. soft
   E. a direct cause of calculus
      1. A, B, D
      2. A, C, D
      3. A, B, D, and E
      4. all of the above

5. Materia alba is
   A. hardened plaque
   B. removed by irrigation or rinsing
   C. bacterial
   D. soft
      1. A, B, and D
      2. B, C, and D
      3. B and D
      4. all of the above

6. Calculus is
   A. a gel-like material
   B. a calcified mass
   C. removed by an ultrasonic cleaning device and curettes
   D. removed by toothbrushing and dental floss
   E. an intermicrobial matrix
      1. A, B, and E
      2. B and C
      3. B, C, and D
      4. C, D, and E

7. Improper toothbrushing can cause
   A. gingivitis
   B. gingival recession
   C. periodontal disease
   D. tooth abrasion
   E. toothbrush attrition
      1. A and B
      2. A and C
      3. B and D
      4. D and E

8. Dentifrices
   A. remove calculus
   B. remove extrinsic stains
   C. remove intrinsic stains
   D. leave your mouth feeling fresh
      1. A and B
      2. A and C
      3. B and D
      4. all of the above

9. Disclosing agents identify
   A. plaque
   B. carious lesions
   C. gingival recession
   D. calculus
      1. A
      2. A and B
      3. B and C
      4. all of the above

10. Which oral physiotherapy aid is most appropriately used to clean interdental areas when large interproximal spaces or open contacts exist?
      1. interproximal brush
      2. dental floss
      3. regular toothbrush
      4. perio-aid
      5. rubber tip

11. The best means of massage for the interdental papilla is the use of a
    1. perio-aid
    2. water irrigating device
    3. balsawood wedge
    4. rubber tip
    5. interproximal brush

12. The function of an oral prophylaxis is to remove
    A. plaque
    B. materia alba
    C. calculus
    D. extrinsic stain
        1. A and C
        2. B and C
        3. A and B
        4. all of the above

13. Using the "heel" or "toe" of the brush is helpful for cleaning which tooth surfaces?
    1. buccal surfaces of molars
    2. lingual surfaces of molars
    3. facial surfaces of anterior teeth
    4. lingual surfaces of anterior teeth

14. Under usual circumstances, a hard toothbrush is
    1. not recommended
    2. highly recommended
    3. used if the patient does not use dental floss
    4. used when teeth are heavily stained

15. The preferred toothbrush is
    1. soft, natural bristled
    2. soft, nylon bristled
    3. medium, natural bristled
    4. medium, nylon bristled
    5. hard, nylon bristled

16. Which of the following toothbrushing methods is designed for massage, stimulation, and cleaning the cervical area and gingiva?
    1. Bass
    2. modified Stillman
    3. Charters'
    4. Scrub brush

17. Which of the following toothbrushing techniques is designed to remove plaque adjacent to and directly beneath the gingival margin?
    1. Bass
    2. modified Stillman
    3. Charters'
    4. scrub brush

18. In which toothbrushing technique are the bristles of the brush pointed toward the occlusal and lingual surfaces?
    1. Bass
    2. rolling stroke
    3. vertical
    4. Charters'

Directions: Match column A with column B.

A

19. Used by a patient with limited dexterity____
20. Used to clean area underneath fixed bridges____
21. Used to clean around gingival margins____
22. Used to clean in between teeth____

B

   1. floss threader
   2. rubber tip
   3. automatic toothbrush
   4. perio-aid
   5. dental floss

23. Which of the following procedures can be included in an oral prophylaxis?
    1. restoring a fractured amalgam
    2. root canal treatment
    3. a full series of x-ray films
    4. polishing of amalgam restorations

24. Fluoride is most effectively used
    A. if ingested in a water supply during the time of tooth development
    B. if ingested in a water supply after teeth have erupted
    C. if present in a municipal water supply in the ratio of 1ppm
    D. if present only in school water supplies for children
        1. A and C
        2. A and D
        3. B and C
        4. B and D

25. When is an occlusal sealant contraindicated?
    1. on primary teeth
    2. when there are deep pits and fissures
    3. on severely decayed teeth
    4. on occlusal surfaces of posterior teeth

26. The sunshine vitamin is
    1. A
    2. D
    3. E
    4. K
    5. B₆

27. The vitamin responsible for proper blood clotting is
    1. A

2. B₁
3. C
4. K

28. Foods that are high caries producers include
    A. syrup
    B. breakfast cereals
    C. vegetables
    D. raisins
    E. citrus fruits
       1. A, B, and C
       2. A, B, and D
       3. B, C, and D
       4. all of the above

29. Which of the following nutrients has been found to be an overwhelming cause of the development of plaque and dental caries?
    1. proteins
    2. carbohydrates
    3. fat
    4. vitamins

30. Under what circumstances are there differences in the recommended daily allowances of food?
    A. child vs. adult
    B. male vs. female
    C. small person vs. large person
    D. pregnant vs. nonpregnant
       1. A and C
       2. B and C
       3. A, B, and D
       4. all of the above

31. Which of the following are considered detergent foods?
    A. apples
    B. rice
    C. raisins
    D. cheese
    E. lettuce
    F. pears
    G. bread
    H. celery
       1. A, B, D, and H
       2. A, E, F, and H
       3. B, C, F, and H
       4. B, C, E, and F

32. Gingivitis involves the
    A. alveolar bone
    B. gingiva
    C. periodontal ligament
    D. cementum
       1. A
       2. B
       3. B and C
       4. A and C

33. Subgingival calculus differs from the supra-gingival calculus in the following ways
    A. color
    B. density
    C. location
       1. A and B
       2. A and C
       3. B and C
       4. all of the above

34. Plaque-control programs should contain
    A. oral physiotherapy instruction
    B. clinical examinations
    C. nutritional counselling
    D. behavioral modification techniques
       1. A, B, and D
       2. A, C, and D
       3. B, C, and D
       4. all of the above

35. Plaque-control programs are given by
    1. dentists
    2. assistants
    3. hygienists
    4. any member of the health care team

36. Which diagnostic test is an indicator of oral bacterial action?
    1. urinalysis
    2. complete blood count
    3. modified Snyder test
    4. scratch

37. The main role of the assistant in preventive dentistry is
    1. curettage
    2. occlusal equilibration
    3. patient education
    4. recontouring defective restorations

38. How often should a patient be recalled?
    1. every 8 months
    2. each year
    3. the time varies with the oral condition of individual patients
    4. whenever the patient decides

39. Which type of patient should not be on a recall system?
    1. an edentulous patient with dentures
    2. a caries-free patient
    3. a patient who brushes and flosses daily
    4. none of the above

40. Immunology refers to the study of
    1. resistance to disease
    2. factors that cause disease
    3. population studies
    4. hyperirritability

41. Population studies of factors that make groups more or less susceptible to disease are called
    1. epidemiology
    2. pathology
    3. ecology
    4. susceptology

42. Some tooth-accumulated materials are
    A. calculus
    B. cementum
    C. plaque
    D. materia alba
    E. saliva
       1. A, B, and C
       2. A, C, and D
       3. B, C, and D
       4. C, D, and E

43. Plaque is
    1. a salivary exudate
    2. a precancerous lesion
    3. the causative agent in aphthous ulcers
    4. an organized bacterial mat

44. Plaque removal should be accomplished at least
    1. every hour
    2. every day
    3. every week
    4. every 2 weeks

45. The aids most commonly used in daily plaque removal are
    1. rubber bands and a toothbrush
    2. a toothbrush and dental floss
    3. an ultrasonic scaler and a toothbrush
    4. water irrigators and dental floss

46. Various toothbrushing techniques include
    A. Stillman
    B. Murry
    C. Charters'
    D. Snyder
    E. Bass
       1. A, B, and C
       2. A, C, and E
       3. B, C, and D
       4. C, D, and E

47. A water irrigator is used
    1. to remove palque
    2. as a substitute for a toothbrush
    3. to remove loose debris
    4. as a substitute for dental floss

48. The optimum amount of fluoride in drinking water should be
    1. 1 ppm
    2. 10 ppm
    3. 100 ppm
    4. 1000 ppm

49. Nutrition is
    1. ingested food
    2. proper diet
    3. the intake of nutrients
    4. the process by which the body assimilates and utilizes food

50. Food is used by the body
    A. for fuel
    B. for growth
    C. to form herpetic lesions
    D. for repair
    E. to produce toxins
       1. A, B, and D
       2. A, C, and D
       3. B, C, and E
       4. C, D, and E

51. Metabolism is
    1. the anabolic chemical reaction
    2. the sum of all the anabolic and catabolic chemical reactions
    3. the cardiovascular reactions
    4. a respiratory difficulty

52. Vitamins are
    1. unnecessary
    2. numbered from 1 to 10
    3. essential for normal body functions
    4. inorganic compounds

53. A deficiency of vitamin A may result in
    1. scurvy
    2. problems in enamel formation
    3. deafness
    4. pulpal necrosis

54. Vitamin C influences the
    1. healing of wounds
    2. enamel formation
    3. formation of periapical lesions
    4. absorption of iron

55. A riboflavin deficiency results in
    1. a malformation of dentinal tubes
    2. caries-prone teenage years
    3. cheilitis
    4. a herpetic lesion

56. Green stains on children's teeth can be the result of
    1. intrinsic staining
    2. excess topical fluoride
    3. trauma
    4. chromogenic bacteria

Answers and Explanations

1. **2** Plaque forms at the gingival margin and on the proximal surfaces of teeth, because these areas are not as likely to be exposed to the self-cleansing process which occurs during normal mastication.

2. **4** Although the precise etiology of periodontal disease is unknown, it is believed that plaque, materia alba, food debris, and calculus contribute to the disease.

3. **1** An acquired pellicle is the first step in plaque formation. Plaque requires 24 hours to mature, but a pellicle or film takes only minutes to form.

4. **3** Plaque is an invisible, soft, gelatinous mass of bacteria and pellicles adhering to tooth surfaces.

5. **2** Materia alba is food debris that can be removed by irrigation. It is soft and bacterial.

6. **2** Calculus is a hardened or calcified material that can be removed only through mechanical means. Common instruments for removal include curettes and ultrasonic cleaning devices.

7. **3** Improper toothbrushing (i.e., scrubbing the gingiva and tooth surfaces too hard) causes gingival recession and tooth abrasion.

8. **3** A dentifrice or toothpaste is an abrasive material that removes extrinsic stain. Dentifrices contain pleasant flavorings that result in a feeling of cleanliness when used.

9. **1** Disclosing tablets stain invisible plaque and consequently let the patient visualize this material. Carious lesions, gingival recession, and calculus can be identified only through clinical examination.

10. **1** An interproximal brush is most effectively used when interdental spaces are sufficiently large. Dental floss is most effective in cases of tight contacts.

11. **4** Rubber tips are best used to stimulate interdental papilla. This process helps keratinize the gingiva and decrease inflammation. Balsawood wedges are used primarily to clean large interproximal tooth surfaces and secondarily to massage the papilla. Wedges are not as effective as rubber tips because they are stiffer and more difficult to manipulate.

12. **4** An oral prophylaxis removes all tooth-accumulated material.

13. **4** The heel and toe of a toothbrush are most effective in cleaning lingual surfaces of anterior teeth since these areas are narrow and curved.

14. **1** In general, hard toothbrushes are not recommended because they can cause abrasion of the gingiva or enamel.

15. **2** The toothbrush most effective in removing tooth accumulated material is soft and nylon. Softness is preferred to decrease the possibility of damage to hard and soft tissues, and nylon has been accepted as a material of consistent quality that is superior to natural bristles.

16. **2** The modified Stillman method is designed for proper hygiene of the cervical and gingival areas. This method gently forces the bristles into the sulcus and against the gingival margin.

17. **1** The Bass technique is the most effective method of removing plaque from the sulcus, because the bristles of the brush actually enter the sulcus.

18. **4** The Charters' technique is used to stimulate the gingiva around each tooth. The bristles of the toothbrush are pointed toward the occlusal surface at a 45-degree angle.

19. **3**

20. **1**

21. **4**

22. **5**

23. **4** Polishing amalgam restorations is a routine procedure during an oral prophylaxis. This procedure can be done by the dentist or an auxiliary if state law permits.

24. **1** Fluoride is most effectively used if ingested during the period of tooth development. Through a complex process, fluoride hardens the tooth matrix, making it more impervious to the decay process. The optimum ratio in municipal water supplies is 1 ppm.

25. **3** Occlusal sealants are used primarily on undecayed tooth surfaces in order to prevent decay from forming. They are not used on severely decayed surfaces.

26. **2** Vitamin D which is largely derived from sunshine is instrumental in balancing the calcium and phosphorus ratio in the body. It is essential for bone and tooth formation.

27. **4** Vitamin K, found in green vegetables and egg yolks, is essential for formation of prothrombin, an agent necessary to promote proper blood clotting.

28. **2** Foods containing high levels of sugars are most responsible for producing caries.

29. **2** Carbohydrates have been found to be the most influential nutrient in causing caries. All carbohydrates are broken down to produce sugars, which interact with oral bacteria to form acids that can cause decay.

30. **4** Recommended daily allowances of foods differ among patients on the basis of such factors as age, sex, body size, and pregnancy.

31. **2** Detergent foods include fresh fruits and vegetables. Their textures actually help perform a cleansing action during the mastication process.

32. **2** Gingivitis is simply an inflammation of the gingiva that does not include involvement of underlying supporting structures.

33. **4** Subgingival calculus is darker and not as thick as supragingival calculus, which forms in an open area.

34. **2** Plaque-control programs are designed to permit patients to take responsibility for their own oral hygiene. Clinical examinations are given before such programs and can determine whether the patient should participate in a plaque-control program.

35. **4** Plaque-control programs can be given by any member of the health care team. Often this task is delegated to an auxiliary.

36. **3** The modified Snyder test is a colorimetric test of the amount of acid-producing bacteria in the saliva. This test is an indicator of the patient's caries susceptibility.

37. **3** The main role of the assistant in preventive dentistry is to educate and motivate patients. The information offered usually includes material about plaque control and proper nutrition.

38. **3** The time between recall visits, examination, and oral prophylaxis varies according to the needs of the individual patient. Patients with a high caries index or those who are susceptible to periodontal disease are recalled more often than are patients who are less susceptible to oral disease. The usual time between recall visits is 6 months.

39. **4** All patients should be seen on a regular recall basis. Edentulous patients should be regularly recalled to examine the soft tissue and occlusion and to repair dentures.

40. **1** Immunology is the study of resistance to disease. Immunity can be acquired or natural: natural immunity is obtained in utero; acquired immunity is obtained after birth as the result of antibodies being introduced by injection or as the result of infection.

41. **1** Epidemiology is the study of causes and factors that make a population more or less susceptible to disease.

42. **2** Tooth-accumulated materials are supra-gingival and subgingival calculus, plaque, materia alba, and stains.

43. **4** Plaque is an organized bacterial mat. As plaque matures there are alterations in the number and type of bacteria. If the bacterial mat is not disrupted it will calcify and become calculus.

44. **2** Bacterial plaque forms daily. To avoid deleterious effects of plaque, it should be thoroughly removed every day.

45. **2** The aids most commonly used in daily plaque removal are the toothbrush and dental floss. The toothbrush removes the plaque and debris from the occlusal, facial and lingual surfaces of the tooth. Dental floss is used to remove plaque from the proximal (mesial and distal) surfaces of the teeth. Other aids, such as toothpicks, can be substituted for dental floss if the particular condition dictates.

46. **2** Various toothbrushing techniques include the following. Stillman: The side of a firm bristle brush is placed against the tooth and the gingival tissue with the bristles pointing gingivally. The brush is pressed against the tissues and pulled coronally. Charters': The side of the brush is placed against the marginal gingival tissue and tooth with the bristle pointing coronally. The brush is pressed against the oral tissues and is moved in small circular motions. Bass: The bristles of a soft nylon brush are placed at a 45-degree angle into the gingival sulcus. The brush is then rotated in small circular motions.

47. **3** Water irrigators are used to remove loose debris. They will not remove plaque or calculus.

48. **1** The optimum amount of fluoride in drinking water is 1 ppm. Excessive amounts of fluoride (more than 2 ppm) may cause alteration in the calcification of enamel resulting in a condition known as mottled enamel.

49. **4** Nutrition is the process in which ingested food is assimilated and utilized by the body.

50. **1** Food is used by the body for fuel, growth, repair, and regulation of body functions.

51. **2** Metabolism is the sum of all anabolic and catabolic chemical changes that food undergoes in the process of nutrition.

52. **3** Vitamins are organic compounds essential for

normal growth, body functions and health. They are catalysts and not made by the body. Vitamins are classified as water soluble (e.g., B and C); and fat soluble (e.g., A, D, E, and K).

53. **2** A deficiency of vitamin A affects structure and function of ameloblasts and causes faulty enamel formation. Vitamin A also affects vision, growth, keratinization, and resistance to infection.

54. **1** Vitamin C has an important role in wound healing. Oral manifestations of a deficiency of vitamin C are poor wound healing, friable bleeding gingiva, and tooth mobility.

55. **3** Oral manifestations of riboflavin deficiency are cheilitis (lips become swollen, crack easily especially at the corners of the mouth) and glossitis (tongue is red and swollen).

56. **4** Green stains on children's teeth are often the result of chromogenic bacteria. This is due to poor oral hygiene. It is an extrinsic stain and can be removed during oral prophylaxis.

Bibliography

Bernier, J.L. and Muhler, J.C. *Improving Dental Practice Through Preventive Measures,* 3rd ed. St. Louis: The C. V. Mosby Co., 1975.

Caldwell, R.C. and Stallard, R.E. *A Textbook of Preventive Dentistry,* Philadelphia: W. B. Saunders Co., 1977.

Carlos, J.P. *Prevention and Oral Health,* Baltimore: DHEW Publication No. (NIH) 74–707, 1973.

Guthrie, H.A. *Introductory Nutrition,* 4th ed. St. Louis: The C. V. Mosby Co., 1979.

Hefferson, J.J.; Ayer, W. A.; and Koehler, H.M. (eds). *Foods, Nutrition and Dental Health,* South Ill.: Pathodox Publishers, 1980.

Newman, H.N. *Dental Plaque,* Springfield, Ill.: Charles C Thomas Publishers, 1980.

Randolph, P.M. and Dennison, C.I. *Diet, Nutrition, and Dentistry,* St. Louis: The C. V. Mosby Co., 1981.

Section on Instructional System Design, Department of Periodontology, School of Dentistry, University of California, San Francisco. *Developing a Plaque Control Program,* Berkley, Calif.: Praxis Publishing Co., 1972.

Section on Instructional System Design, Department of Periodontology, School of Dentistry, University of California, San Francisco. *Plaque Control Instruction,* Berkeley, Calif.: Praxis Publishing Co., 1978.

Silverstone, L.H. *Preventive Dentistry,* Fort Lee, N.J.: Update Publishing International Inc., 1978.

7

Behavioral Sciences

Course Synopsis

Introduction

Dental assisting is a profession that involves working with people. As a member of the treatment team, the assistant functions as an important extension of the dentist. In most busy offices, the dental assistant is the first member of the dental team the patient meets and the last person the patient sees before leaving. The philosophy, rules, atmosphere, and concern of the care providers is transmitted during these encounters. The assistant will usually greet, escort to the treatment room, and prepare the patient for treatment. During treatment, the assistant often stays with the patient when the dentist is out of the operatory and at the conclusion of treatment, the auxiliary dismisses the patient. In addition, the auxiliary can arrange appointments, negotiate payment arrangements, and conduct other office or treatment business with the patient. During these interactions, the assistant may be called upon to calm the patient, provide support or understanding, and clarify patient perceptions of office expectations.

A well-functioning office requires a well-functioning team in which each member knows his or her job, works well with others, and communicates both quickly and clearly. On a daily basis, interpersonal misunderstandings and conflicts occur and should be resolved productively. From the initial interview before accepting a job in the dental office to daily on-the-job performance, and even at the point terminating employment, it is essential that the dental assistant be aware of the demands and characteristics of work group dynamics.

The dental assistant who is able to function as a professional in health care delivery combines the knowledge of the psychology of individuals and groups, specific interpersonal skills and techniques, and a knowledge of and the ability to use himself or herself as a therapeutic instrument.

Starting With The Self

An important aspect of the dental assistant's job is providing the emotional support and information necessary to the patient for accepting and cooperating with dental treatment. It is not required that the auxiliary be a psychotherapist, but it is important that he or she be able to understand, guide, and relate to the patient's behavior. The behavior of others can be modified by changing ones's own behavior and perceptions. Although the assistant cannot control the patient directly, he or she can change the expectations of the situation. Self-knowledge and social skills are the tools the dental assistant applies when working with others. Dental care often makes people anxious, frightened, and confused. In these states, people often behave in ways that can cause problems during treatment. The assistant must respond to this behavior in ways that are helpful to the patient. Several areas of personal functioning are important in this activity:

1. *EFFECTIVE PRESENTATION OF SELF IS CRUCIAL TO PROFESSIONAL FUNCTIONING*. People learn something about each other when they first meet. They use the clues that are given to determine who others are and how they should behave. The assistant can control the messages he or she provides by paying attention to dress, posture and movement, eye contact, and personal tempo.

   The clothes people wear and how they wear them reveal information about themselves. For example, a white uniform informs the patient that the auxiliary is a part of the treatment team and is engaged in an efficient, no-nonsense activity.

   Upright posture and purposeful, directed activity conveys to the patient that the auxiliary is engaged in important work, is conscientious, and knows what he or she is doing.

   Direct eye contact conveys interest, alertness, and attention. Through appropriate eye contact with the patient, the auxiliary begins to establish or continue the relationship with the patient.

   Professional speech, whether on the phone or in person, should be modulated, calm, and clear. In the office, conversation should be to the point and appropriate to the interaction.

2. *THE DENTAL ASSISTANT SHOULD BE CENTERED WHEN INTER—ACTING WITH PATIENTS*. Since the dental patient is often anxious, feeling a little out of control, and not thinking clearly, it becomes the auxiliary's responsibility to preserve the stability of the situation. The auxiliary must avoid being "thrown off balance" by the patient's misperceptions, upset, or inappropriate behavior. Ceramicists speak of "centering" their clay on the potting wheel so that the clay will respond only to the pressure of their fingers and will not wobble because it is unbalanced. In much the same way, the auxiliary must "center" himself or herself within the treatment situation and create an internal calmness and receptiveness so that the only response given is to the actual behavior of the patient. The auxiliary's response should not be amplified or distorted by the concerns brought from home or from previous patients. It is important to react directly to the actual.

3. *ESTABLISHING A CLEAR AND ACCEPTABLE INTERPERSONAL CONTACT IS AN IMPORTANT KEY TO PATIENT MANAGEMENT*. A contract is the expectation for certain behavior or behaviors that one person develops concerning the other. These contracts are not legal or written, they are psychological. Often the expectations are not even shared with the other. Whether the contract is explicit (shared) or implicit (not discussed), when it is broken the other party feels betrayed and hurt. The dental assistant can be very helpful by negotiating clear, explicit contracts. The patient should be told exactly what is expected of him or her in the office. In the same way, the auxiliary should try to discover the patient's expectations of the staff and office and clarify them if they are unreasonable or unrealistic.

Communication

Almost all interaction taking place in the dental office is based upon communication. To be effective, the assistant must exchange clear and accurate messages with the dentist, other auxiliaries and patients. In the busy office, patients often depend upon the auxiliaries to convey their needs, concerns, messages, and questions to the dentist; in turn, the dentist may depend upon the staff to be the liaison for important communication with patients. To be effective in this job duty, the auxiliary must understand the nature of the communication process.

Primary Functions of Office-Based Communication

The auxiliary must convey information to the patient in the form of instructions and explanations. Besides telling the patient when to come to the office, how to pay for treatment, where to sit, etc., the assistant may also provide oral health care instruction and answer patient's questions regarding office policy, dental insurance, and office records. The auxiliary must elicit and clarify information presented by the patient. Often the auxiliary requests basic personal information from the patient before or during an initial appointment. In addition, the auxiliary will listen to, clarify, and transmit patient's concerns to the dentist. Often communication is intended to influence or modify behavior. The auxiliary through proper selection of words and tone of voice can praise a patient, punish a patient, or encourage a desired behavior.

The dental assistant will want to support the patient by sharing feelings. The right gesture or words often provide the patient with the support necessary to survive an anxious moment. The ability to express empathy is a key factor in the assistant's attempts to be helpful.

Finally, communication is a part of creating and modifying personal relationships. The very act of communication bonds people together and most relationships are defined by the quality of their communications.

Communication is the development of a shared meaning. Communication is a process, not an event. Many individuals believe that they are engaged in an act of communication when they speak to another person. But, often they are wrong. It is not enough just to send a message. The message must be perceived and understood. The receiver, rather than the sender of the message, defines both the quality and the meaning of the message.

There are a number of techniques that increase the likelihood that the receiver will understand messages. Some of these techniques will be reviewed in this chapter.

Methods of Communication

It is possible for the dental assistant to increase the probability that accurate communication occurs. Some of the obvious methods are knowing the subject being discussed, using words the other person understands, and listening carefully.

BUILD REDUNDANCY INTO MESSAGES. The same message can be given in different forms. For example, the auxiliary might not only tell the patient how to brush but could also demonstrate the techniques. Often, providing the patient with written as well as verbal information will help ensure that the message is received.

FOCUS THE ATTENTION OF THE RECEIVER. Before providing information, tell the receiver what you plan to present. Help your listener to decide on what to focus his or her attention.

REQUEST FEEDBACK. After the message has been sent, ask the listener to tell you what you have said. At times, you might want the patient to demonstrate a skill you have just presented.

UTILIZE ACTIVE LISTENING. Active listening is a method used to help the message sender increase the ability to be understood. As a dental assistant, you will want to ensure that you accurately understand the patient's message and that the patient feels he or she is being heard and receiving attention. Active listening was developed as a therapeutic skill by Dr. Carl Rogers (a psychotherapist), but it works well for the auxiliary. There are three types of receiver activity involved: restatement, reflection, and clarification.

Restatement. The reciever tells the message sender what he or she has just heard. The reciever does not add information but merely, in his or her own words and those of the sender, repeats the message received.

Reflection. The receiver tells the sender the feelings are being received. In other words, the receiver provides his or her own interpretation of the emotional meaning of the message.

Clarification. The receiver asks the sender to add information in areas that were unclear in the original message. Thus, the sender is given the opportunity to expand and explain those elements of the message that were originally unclear.

PROVIDE CLEAR INSTRUCTION. The dental assistant is often called upon to provide patients with home care instruction. There are specific guidelines for providing clear, usable instructions.

Begin by giving the patient a clear overview of the task. The patient should be told what the task is supposed to accomplish and what the patient is to learn.

The second step is to determine the receiver's perception, expectations, and knowledge of the required task. The instructor should determine the receiver's readiness and willingness to undertake the task. The instruction should be tailored to the needs of the receiver.

Allow time for questions, feedback, and correcting misconceptions. Build in redundancy. The best instruction should not only be verbal but also visual.

The instructor should be open to the receiver's ideas and perceptions. If the instructor listens to the receiver, he or she is more likely to be clear and helpful.

BE SPECIFIC WHEN GIVING INSTRUCTION. Use the correct name for objects and avoid vagueness in terms and instructions. When steps are involved, they should be numbered and given in order.

DO NOT OVERLOAD THE RECIPIENT. A person can learn only so much in one sitting. At the same time, evaluate the receiver's knowledge. Where possible, allow the receiver to demonstrate his or her knowledge and understanding.

Finally, give reinforcement, praise, and encouragement.

The Psychology of the Patient

The psychological needs and concerns of the patient influence his or her perception of and reaction to dental care. Often, members of the treatment team fail to recognize the patient's concern until problems arise. Mishandling or ignoring these needs can result in behavior that creates difficulty for the treatment team and for the patient. If the dental assistant is aware of and responsive to patients concerns, he or she can prevent problems as well as help patients to accept treatment calmly and cooperatively.

Dental patients can be separated into four age groups: children, adolescents, adults, and the elderly. Each age group faces social, emotional, and intellectual challenges and opportunities as a result of their level of physical, psychological, and societal maturation. As a result, each group presents different concerns in the office and requires different management strategies.

Children are focused on their actual experience. A child's thinking and understanding is concrete. The word and the experience are perceived as being the same, that is, a child takes what is said literally instead of symbolically. For example, when a child hears that the dentist is going to use a hatchet, he or she pictures teeth being chopped. It is therefore important that the dental assistant select words carefully to convey nonthreatening, familar images to the child. Thus, the injection or shot might be referred to as "sleepy water," which will be squirted near the tooth or gums to "put the tooth to sleep." In addition, young children often make a direct causal connection between discomfort experienced as the dentist works and punishment. A child feels that he or she has done something wrong if he or she is being hurt. (This thinking, called "imminent justice," is preserved in our language in the form, "It serves you right".) It is very important for the dentist and auxiliary to clarify for the patient that the dental treatment is not punishment and that the child has not done something bad or wrong in taking care of his or her teeth. Parents should not be allowed to use the dental visit as a threat or punishment to force a child to adopt desired oral care habits.

A related issue for children is "body integrity." A child believes that each part of his or her body is crucial to personal identity. Loss of a body part or a change in appearance (such as the loss of a tooth) can be upsetting. Fear of mutilation, such as having a tooth drilled, is more threatening than the possibility of pain. Providing a child with a mirror so that he or she can see that the dentist is not causing damage is an effective strategy for calming the child's anxiety. If a tooth must be extracted, it is a good idea to allow the child to bring it home and to control its disposal.

A third crucial issue for a child is competence. Children judge their own worth in terms of what they can do. Actions are concrete demonstrations of one's value. Because a child has acquired the cognitive and physical capacity to perform tasks by the end of nursery school, teachers and peers expect the child to demonstrate a level of competence. Children feel they must earn the approval of peers and adults. The auxiliary, in giving instruction and correcting behavior, should concentrate on what a child does well, rather than on what he or she does wrong. Success leads to success. Children's behavior is best controlled by telling them exactly what is expected. A child should be guided step by step through the visit. The desire to do things correctly is a powerful motivator. This developmental period is also an excellent time in which to instill positive oral habits.

Related to a child's concern with competence is his or her concern with self-control. Children often panic when they feel out of control. It is therefore important to avoid restraining or immobilizing a child unless it is necessary for treatment or to prevent the child from "acting out." By carefully explaining what is going to happen, the auxiliary can help the child retain a sense of control. A good technique is the method of tell–show–do:

EXPLAIN TO THE CHILD WHAT IS GOING TO BE DONE.

FAMILIARIZE THE CHILD WITH THE SETTING, INSTRUMENTS, AND PROCEDURES.

PERFORM THE PROCEDURES, TELLING THE PATIENT WHAT IS HAP—PENING.

A final note regarding children is in order. Research shows that the dental habits and feelings about dentists expressed by adults are often the result of childhood experiences with treatment. Positive experiences as a child can be the key to positive dental health in adulthood.

Adolescents tend to be focused on themselves. In psychological terms, the adolescent is considered egocentric. That is, an adolescent perceives and judges the world in terms of his or her own needs and philosophy. Because he or she has developed physically into a "mature body" and intellectually to the point of being able to think abstractly and for the long term (like an adult), the adolescent starts to assume adult status. Thus the adolescent is beginning the process of establishing himself or herself as an independent entity separate from parents. Two psychological–patient management issues become critical. First, although adolescents desire independence, parents are very much concerned with both the economic and dental-medical aspects of treatment. Involving parents in the dental treatment is a tricky problem. On the one hand, the parents are paying the bill. They are also legally responsible for their child's welfare. Often, problems of living (e.g., sexually transmitted diseases, signs of stress, changes in health status) are revealed in the dental examination. On the other hand, the adolescent wishes to preserve autonomy and privacy. Developing an alliance with the parents can place the treatment team in the center of a family power struggle. As a general rule, it is better to work directly with an adolescent patient. Rather than ask parents to reinforce appointment-keeping or home care compliance, it is more effective to form a therapeutic alliance with a patient. To do this, it may be necessary to consider very carefully an adolescent's need for privacy before involving parents in the resolution of social and medical problems discovered in the course of treatment.

A second psychological–patient management issue is also related to the adolescent's search for an autonomous identity. Since adolescents are questioning their parents' standards and values, they must look elsewhere for new criteria, often to the judgments of peers and other nonfamily adults. Other people's judgment determines an adolescent's standard of personal value. Appearance becomes very important. A primary issue for adolescents is whether teeth are straight and pretty and whether speech is clear. Also, the approval of others is crucial. An adolescent is less concerned with how well he or she does than with whether people judge him or her as intelligent, nice, special, etc. When giving health instruction or responding to an adolescent's questions and requests concerning treatment, it is important the adolescent not feel patronized or negatively perceived. It is helpful to tell the patient what he or she is doing correctly and incorrectly; it is important to convey the impression that whether the action or request is correct or not, you respect the person. Negative statements should be avoided.

Adolescents can be extremely provocative as they test to see whether others will reject them or become involved with them. Some patients will become hostile and very touchy. Others will become seductive or intrusive or both. The auxiliary's patience and tolerance will be challanged. The appropriate stance with an adolescent is to maintain an accepting, warm, but nonpersonal manner. It is important to maintain a nonjudgmental, professional attitude and to avoid becoming overinvolved in the adolescent's very intense life struggles. One can listen, offer support, and accept the person without becoming a major actor in the drama. It is important to create the type of atmosphere that will allow the patient to cooperate with and benefit from dental treatment.

Adults tend to be focused on time, convenience, and function. The primary pressure faced by an adult patient is getting done all the things for which he or she is responsible. Job pressures, family responsibilities, and social relations tend to take precedence over dental care. Patients are usually more concerned with how long the treatment will take, how much their daily functioning will be impaired, and how much treatment will cost them than they are with esthetics, the dental staff's opinion, or treatment discomfort. To meet the dental patient's need and to elicit cooperation, the auxiliary must enter into a clear exchange with the patient regarding expectations. The office hours and office policies regarding punctuality and payment must be clearly discussed. After the treatment plan is presented by the dentist, the schedule of office visits and payments should be discussed by the auxiliary with the patient. Treatment is likely to fail and the relationship with the patient to sour if the expectations of both the dental office and the patient are not clearly defined. Appointments should be arranged that will fit within the patient's work and family obligations. Financial arrangements must be consistent with the patient's ability to pay. Adults will require information concerning their insurance benefits and accurate documentation of their treatment and its cost.

In providing patient education, the auxiliary should focus upon the immediate and long-term effects of oral functioning. Adults can plan ahead and will be concerned with their long-term health and the economic consequences of noncompliance. They recognize that they will suffer for their mistakes and benefit from their diligence. They will be able to accept short-term inconvenience in the hope of long-term benefit. For adults, dental health care is an investment. The auxiliary must convince an adult that the investment is worthwhile.

An elderly patient is concerned with loss of function and loss of social identity and importance. Old age is more a function of social expectations (social age) and current physical state (physical age) than it is of the passage of years (chronological age.) Socially, retirement, reduced financial ability, and family status changes (children marrying and leaving home, birth of grandchildren, and death of family members and close friends) define a person as getting on in years. Physically, decline in fitness or flexibility of cognitive functioning is an indicator of "aging." As the individual enters old age, his or her ability to do things for himself or herself decreases. For example, the loss of teeth and the necessity of wearing dentures will affect the patient's ability to talk and eat as well as appearance and self-concept. The loss will have an impact on all aspects of the individual's functioning. Chronic illness is both the cause and the result of a gradual physical deterioration of the body.

Dental illness is a chronic disease related to aging. Once the body functioning is disrupted by chronic disease, it is not unusual for the entire social and physical functioning of the individual to decline. The result of these changes is an increased dependence on others.

Two problems faced by the auxiliary who works with the elderly patient are hypochondriasis and depression. Hypochondriasis is an excessive anxious concern with the functioning of parts of the body. The patient will become very concerned with small lesions, the way their various dental prostheses fit and look, and their general oral health. They will experience a greater need for sympathetic attention and concern.

Depression is a morbid sadness and feeling of loss. In an elderly person, it is usually the result of the loss of self-esteem that occurs when the individual is unable to contribute to his or her own and other's welfare. The aging person feels useless and a burden to those around; he or she experiences a loss of purpose that was provided by a defined job and family role.

In both these cases, the auxiliary can provide relief by according the patient special attention. It is helpful to allow the patient to share his or her experiences. Listening respectfully to the patient's opinions and advice is beneficial to the patient and may even be of help to the auxiliary. Secondly, reminiscence is therapeutic to elderly persons. It allows them to reinstate social roles and contributions. Finally, the dental visit, because it is a personal process of taking care of one's needs, is often an important event in the elderly person's life. It involves planning and getting ready for the visit and receiving focused concern and attention; it is often an important topic of discussion with friends.

Because of the changes in cognitive and emotional functioning in older people, elderly patients may need special support in the dental setting. Dental treatment can be demanding physically. Patients may become disoriented and confused. It is often helpful to suggest that the patient arrange to be accompanied by a friend or member of the family when he or she comes for treatment. It may also be necessary, if the patient does come to the office alone, to ensure the patient gets home safely by arranging transportation.

Secondly, elderly patients have some difficulty adapting to new ideas or demands. It is helpful if the auxiliary builds upon the patient's past experiences, beliefs, and habits when giving instruction in necessary home care techniques. New procedures and methods as well as appointment times and directions should be written out and given to the patient to take home. Providing this support will enable the patient to cooperate satisfactorily with treatment.

Finally, it is important to encourage and support the patients' striving to maintain a high quality of life. Many people, including elderly patients, see old age as a period in which one is simply waiting for death. They hesitate to invest time or economic resources in improving the opportunity to live a full life. With the increased ability of modern medicine to preserve life, this attitude is inappropriate. The elderly patient in the dental office can radically improve the quality of life by increasing the functional efficiency of his or her oral apparatus and by improving his or her appearance and speech. It is the dental assistant's responsibility to support this effort.

The Patient's Psychological Concerns

Dental treatment often elicits an anxiety reaction in patients. Anxiety is different from fear in that fear is usually a focused response to a specific, observable threat, while anxiety is a generalized response to a situation. Anxious patients often hyperventilate and may even faint. They may also exhibit behavior that creates patient-management problems. In addition, the anxious patient's psychological and physiological responses may increase resistance to anesthesia, making it more difficult for the dentist to comfortably perform treatment. The auxiliary can often help the patient cope with and/or decrease the anxiety response by awareness of behavioral and psychological issues involved:

An important issue is the patient's need for control. Depending on upbringing and experience, people exhibit characteristic needs to control their social and physical experience. Some people cope with their anxiety in the dental office by demanding to know everything about their treatment and requesting that they be consulted on every decision. Others go to the other extreme, desiring to turn everything over to the dental team and avoiding being given any information. Often this second group will voice the wish that they could be put to sleep and awakened when everything is over. Of course, most people fall along the continuum between these two extremes. It is important that the auxiliary be aware of the patient's needs and responsive to these concerns. The overcontrolling patient will be less of a problem if he or she is given complete information and allowed to participate in treatment planning within clearly defined limits. The patient should understand that the dental team must set certain rules if successful treatment is to be accomplished, but the auxiliary should realize that this patient will initiate fewer problems when kept fully informed. The patient who desires to give up all control and avoid knowledge may be even more of a problem. This patient often fails to fulfill home care instructions and, at times, may fail to provide informed consent to treatment. This patient also needs information to decrease anxiety, but, in this case, the patient should be educated slowly and carefully. Where possible, the patient should be encouraged to ask questions and participate in decision-making. Often, the overtly compliant patient will secretly resist treatment and express hidden resentment at being controlled by failing to understand directions and becoming helpless in the chair.

A second issue is the way in which the patient perceives the events occurring around him or her and interprets the sensations felt in treatment. Besides the patient who has a firm hold on reality and who perceives accurately the events occurring in treatment, there are other types of patients. Some patients amplify every sensation they experience. Mild pressure or discomfort may be classified as pain. Every experience is magnified out of proportion. In their response to anxiety, these patients increase their vigilance. In contrast, some patients deny that they feel or experience anything. They report to the dentist that they are not feeling any pain and that he or she can proceed even without anesthesia. These patients may be so anxious about their pain and discomfort that they pretend that nothing is really happening. Unfortunately, when pain becomes overwhelming or the anxiety too great, the defense breaks down. The patient can no longer deny his or her experience and may panic. Another type of patient may distort the actual reality of the situation. For example, a very suspicious patient seeing two auxiliaries talking may assume they are talking about him or her.

With each of these types of patient, the auxiliary and dentist must work to improve the ability to perceive reality clearly. For example, the hypersensitive patient can be helped to distinguish between pressure and pain so that he or she can clearly determine what is actually being experienced. This clearer perception will reduce concern over treatment. The denying patient can be guided to recognize and accept the experience of treatment and to allow the dentist to provide appropriate anesthesia. The distorting patient should be given more information before and during treatment. At each point in treatment what is occurring should be explained both carefully and slowly.

The third issue is the patient's perception of the dentist and the treatment team. Most people use their past experience to guess how new people will behave and think. They project characteristics about others. In the dental situation, the anxious patient often sees the members of the dental team as authority figures. The patient then irrationally expects them to have special powers, knowledge, or abilities. This psychological process is called transference. Often the patient will react to the dentist or dental team members positively or negatively in terms of these perceptions. The dental assistant should be alert to these magnified expectations and help the patient develop a more appropriate understanding of the treatment situation.

Patients With Specific Handicaps

Some patients will present themselves in the office with physical problems. Some patients are confined to wheelchairs or are unable to control their body motions (for example, cerebral palsy patients). Other patients may be emotionally disturbed. In each case, it may be necessary to make special provisions for these people. The dental auxiliary can make it easier for these patients by making the necessary provisions in advance of the patient's arrival or introduction into the treatment room. The auxiliary should review the patient's chart prior to treatment and make any needed preparations so that the patient will not be forced to be embarrassed.

Patients who experience psychological or emotional difficulty may require that the office environment be simplified. The staff should decrease the activity level of the treatment room for the disturbed patient. Too much stimulation can confuse the patient and make him or her more anxious or disoriented. Patients who are easily confused or upset should be placed in quiet environments and focused onto the treatment taking place. Because they become easily disoriented and may panic, they should be guided carefully through each step of treatment.

Patients with physical handicaps might require special modifications of the treatment apparatus. Patients in wheelchairs may have to be treated in their chairs if it is too difficult to transfer them to the dental chair. Many patients with physical handicaps needlessly avoid treatment because of embarrassment or feeling that they are unacceptable for treatment.

Patient Management

Often the dental assistant is called upon by the dentist to help educate or manage a patient. Several approaches for assisting the patient are discussed below.

Motivation

Action is the result of the interaction of knowledge, ability, and motivation. If an individual is to perform a task, whether it be as a patient fulfilling home care instruction or as an employee meeting job expectations, the person must understand how he or she is supposed to behave. In addition, the individual must be willing to perform the task. This willingness to act is called motivation.

Motivation is the result of personal impulse or desire to obtain a particular object or experience. This impulse or desire is called a drive. Primary drives arise out of a biological need for food, water, sex, or stimulation. Secondary drives are learned needs which grow out of the primary drives. These needs might be for attention, love, respect, safety, etc. Abraham Maslow, a psychologist, has described a heirarchy of needs. He states that one must satisfy lower-order needs before being gratified by higher-order needs. The first level of need is related to survival concerns. The individual ensures that he or she will not starve, die of thirst, suffer terrible pain, or be physically attacked before being able to focus on the next level of concern. For example, if a patient presents in pain, the pain must be relieved before the patient will listen to discussions of oral hygiene, reliability, or long-term treatment plans. The second level of need is for acceptance and approval. Patients are often concerned about whether the dental staff accepts, respects, and approves of them. The third level of need is to do things well and properly. People feel good when they see that they are doing things correctly. The highest order of need is to grow and to develop one's potential to the highest order.

Fredrick Hertzberg, another psychologist, has divided needs into deficiency needs and sufficiency needs. When one meets a deficiency need, the drive is fulfilled and the motivation to act ends. For example, when a hungry individual is fed or a person in pain is relieved, he or she stops striving to meet the goal. On the other hand, when one satisfies a sufficiency need, one tends to work even harder. For example, the more skillful a person becomes the harder he or she tries to improve skills. Patients who come to the dentist in an effort to maintain their health and appearance are generally more reliable than those who appear in emergencies for relief of pain.

The dental assistant cannot motivate a patient to brush his or her teeth, keep appointments, or pay on time. One person cannot motivate another; motivation is an internal state. The dental assistant can elicit the patient's motivation by creating situations in which the patient's needs can be fulfilled by responding to the dental assistant's requests. Furthermore, if the dental assistant focuses on the patient's sufficiency needs (higher-order needs, such as oral health, reliability, responsibility) rather than on the patient's deficiency needs (lower-order needs, such as fear of pain or loss), the patient is most likely to develop positive dental habits.

There are three steps in eliciting a patients' motivation. The first is helping the patient assume ownership of the particular task or problem. If the patient is to take responsibility, he or she must recognize that a problem or need exists, see what can be done to resolve the problem, and exhibit a readiness to act. The second step is to show the patient that there is a reasonable probability of success following action. And finally, once the patient acts, the behavior should be reinforced.

Behavior Modification

Behavior modification is a technique that developed from observing how all organisms, including people, learn. Behavior modification is generally used to meet one of three objectives: to increase the rate or frequency of a desired behavior, to decrease the rate or frequency of an undesired behavior, or to substitute a new behavior for an existing undesirable one.

When an individual is reinforced (rewarded) for a particular response, he or she is more likely to exhibit the same response to that stimulus in the future. However, when the response is met with punishment, the individual is less likely to exhibit the same behavior. By controlling the outcomes or contingencies to a patient's behavior, the dental assistant can increase the probability the patient will behave appropriately. All individuals, in part, learn how to behave by observing the consequences of their behavior.

Shaping

Shaping is a technique based on the principles of behavior modification. It was developed by Dr. B. F. Skinner. It is a useful method of improving patient behavior. When an individual who has developed a particular response to a stimulus does not receive his or her usual reinforcement (reward), he or she tends to repeat the behavior in a more intense form. For example, if a patient whose behavior is usually met with a smile suddenly receives silence or indifference, he or she will usually repeat the behavior. If the behavior continues to be met with no response (negative reinforcement), the person tends to stop. However, if the repeated, stronger behavioral response does not receive a reinforcement (e.g., attention), the individual will adapt the new (more extreme) behavior. By strategically rewarding and withholding rewards, the auxiliary can guide the patient into modifying his or her former behavior. This method is helpful but also indicates the possibility of making behavior worse. For example, ignoring a problem patient until you can no longer stand his or her provocative behavior and then exploding (giving attention) may lead to worse behavior. An important rule to remember is that when one witholds reinforcement (e.g., ignores behavior), the behavior becomes more extreme before it disappears.

Desensitization

Sometimes the patient's primary response to the dental situation is fear, avoidance, and anxiety. This reaction may block the patient's ability to cooperate with treatment. Desensitization is a technique used to decrease the likelihood of this response. This is done by teaching the patient a new response that is incompatible with the frightened or anxious response. For example, the patient can be taught to relax and think pleasant thoughts in response to a signal. Then the patient is gradually introduced to aspects of the dental situation and signalled to relax when he or she perceives each aspect. Gradually, a new response (the relaxation and thinking pleasant thoughts) that is incompatible with the phobic response (getting anxious and frightened) is substituted for the old one.

Working in the Dental Team

An important responsibility of the dental assistant is functioning as a productive member of the dental team. All work groups have certain characteristics in common.

Conflict

Interpersonal conflict is an issue in any work group. Conflict is often attributed to personality differences, but it is seldom this simple. In a work group, conflict is most likely to arise out of the structure of the working situation itself. There are two types of conflict. The first is called zero-sum conflict. This type of conflict often arises when two or more people are competing for the same object. This object could be desk space, the right to provide patient education, or priority on vacation time. What is important is that the individuals are in conflict because they want the same thing—not because of feelings about each other. This type of conflict is best resolved by negotiation, compromise, and the addition of new resources. Clarifying the conflict is not helpful, since it only serves to make the competition more open and intense.

A helpful method of breaking the impasse and developing interdependence and trust is for one party to give to the other something the other values but which does not cost the giver. This is known as the Osgood Solution and is a commonly used strategy even between nations.

The second type of conflict is more personal and usually involves feelings of betrayal. This conflict arises when one individual fails to meet the expectations of the other. The results of contract violation lead to a desire to punish. In this situation, the parties involved must sit down, clarify their perceptions and feelings, and work out their differences.

The number of individuals in the work group is important. Groups of fewer than five have special properties because of the possibilities of becoming imbalanced. Groups of three and five tend to be unstable because of the probability of uneven numbers in each subgroup.

Power

Power is the ability to control or influence the behavior of others. In most groups, an informal pecking order is established that determines who influences whom. In the dental office, four sources of power exist. Expert power is derived from having the knowledge and skills necessary for accomplishing a task. In the office, every member at one time or another will assume leadership because of the possession of some special knowledge. However, the people who have been in the office the longest and know the most about the way things are done tend to control office activity. Reward power is derived from being able to control the rewards available. For example, the person who holds the purse strings of the office or who is in charge of hiring and firing is often quite powerful in day-to-day activity. The receptionist who controls the patient's access to the dentist has this power over the patient. Position power is based on each individual's formal job title. For example, the office manager, by virtue of the job title is able to control the office. Finally, referent power is a form of social power that stems from one person's identification with another. In terms of optimum functioning, expert power, because it supports the organizational structure, is the most legitimate source of power.

Question Section

Directions: Each of the questions or incomplete statements below is followed by four suggested answers or completions. Select the BEST answer in each case.

1. A patient has been treated at a dental office for many years. The assistant has never had a chance to talk with the patient, and when she arranges an appointment, she tells the assistant that she must have a long appointment, because, as a practicing lawyer, she is very busy and can afford only one afternoon for her dental care. The patient's insistence is probably her way of
   1. indicating that she is anxious and wants special treatment
   2. credentialing herself
   3. making conversation
   4. making a nuisance of herself

2. A 26-year-old patient who has been coming to the office for about 3 years has been sitting in a relaxed position in the reception room. When the dental assistant enters the room and informs the patient that she should come into the operatory, the patient arises very slowly and walks with short, tight steps. When the assistant places her in the chair, she crosses her legs tightly, pulls back into the chair and talks in a low whisper. The patient is probably feeling
   1. physical discomfort
   2. very cold
   3. concern about her treatment
   4. fright

3. An 80-year-old man who has been a patient of the same dentist for a long time is having problems with his dentures, which were constructed two years ago; they just don't feel right to him. The doctor has told the patient that there is nothing really wrong with the dentures and suggested that the patient likes the attention and expects special treatment, since he has been a patient for many years. The patient has just called for a long appointment because he feels that his dentures need a lot of adjustment. The assistant checks the doctor's schedule and discovers that the next available appointment is two weeks away and informs the patient, who becomes very angry, refuses the appoint-ment, and demands to speak to the dentist. What probably went wrong?
   1. the patient is just a general problem and the assistant should not have had to deal with him
   2. the patient is getting senile and doesn't understand that the doctor is very busy
   3. The patient doesn't feel that the assistant is giving him the attention and concern he deserves
   4. the patient expects that he will be taken immediately and cannot stand the frustration of being put off for so long

4. A 35-year-old female patient is having trouble disciplining herself to comply with appropriate oral care activities. The assistant and patient have decided to develop a "behavior modification" protocol to help her establish new habits. After establishing that she desires to change her present behavior the first step for the assistant is to
   1. specify the behavior she wants to change
   2. develop a very special rapport with the patient
   3. give the patient encouragement
   4. tell the patient how great her mouth is going to feel when she develops new oral habits

5. A patient has come into the office with a troubled look on his face and a complaint. He begins his conversation with an insult and then begins to criticize everything about the office and the dentist. The assistant's most appropriate response at this point would be to
   1. ask the patient to leave
   2. provide an explanation or apology for each complaint
   3. engage in active listening
   4. become occupied in some paper work or other work until the patient calms down and behaves more appropriately

6. A dental assistant has been talking to a quiet, withdrawn woman about 24 years old concerning oral health self-care, and is concerned about her responses. Since the patient doesn't talk much, the assistant is uncertain as to whether she is really listening. How might the assistant discover whether the patient is involved?

1. observe how the patient positions her body relative to the assistant
2. check to see whether the patient maintains eye contact
3. ask the patient whether she understands
4. watch to see how often the patient says, "I understand," "Okay," "Yes," and other such comments

7. Two auxiliaries in the office have managed to get hooked into a competitive struggle over who is going to do patient education and work chairside. It seems that one person—the one who works with patients—gets all the interesting jobs, while the other always ends up doing paper work and answering phones. The conflict is beginning to interfere with performance. A good approach toward ending the conflict would be for each auxiliary to
   1. sit down with the other and talk it out
   2. go to the dentist and tell him or her to choose between them
   3. ignore the other
   4. accommodate the other without inconveniencing himself or herself

8. A patient is always 15 minutes to a half-hour late for her dental appointments. Each appointment the assistant reminds her to come on time, but she continues to be late. What might the assistant do to reduce the probability that the patient will continue to arrive late?
   1. try to find out why the patient always comes late
   2. threaten to not give the patient an appointment if she comes late again
   3. cancel the patient's appointment if she is more than 5 minutes late
   4. give the patient an appointment time that is really 20 minutes earlier than the scheduled treatment time

9. A 6-year-old boy begins to cry and says he is afraid of the dentist, the moment his mother brings him into the office. He does not calm down even after sitting in the reception room. The assistant suggests to his mother that another patient be treated first while she tries to calm him down. Since he continues to cry, the assistant suggests to the mother that she take him home and bring him back when he is calmer. At his next visit, he begins crying when he comes into the office. The assistant and mother decide to be firm and to prepare him for treatment. When the assistant attempts to bring him into the treatment room, what is he most likely to do?

1. become hysterical
2. become cooperative
3. become very quiet and docile
4. continue to cry softly but accept treatment

10. To the job applicant for a dental assistant position, the most important outcome of the job interview is
    1. whether or not he or she gets the job
    2. getting a clear view of the job requirements
    3. whether or not the dentist is impressed with his or her qualifications
    4. demonstrating how much he or she knows and is able to do

11. The most effective method of decreasing a zero-sum conflict is to
    1. clarify expectations
    2. develop interdependence
    3. make people agree to get along
    4. ask each person to be more tolerant of the other

12. When working with the very passive, withdrawn patient, it is important for an auxiliary to be
    1. very supportive and reassuring
    2. quiet and unobtrusive
    3. friendly, talkative, and enthusiastic
    4. clear and willing to give explanations

13. A patient persists in exhibiting inappropriate behavior in the office each time he comes. He makes wisecracks at the auxiliaries and goes into the office in which he doesn't belong. The dental auxiliary can help this patient by
    1. reminding him firmly of office rules
    2. asking the doctor to offer him premedication (sedation)
    3. yelling at him and threatening to throw him out of the office
    4. calling his wife and requesting that she deal with him

14. A local executive has for the third time had his secretary call to confirm the time of his appointment. When the appointment was first made, he made a great show of checking his calendar and negotiating a time that would be convenient to him. He also made sure to leave his business card with the receptionist so that she would have his office number in case she had to reach him. All this probably occurred so that
    1. he can be sure that he wastes no time
    2. he can feel sure that the receptionist knows how important he is

3. he can make sure that he doesn't miss his appointment
4. he can make sure that he can be reached if a problem with his appointment time arises

15. An important method of improving the quality of an interpersonal contract is to
   1. continually enforce the elements of the contract
   2. make explicit expectations of the other
   3. make the rewards more attractive
   4. increase the dimensionality of the contract

16. When meeting the patient for the first time, the auxiliary should be aware of his or her tendency to
   1. want to take care of the patient
   2. stereotype the patient
   3. like the patient
   4. accept what the patient says

17. A 58-year-old man has been told that because of periodontal problems and resultant bone loss, he is going to lose several teeth. His primary concern is likely to be
   1. that he is going to look bad
   2. that he is losing health and vitality
   3. that his body is going to suffer harm
   4. that the dentist disapproves of him for allowing this to occur

18. One of the most important tasks of the auxiliary when attempting to support an anxious patient is to
   1. be efficient
   2. be calm and cool
   3. be centered
   4. be strong

19. A mother has brought her 5-year-old son to the office because one of his primary teeth was slow to fall out; the dentist had to remove the tooth. It would be helpful to allow the child to take his tooth home because having the tooth will allow him to
   1. make money from the tooth fairy
   2. relieve his sense of body harm or loss
   3. bring a gift to his mother
   4. remember what went on in the office

20. A problem that most auxiliaries face in the dental office when wearing a uniform and being placed in charge of seating the patient is
   1. the patient thinks the auxiliary is knowledgeable about the situation
   2. the auxiliary lacks information to give to the patient

3. the auxiliary is seen as a punitive figure
4. the auxiliary has to deal with the patient's anxiety

21. The primary requirement of a "reinforcement" when used to modify behavior is that it is
   1. visible and tangible
   2. simple for the auxiliary to administer
   3. inexpensive and easily obtained
   4. adequate to elicit the behavior

22. During the job interview, when the assistant is asked by the dentist about knowledge of dental procedures and skill development, it is important that the assistant be both positive and honest. The assistant should not
   1. reveal what he or she doesn't know
   2. state that his or her expectations include working at chairside at least 50% of the time
   3. ask specific, direct questions about how the office functions
   4. pretend that he or she knows something that he or she doesn't

23. When giving a patient instructions or discussing payment plans, the auxiliary should try to create an interpersonal distance of
   1. 1 foot
   2. 3 to 4 feet
   3. 6 to 8 feet
   4. about 10 feet

24. People who don't face the person to whom they are speaking are often
   1. being rude
   2. avoiding intimacy
   3. not involved in the discussion
   4. in a hurry

25. Active listening involves
   1. being alert and attentive
   2. checking perceptions
   3. leaning forward and showing interest
   4. being a concerned listener

26. After his second visit, a 73-year-old patient begins to give an assistant advice about how to run the practice. As a former businessman, he feels qualified to help put the business in order. He is probably concerned with the following personal issue
   1. he is seeking approval
   2. he wants to maintain his dignity and former occupational status in the eyes of the assistant

3. he is upset and hopes by one-upping the assistant that he can gain control of his dental experiences
4. he is trying to reduce his fear by intellectualizing

27. A 15-year-old orthodontic patient is not properly or consistently cleaning his teeth and oral tissues under his appliance. Despite reminders from the dentist and continual pressure from his parents, he continues to neglect his care instructions. To increase compliance, the dentist should
    1. check to see whether the patient has friends who are telling him that it's unnecessary to be so worried about his teeth. If so, provide him with better instruction and education
    2. check to see whether the parents are using correct terminology when speaking with their son and to see whether they fully understand what is to be done
    3. attempt to establish an agreement with the adolescent concerning the self-care needed and the probable outcome of neglect
    4. threaten to discontinue treatment if the adolescent doesn't shape up

28. When treating a pedodontic patient, the dentist's first concern should be
    1. to establish a rapport with the parents
    2. to obtain a thorough dental–medical history
    3. to establish a rapport with the child
    4. to ensure that both parents and child know the dentist is the boss while the child is at the dental office

29. The patient who is most likely to want to spend more time with the dentist in the dental office is
    1. the five-year-old child after the second visit
    2. the eight-year-old child
    3. the 24-year-old housewife with a small child at home
    4. the elderly patient

30. The dental assistant's primary responsibility in patient management and the application of dental psychological principles is to
    1. enable the patient to accept and tolerate dental procedures
    2. help the patient resolve psychological problems
    3. keep the patient still and quiet until the treatment is completed
    4. maintain his or her own sanity

31. Sometimes a patient will elicit strong anger in an assistant. At those times, the assistant will probably be most effective if he or she
    1. swallows the anger and gets on with the job
    2. punishes the patient and gets it over with
    3. recognizes the anger and tries to understand what it is that leads to the reaction
    4. recognizes that since he or she gets along with most patients, there is probably something wrong with the patient

32. The most difficult type of behavior to change is
    1. approach behavior
    2. habitual behavior
    3. escape behavior
    4. aggressive behavior

33. A major source of office conflict in a busy office is
    1. laziness on the part of some of the staff
    2. intolerance of interpersonal differences
    3. tension resulting from working with many patients
    4. unclear job roles and duties

34. In the office, feedback to other auxiliaries or to patients is most likely to be helpful when it is
    1. given gently
    2. given nonjudgmentally
    3. given firmly
    4. very tactful

35. One of the best cues for discovering how receptive one person is to another is to observe
    1. the amount of eye contact that occurs
    2. body posture
    3. the number of statements of interest
    4. the amount of body movement that takes place

36. A dental assistant is charged with the responsibility of providing support to anxious patients and he or she must always remember that
    1. fatigue causes depression and feelings of helplessness
    2. if fears and anxieties are not focused upon, they will go away
    3. feelings are real
    4. everyone is motivated by their unconscious

37. In managing the hostile-aggressive patient, the auxiliary is most likely to be successful if he or she

1. directly challenges the patient and threatens to dismiss him or her
2. gives up, backs down, and lets the patient have his or her way
3. establishes clear but limited options for the patient
4. refuses to see the patient until the patient agrees to behave

38. An assistant has been providing oral health instruction to a 16-year-old girl who is receiving periodontic treatment. Her mother comes with her at each visit. The assistant notices that despite the amount of education he or she provides, the girl's oral health status does not improve. What might the assistant do?
    1. inform the mother that she should remind the girl to take care of her mouth
    2. tell the girl that if she doesn't begin to develop oral hygiene habits, she will lose her teeth
    3. yell at the girl for being so uncooperative
    4. teach the girl how to assess the health of her oral cavity

39. One important aspect of communication is perception of the message being sent. What is one of the major influences affecting message perception?
    1. the intentions of the sender
    2. the expectations held by the receiver
    3. the length of the message
    4. the complexity of the message

40. Effective communication can take place only when
    1. the sender (speaker) has presented himself or herself in a clear and concise manner
    2. the message being sent is clear
    3. the receiver understands the message being sent

41. A major determinant of how a particular behavior is interpreted is
    1. the setting in which the behavior takes place
    2. the level of anxiety of the receiver
    3. the level of calmness of the sender
    4. the timing of the behavior

42. It is often stated that the best age group for teaching preventive care is 7-12. What is unique about this group in terms of preventive management?
    1. they are less likely to be counterdependent
    2. they are very concerned with doing things right

3. they identify with the dentist and want to please him or her
4. the disease processes have not really begun

43. The major purpose of giving feedback to another person is
    1. to induce the other to change behavior
    2. to provide information for decision-making
    3. to correct behavior that has gotten out of hand
    4. to let the other know that he or she is being heard

44. One reason that the use of restatement will help stop an argument is
    1. the persons involved are forced to listen to one another
    2. the persons involved can distinguish between understanding and agreement
    3. it slows down the pace and forces the participants to think
    4. it forces each party to more closely examine the other's ideas

45. One fairly reliable indicator of lying is
    1. voice pitch
    2. unwillingness to look another person in the eye
    3. stammering and hesitancy of speech
    4. body rigidity

46. A useful measure of the success of a helping relationship is
    1. the number of options discovered or explored
    2. the number of clear solutions developed
    3. how satisfied the person being helped feels
    4. how satisfied the helper feels

47. An average-looking 16-year-old girl has been scheduled for restorative work. When the assistant talks to her, he or she discovers that she hates to smile because she is embarrassed about her mouth and the way it looks. She feels that there is a huge gap between her two front teeth. In reality, there is a slight, but not unsightly, gap between the two anterior teeth and a slight protrusion. Her mouth is not really unattractive in the assistant's opinion. What might the assistant say to her?

    1. "You are making a mountain out of a molehill and to me, you look fine. Stop being silly."
    2. "Lots of people look far worse than you do. Why don't you find something important to worry about, like your school grades."

3. "You look okay to me, but I can understand that you would like to have perfect teeth. What do your friends say?"
4. "I am sure everyone likes you no matter how you look."

48. A patient always does exactly what she is told. She never asks questions or makes any requests. How can an assistant help her to increase the likelihood that her treatment will really meet her needs?
   1. give her very clear instructions and always be firm in expectations
   2. encourage her to ask questions and to express her doubts
   3. request the dentist to take very special care of her
   4. ask her to bring in someone else with her to be present when you give her information or education

49. In a dental office, a characteristic of the work group that is very likely to be noticed by the patient, but not by the people working in the office is
   1. a special language that has developed among the staff
   2. a set of norms and rules that has developed among the working staff
   3. a set of power hierarchies that have developed
   4. the efficiency and interest of the working class

50. The first step in eliciting a patient's compliance with a home care regime is
   1. telling the patient that he or she must take better care of his or her oral tissue
   2. educating the patient how to care for his or her teeth and other oral tissues
   3. helping the patient recognize that home care is necessary for healthy teeth
   4. warning the patient that if the oral tissues are not taken care of, he or she will lose all of his or her teeth

51. A patient in the office is a professor of biology. Although the assistant has given him attention and time, he constantly criticizes, comments, and questions the treatment plans for his mouth. The assistant finds that the more attention that is given to him, the more trouble he becomes. How might the assistant turn this situation around?
   1. get rid of him
   2. tell him that he or she does not have time to argue
   3. ask him a question about some aspect of the ecology of the oral cavity

4. tell him that he or she is usually very busy, but since he is so concerned, a special session will be scheduled to discuss his concerns about his mouth

52. Most defensive behavior represents
   1. basic personality structure
   2. learned behavior
   3. difficulty in accepting treatment
   4. an inability to relate to authority

53. Often when someone tries to help another who is having a problem in his or her life, he or she finds out later that the other is not grateful and is, in fact, a little resentful. What is likely to cause this problem?
   1. the helper has given the other bad advice
   2. the helper is seen by the other as an evaluator
   3. the helper did not show the other enough sympathy and concern
   4. the helper did not provide enough advice, and the other had to solve the problem on his or her own

54. A very effective method of lowering patient anxiety is to
   1. sing to him or her
   2. use a quiet voice and show a calm manner
   3. give clear explanations
   4. ignore the upset and work slowly giving the patient time to calm down

55. A 52-year-old, neatly groomed, gentleman has presented in the office with moderately severe gingival problems. Several teeth have become loose and will have to be extracted and replaced. When the dentist explains this to him, he becomes overly (in the dentist's judgment) upset and seems quite shaken. What is likely to be his primary concern?
   1. that he will suffer a lot of pain
   2. that his appearance will suffer
   3. that he is losing his health
   4. that he has not exercised proper dental health care

56. It is very important that the dentist elicit the patient's most mature level of coping with the anxiety raised by the dental visit. One form of coping that can create real problems with treatment is
   1. denial
   2. aggression
   3. countertransference
   4. transference

57. A patient in the office is a very intense 7-year-old. She asks the assistant many ques-

tions about her teeth and seems to be very interested when the assistant teaches her how to brush her teeth. In fact, the dentist had to fill cavities in four different teeth and would like to get her to brush more often. How might the assistant encourage her to become more involved in her home care?

1. tell her that she will have more cavities if she doesn't brush
2. promise her a prize if she has no cavities on her next visit
3. give her a new toothbrush
4. provide her with disclosing tablets and teach her how to use them

58. A major fear that many handicapped patients feel when coming to the dental office is
   1. that they will not be able to tolerate treatment
   2. that the dentist will not want to treat them
   3. that they will be further mutilated
   4. pain

59. Active listening involves a variety of techniques designed to help the patient better communicate with the health provider. These techniques are
   A. restatement and reflection
   B. agreement and disagreement
   C. clarification
   D. leaning forward and expressing positive interest
      1. A and B
      2. A and C
      3. C and D
      4. B and C

60. One effective way of stating one's role and privileges in the dental setting is to
   A. wear a name plate or badge
   B. act formal and stand up straight
   C. wear a white coat
   D. charge high fees or demand formal appointments far in advance
      1. A and C
      2. B and D
      3. A and B
      4. D only

61. A very experienced dental assistant has gained a position of power and influence in an office after being there for only a short period of time. What has likely led to her position of influence and power?
   A. she offers to help out wherever she can
   B. she keeps quiet and waits to be asked to participate in office activities; she is not pushy

   C. she is very experienced and lets everyone know
   D. she takes the time to find out what is going on in the office
      1. A only
      2. B only
      3. C and D
      4. D only

62. Children and adolescents are similar in some ways but very different in others. Which patient management strategies tend to be different for adolescents and children?
   A. the use of praise
   B. enlisting the parents' support and cooperation
   C. avoiding particular words
   D. showing interest and concern regarding the problems
      1. A, B, and C
      2. A and B
      3. B and C
      4. C and D

63. Being able to provide appropriate and helpful feedback is an important skill for the dental assistant to possess. Feedback is likely to be most effective when it is
   A. used to alert or reassure the patient that the assistant is paying attention
   B. used to describe a particular behavior just exhibited by the patient
   C. used tactfully to tell a patient that he or she has stepped out of line
   D. used to inform the patient about a problem that was the result of his or her behavior
      1. A and D
      2. B and D
      3. C and D
      4. A and C

64. Letting a child hold a mirror and watch what the dentist is doing in his or her mouth is based on the notion that
   A. children will be distracted from their concerns by playing with the mirror
   B. children fear mutilation and are calmed by seeing that they are not being extensively damaged
   C. children have a need to actively participate in their treatment
   D. children need something to do while they are being treated
      1. A and B
      2. A and C
      3. B and C
      4. A and D

Answers and Explanations

1. **2** This patient wants to assure herself that the assistant knows how important and busy she is and that she will be treated appropriately. For example, she may really be telling the assistant that she should be billed (she is reliable and important) rather than required to pay each time. Credentialing is an important aspect of the interpersonal process. One of the purposes of introducing oneself is to indicate to others how we expect to be treated.

2. **4** The types of behavior described are common body language signals of fear or anxiety.

3. **3** The patient believes that he has developed a special relationship with the office and the dentist. In his mind, the contract calls for special attention. He, therefore, feels the assistant is violating this contract and treating him unfairly. If he felt that the assistant was aware and respectful of his special status, he would probably accept the appointment offered.

4. **1** All behavior modification protocols begin with a specification and measurement of the actual target behavior. Behavior is the focus of the effort rather than an attempt to change attitudes or feelings.

5. **3** Some people react to feelings of anxiety with aggression and/or hostility. Active listening will enable the dental assistant to identify and respond helpfully to the anxiety or concern presented by the patient. Hostility or defensiveness tends to provoke more hostility. Ignoring the patient is a form of aggression.

6. **1** Body language is less amenable to conscious control than verbal reactions. Eye contact is often not a good indicator because many people are taught to make eye contact when speaking to an authority and do so in the absence of real attention.

7. **4** Since the conflict is not related to a violated expectation or a betrayal, but is related to a competition for scarce resources, it is more effective to engage in trade-offs and bargaining. The Osgood Solution is an effective strategy for zero-sum conflicts.

8. **1** It is more effective to remove the cause of the resistance than to try to overcome the resistance. For most people, the most common reaction to being pressured is to get angry or to resist more. If the patient is appointed earlier than the scheduled treatment time, and she finds out that she is not really expected at that time, she will probably become even more casual about her appointments.

9. **1** If a particular behavior has been reinforced in the past, the individual is likely to repeat the behavior with greater intensity. Since crying worked before, the child is likely to assume (it is important to recognize that this assumption may not be a conscious process) that on the second occasion he just wasn't crying hard enough.

10. **2** Self-selection (honestly done) tends to be the best predicator of job success and satisfaction. It is important for the prospective dental assistant to select a job that is appropriate and acceptable.

11. **2** Zero-sum conflicts are the result of competition. Competition is reduced when the parties are invested in each other's position outcomes.

12. **4** It is important that the patient become an active partner in his or her dental therapy. Often the patient's passivity is perceived as acceptance and cooperation rather than a lack of ownership of the decisions being made. Since passivity is often a result of feeling helplessness or inadequacy, the patient should be given the understanding of what is being done so he or she can participate.

13. **1** The patient's inappropriate behavior is probably due to his anxiety concerning dental treatment. The dental assistant can help him control his anxiety by more clearly structuring the situation for him. Punishing him is only going to increase his anxiety; sedating him will only increase his sense of helplessness and confusion.

14. **2** The patient's activity primarily serves to credential him as a business executive who is very busy and important. He is signalling that he expects the office to be concerned about the use of his time.

15. **2** The quality of the interpersonal contract is based on the clarity and mutual understanding and acceptance of its provisions.

16. **2** In an effort to predict the patient, the auxiliary is likely to project personal characteristics upon the patient that he or she has observed in similar patients in the past. Everyone uses experiences to prepare for new situations. Wanting to take care of the patient, liking him or her, and accepting what he or she says are actions resulting from the auxiliary's stereotyped impressions of the patient.

17. **2** In middle age, the individual becomes aware of his or her own mortality. The loss of teeth often is seen by the patient as a signal of loss of vitality or health. It is important to reassure the patient that the progress of disease can be halted and the loss of teeth is not a sign of a general body deterioration or aging.

18. **3** The anxious patient needs to test reality. The auxiliary must give the patient his or her complete attention and not become distracted by other events occurring in the office. In addition, the auxiliary must be careful not to bring his or her problems from home into the office. The reaction to the patient's behavior should be to that behavior and not due to a delayed reaction to a problem at home.

19. **2** A primary concern of the young child is body integrity. The child sees the alteration or loss of any body part as an assault on the body's integrity. The lost tooth is an important (psychological) part of the child's body.

20. **1** A uniform in the medical–dental situation acts as a credential of knowledge. The patient assumes special knowledge and training when he or she sees the uniform.

21. **4** Unless the reinforcement is attractive enough to elicit the behavior desired of the patient, it will not be adequate for use in a behavior modification protocol.

22. **4** The dental interview is the first step in building an effective working contract. If the dental assistant misleads the dentist, he or she will create expectations that cannot be fulfilled. The primary source of interpersonal conflict is a feeling of betrayal.

23. **2** An interaction such as giving instructions or developing an interpersonal contract should occur in personal space. Less than 1½ feet is intimate space. More than 5 feet is social space.

24. **2** Body orientation is an indicator of psychological attention. Often when an emotional reaction to the interaction is too intense for the participant, he or she will turn away to decrease the sense of contact.

25. **2** Active listening is by definition a process in which the listener works with the speaker to create meaning. In the process of checking perceptions, the listener clarifies and corrects his or her perceptions. Signalling or pretending that one is paying attention is not active listening.

26. **2** Often persons who have defined themselves by their employment feel a loss of social identity after retirement. In our culture, people gain importance through their contributions to society. This patient is asserting his past occupational status and trying to regain the sense of importance he once felt.

27. **3** The most effective method of working with an adolescent is to establish a therapeutic alliance in which the adolescent's need to be appropriate and responsible is elicited. Adolescents are concerned about the quality of their relationships with important others. By building a positive relationship, the dentist can increase the patient's need to comply with treatment.

28. **3** Children are very self-centered. The dentist must begin by establishing a positive relationship with the patient so that the patient will want to please him or her.

29. **4** For the elderly patient, the dental office visit is an important event in his or her life. Health care is a critical issue for the elderly because of the increase in susceptibility to chronic illness that occurs in old age. In addition, the dental visit is a responsibility that provides something important and essential for the elderly person for whom leisure might be a problem.

30. **1** The goal of the dental assistant is to decrease patient problems during treatment. Just keeping the patient quiet is not enough as it is important for the patient to participate in his or her treatment. It is not the dental assistant's job (or training) to resolve psychological problems that arise in the office.

31. **3** The anger is the result of a reaction to the behavior of another. The behavior is not the cause of the anger. If the auxiliary understands the source of the anger, he or she will be better able to adapt suitably to the patient's behavior.

32. **3** Escape behavior is self-reinforcing and therefore beyond the control of the auxiliary. The outcomes of approach behavior and aggressive behavior are usually accessible to the auxiliary, and habits can be intercepted or modified by presenting alternative behavioral possibilities.

33. **4** A sense of resentment and betrayal is often a result of a confusion over who is to do what. Most office conflicts are not a result of personality clashes or personal problems but rather are a result of a lack of cooperation among staff in getting work done.

34. **2** Feedback is intended to be informational. Its goal is to provide information that can be used in self-change. If the feedback is judgmental, regardless of how tactfully or gently it is given, it will evoke the patient's need to defend him/herself.

35. **2** Body posture is a form of body language. Body orientation and the way the body is held (e.g., tense, alert, slumped) provide important clues to the person's emotions, concerns, and interests.

36. **3** For the patient, the feelings he or she experiences are current reality. To deny the feelings is to

deny the patient's experience. It is the auxiliary's job to help the patient to clarify his or her perceptions of the dental office experience.

37. **3** Establishing clear but limited options is a method of guiding the patient in a nonhostile or nondefensive way. Attacking the patient or giving in to the patient is not likely to produce a productive outcome for the office or the patient.

38. **4** An adolescent needs to feel respected by adults. By enlisting the patient in her treatment, the auxiliary signals his or her feeling that the patient is capable and dependable. Attacking the patient will further alienate the patient. Since adolescents are trying to develop independence from their parents, enlisting the parents is likely to cause more problems than it solves.

39. **2** The receiver interprets what he or she hears, feels, and sees. The human organism is an information processing organism and all information is interpreted in the light of its meaning for the receiver. Therefore, expectations (e.g., suspicions, hopes, fears) will determine the importance and meaning of the information received.

40. **3** Communication success is ultimately determined by the receiver's ability to understand the message sent, not by the sender's skill in sending the message. Communication is, by definition, the development of a shared meaning, not simply sending a message.

41. **1** Behavior always occurs within a social context. The context determines, in large part, the appropriateness and meaning of a behavior.

42. **2** A primary psychological need of the child is competence (being able to do tasks correctly). Children judge their worth by what they can do well and poorly. They are very motivated to perform well. Teaching them how to keep their oral structures healthy is likely to be very successful.

43. **2** Feedback is, by definition, a process of mirroring an individual's behavior. Feedback is information about the outcomes of one's behavior.

44. **1** In order to restate another's comments an individual must be able to understand and formulate what he or she said. In addition, this process makes clear to the other that the disagreement is not due to lack of understanding but a different perception of the situation.

45. **1** When a person lies, the throat unconsciously constricts, raising the voice pitch. Many individuals can lie while maintaining eye contact, speech fluency, and a relaxed manner.

46. **1** The helping relationship is most effective when the individual being helped not only finds a solution to the current problem but also becomes more effective at problem solution. Often, an individual accepts another person's solutions as a way of avoiding taking responsibility for his or her decisions.

47. **3** The auxiliary is clarifying reality, while at the same time not judging the patient. Implied criticism can elicit a defensive reaction from the patient.

48. **2** Often, anxious or highly dependent patients give up all decision-making and control to the dentist. This can be a problem both legally and in terms of self-care. One way to elicit ownership of a patient's dental problems and his or her care is to support the patient in questioning and raising issues about his or her state of oral health.

49. **1** In all groups, norms, rules, and power relationships are developed and explicitly supported by their members. The office members introduce patients and new members of the office to these characteristics. However, as people work together, their working vocabulary changes; they adopt special words and phrases that speed up communication. These code words become commonplace to the group members and go unnoticed by them; however, the patient will be aware of these words because of their unfamiliarity in general discussion.

50. **3** All efforts to elicit a patient's motivation begin with having the patient recognize that a problem exists and that the patient's activity will make a difference. Just telling a patient that he or she should be concerned, or threatening the patient with long-term punishment, is not likely to be effective. Education in method should occur after the patient's interest is elicited.

51. **3** The patient is attempting to assert his importance and worth by reminding the staff that he has expertise. If members of the staff explicitly recognize his capability and knowledge, he will have less of a need to credential himself by criticizing.

52. **2** Most situational behavior as defensive behavior is a result of past experiences.

53. **2** People often disclose a lot about themselves when they are upset. If the listener acts like a parent and gives advice and comfort, he or she is likely to be perceived in the parenting role. Often, people retain their feelings of being evaluated and given disapproval by their parents. This process is called "transference."

54. **3** Anxiety is a fear of something fantasized or unknown. The explanation will serve to focus the patient's concerns and enable him or her to apply specific skills.

55. **3** People during their middle years become aware of their mortality and are concerned with preserving their health and well-being. Often, dental problems that require repair or loss of teeth serve as a signal to the patient that he or she is getting old.

56. **1** Denial is a way of fending off anxiety. However, when pain or discomfort becomes too in-

tense to deny, the patient is likely to feel out of control and panic. Countertransference is not a form of coping. Aggression can be easily controlled by clear limits and firmness. Transference is a valuable support for therapeutic alliance as long as distortions are clarified.

57. **4** Since the child is seven, she is likely to be concerned with her ability to do things and very concrete in her thinking. Disclosing tablets will enable her actually to see the problem of plaque and recognize when she has been successful in cleaning her teeth. Threatening her or promising a prize are external motivators and less likely to be effective on a daily basis.

58. **2** Handicapped patients often pose special problems of logistics in delivery of treatment. These problems might previously have led health providers to reject the patient.

59. **2** Active listening involves the use of restatement, reflection, and clarification.

60. **1** Uniforms serve as indicators of status. In this society, clothes and badges often signal rank and privileges.

61. **3** Knowledge is a primary source of power. People tend to listen to the individual who appears to have the knowledge necessary to complete the current task. The auxiliary who either enters with technical knowledge or has acquired information about the office is most likely to be able to influence the outcomes of others.

62. **1** Since children are very concerned with competence, the dental assistant should avoid criticism; adolescents, being more concerned with how the dental assistant feels about them, are more likely to benefit from a balance of praise and criticism. Parents will play a strong part in the child's treatment but the treatment will probably be more effective if the parent is not included. Including the parent may elicit the normal power struggles of adolescence. Children are more sensitive to loaded words than are adolescents.

63. **2** Feedback should be presented nonjudgmentally and serve the function of providing factual information a patient can use to modify his or her behavior.

64. **3** Children are very concrete in their thinking. Their fantasies are more frightening than reality. Being able to see exactly the limits of what is occurring will allow them to appropriately cope with their fears. Children also feel more comfortable if they are actively participating rather than being passive. It is important to tell the child what to do rather than what not to do.

Bibliography

Berni, R. and Fordyce, W. *Behavior Modification and the Nursing Process,* 2nd ed. St. Louis: The C. V. Mosby Co., 1977.

Dworkins, S.F., Ference, T.P., and Giddon, D.B. *Behavioral Science and Dental Practice,* St. Louis: The C. V. Mosby Co., 1978.

Froelich, R.E.; Bishop, F.M.; and Dworkins, S.F. *Communication in the Dental Office: A Programmed Manual for the Dental Professional,* St. Louis: The C. V. Mosby Co., 1976.

Giddon, D.B. and Hittelman, E. "Psychological aspects of prosthodontic treatment for geriatric patients," *Journal of Prosthetic Dentistry* 43:4 April 1980 374–379.

Goffman, E. *The Presentation of Self in Everyday Life,* New York: Doubleday and Co., Inc., 1959.

Havinghurst, R. *Developmental Tasks and Education,* 3rd ed. New York: McKay Publishers, 1972.

Hirsch, S. and Hittelman, E. "Effective Communication," *General Dentistry* 26:4 July–August 1978 38–43.

Ingersoll, B. *Behavioral Aspects in Dentistry,* New York: Appleton-Century-Crofts, 1982.

Malamed, B. and Siegel, S. *Behavioral Medicine: Practical Application in Health Care,* New York: Springer Publishing Co., Inc., 1980.

Mayerson, E. *Putting the Ill at Ease,* New York: Harper & Row Publishers Inc., 1976.

Morton, J., et al. *Dental Teamwork Strategies,* St. Louis: The C. V. Mosby Co., 1979.

Morton, J.C. and Rickey, C.A. *Building Assertive Skills,* St. Louis: The C. V. Mosby Co., 1980.

Smith, F. "Management of the Child Patient and the Handicapped Patient," *Clinical Dentistry* Vol. 1, Chapter 33.

Weinstein, P. and Getz, T. *Changing Human Behavior: Strategies for Preventive Dentistry,* St. Louis: The C. V. Mosby Co., 1979.

8

Practice Management

Course Synopsis

Introduction

Dentistry is both a profession and a business. Combining the business of dental practice with clinical expertise is a task that cannot be accomplished solely by a dentist. It is the dental team, comprised of the doctor and auxiliaries, working together, that ensures the delivery of optimum patient care. This environment, created by a cohesively working team, usually results in above-average professional and personal fulfillment for everyone in the dental office.

Practice administration, as it is perceived in the world of modern dentistry, is crucial to establishing an efficient, effective practice. A dental practice cannot be effective unless it is efficient, and both can only be accomplished when the entire dental team uses specific methods and systems which apply to patient and office management.

In an office in which only one auxiliary is employed, that individual must have the ability and flexibility to interchange roles as the need arises. In multiauxiliary practices, where every auxiliary has a specific role with a specific job description, it is especially important for the dental assistant to be knowledgeable about all office duties. It is this cross-training that permits auxiliaries to function smoothly as a team and to interchange roles when necessary.

The following are the basic responsibilities of the business assistant:

1. SCREENING AND RESPONDING TO ALL TELEPHONE COMMUNICATION INCLUDING THE DOCTOR'S PERSONAL AND BUSINESS CALLS AND INQUIRIES RELATED TO FEES AND SERVICES

Every assistant should be aware that the telephone is an essential piece of equipment in the dental office. Without it, and more importantly, without using it properly, a dentist cannot practice effectively. More than 95% of a dentist's business results from telephone calls and the majority of new patients make the initial contact by telephone; therefore, it is imperative that the telephone image conveyed by the auxiliary encourage a friendly, trusting attitude in the caller.

The production of dental services is the main function of the dentist. To maximize the delivery of services, it is necessary to keep delaying factors at a minimum level. Delaying factors include most telephone calls from patients, unexpected salespeople, family and friends. All calls should be screened so that the doctor speaks only to patients who cannot be helped by the assistant.

When a caller questions fees, his or her concern should be addressed by an explanation that fees are contingent on procedures involved. Since a diagnosis cannot be determined over the telephone, a patient inquiring about fees should be scheduled for an examination and told that the dentist will discuss all fees before rendering any treatment.

If a telephone answering machine is used when the office is closed, the recorded message should be clear and understandable. The speaker should request pertinent information (e.g., name, telephone number, including the area code, and purpose of the call) and provide the caller with a clear understanding of what will happen as a result of the call (e.g., the call will be returned, the caller should contact the doctor at another number, or the caller should contact another doctor who will see patients in emergency situations). It is the business assistant's responsibility to connect the answering machine before the office closes and to disconnect the machine during business hours. The assistant should listen to each message and return all calls.

In all telephone communication, the assistant's courtesy, diplomacy, and poise can make the difference between a steady stream of loyal, cooperative patients and a steady stream of frustration and problems.

2. GREETING PATIENTS UPON ARRIVAL AND MAKING THEIR PRESENCE KNOWN

The business assistant is the key public relations member of the office team because he or she makes the first contact with patients, both on the telephone and in the reception area. During the initial interaction with new patients, first impressions often form lasting impressions, and consequently the assistant should make efforts to be courteous and pleasant at all times. The first meeting is a time for exchanging information and familiarizing the patient with office procedures. A warm friendly greeting by auxiliaries can engender the same feelings toward the doctor, even before the patient and doctor meet.

The reception area must be clean and patients should be greeted promptly upon arrival. Patient arrivals should be made known to the doctor as quickly as possible via a signal system. If the dentist is delayed, patients who are waiting should be notified and told approximately how long it will be before they will be seen by the doctor. This information will clarify to all patients that the office has respect for both their time and the doctor's, and this consideration is always appreciated.

3. MAINTAINING AN ACCURATE RECORD AND BOOKKEEPING SYSTEM

A record and bookkeeping system encompasses all paperwork pertaining to the dental practice, ranging from the appointment book, which is usually the first place that the patient's name appears, to collection control, which is often the last. The system must be completely standardized and organized since accurate and adequate records provide a comprehensive history of past and present patient treatment, production records that enable the dentist to assess expenses periodically through cost accounting, and precise tax information. These records can also prevent or resolve malpractice involvement. The following are components of this system that directly involve the business assistant.

A. The Appointment Book

The appointment book is the control center of office activity. A mismanaged appointment book can destroy a potentially fine practice by wasting the doctor's productive time or by creating a schedule that results in the reception room becoming a waiting room filled with unhappy patients. For optimum control, the appointment book should be the responsibility of the business assistant, who has an overview of all doctor-patient activity, knowledge of patient availability in relation to office availability, and an understanding of the amount of time necessary for treatment planned.

Time and motion studies have shown that the most efficient format of an appointment book is the week-at-a-glance style. The format enables the assistant to balance the workload appropriately by noting available time during the week. The patient's name and procedure scheduled for that time slot should be printed in pencil to provide easy reading and to allow any changes to be entered neatly.

In advance, certain periods of time should be blocked out (e.g., lunch and dinner hours, holidays when the office will be closed, vacation time, and professional meetings when the doctor will not be in the office).

Time should be prioritized to reflect the periods of the day that are valued most highly and the type of patients who will be appointed during that time. The preferences of the doctor and working schedules of business people should be reflected in this determination. Elderly patients and young children should be scheduled early in the day, a time when they will be most cooperative. In addition, a philosophy for emergency patients should be developed; some offices reserve buffer periods for unexpected emergencies, while others work them into existing schedules.

Broken appointments and cancellations may disrupt the most organized office. Patients who repeatedly break appointments or cancel them with insufficient notice should be made aware that this is unacceptable behavior. Time created, however, should be used efficiently, and a call list which contains patients' names, telephone numbers, and times they are available on short notice should be created for maximum use of office resources.

Most efficient offices schedule patients in time units. The most frequent unit selected is a period of 15 minutes; therefore, a patient being appointed for a procedure requiring 45 minutes would be scheduled for three units of time in the appointment book. Unit scheduling provides a realistic mechanism for controlling the work load and allows the dental team to adhere to the schedule throughout the day. Scheduling a patient for a 15-minute appointment when the actual time needed is a half-hour is one of the reasons that some offices consistently work overtime. To alleviate improper scheduling and to ensure that each patient will be appointed appropriately for the next visit before he or she is dismissed, the doctor or the chairside assistant must provide the person controlling the appointment book with information about the procedure planned and units of time required for the patient's next appointment.

B. The Day Sheet

The day sheet is a replica of the appointment book for that day and should be placed in each treatment room. This schedule provides the dentist and auxiliaries in the operatories with the information necessary to eliminate checking the appointment book to determine who is expected, when he or she is expected, and the treatment planned. The day sheet also enables the staff to plan ahead and minimize delaying factors by preparing the next patient in the treatment room with necessary instruments and materials.

C. Patients' Records

A series of records should be maintained for each patient. A case history form that includes the patient's past and present medical and dental health histories should be continuously updated to avoid problems. Diagnostic materials include x-ray films, information noted at the clinical examination, and study models. A patient information sheet contains the record of existing conditions and a prioritized treatment plan designed for each patient on the basis of diagnostic materials gathered from and about the patient. The plan enables the dentist to systematically meet the dental needs of the patient and enables the business assistant to facilitate the course of treatment by knowing the procedures required, the order of procedures, the person who will perform each procedure (i.e., the dentist, an assistant, or a hygienist), the time required for each procedure, and the total fee for services to be rendered. Permanent record cards are maintained for each patient and contain specific notations of all treatment performed, the date on which it was performed, materials used, the prognosis, and other relevant information.

Individually and collectively, these records protect both the patient and the dentist should treatment discrepancies arise. Patient records are confidential histories of financial and treatment experiences that cannot be released or made public without the patient's permission. Additionally, before any records leave the office (e.g., for insurance purposes or consultation with a specialist), duplicate copies should be made for legal protection.

D. The Recall System

A responsive recall system is essential to every dental office; it reflects a supportive attitude that encourages patients to maintain proper oral health for a lifetime. At the end of each series of treatments the dentist or the assistant should remind the patient that he or she should return for an examination after a given interval of time. The atmosphere created should be positive and reflect concern for the patient's health, but it should be clear that maintenance and recall are a dual responsibility, and patients who fail to respond may compromise their oral health.

Recall methods vary; some offices telephone patients, others send written reminders, and others us a combination of telephone and mail notices. Once the method of recall is chosen, a file that can be used and updated easily should be established. A patient's recall card should be separated from his or her clinical chart, and each family member should have an individual recall card, since the length of time between examinations may vary.

The most efficient method of recall is a two-card system for each patient; one card is designated by the month during which the recall visit should occur, and the other is alphabetical. For reference, the monthly card should be filed in a box divided in the same manner. Each card should include the patient's name, complete home and business addresses and telephone numbers, preferred type of reminder (written or phone), and an area for response to allow easy recognition of his or her recall pattern.

Alphabetical cards can be filed on a revolving desk file and should include the patient's name, type of reminder preferred, and date of the last appointment. This file also serves as a tickler file and is easily accessible if a patient should call to inquire about recall or to request treatment earlier then the scheduled time. Some newer recordkeeping systems eliminate the tickler file, since the patient's chart has an area designated for recording the month of recall. Most offices give patients the benefit of three recall notices at six-month intervals before the patient is perceived as inactive.

E. Financial Recordkeeping, Payment Arrangements, and Collection

Accurate financial records must be maintained for both efficiency and legal protection, and the actual bookkeeping is only as valuable as the detail and accuracy with which it is maintained. The simplest system is single-entry bookkeeping, which records only payments. The double-entry system records both the debit (charges) and credit (payments) for each office transaction. The two entries provide the necessary information to balance the financial records and provide duplicate records in the event that a patient's card is lost or destroyed. Many offices use a pegboard system, a form of double entry that allows two or more office records to be written at one time through the use of carbon paper and pegs that stabilize punched forms in the correct position. Some large dental practices use electronic data processing systems involving computers to record production and financial data, recall dates, and any other desired information.

Every office has a policy regarding payments. A dental practice cannot survive if there is an inordinate amount of accounts receivable (money owed to the dentist for treatment completed). Fees charged for services rendered represent the dentist's earnings, but only payments actually received constitute income. For the practice to be profitable, income must exceed overhead, which is the cost of the resources needed to produce dentistry, including rent, salaries, supplies, laboratory procedures, and so forth.

Credit experts indicate that delinquent accounts over 90 days old are the most difficult and often impossible to collect. In order to minimize accounts receivable, all patients should be informed of the exact financial obligation before treatment is begun. Various payment policies and methods should be offered as a means of making the responsibility less burdensome. While there are many payment policies, the following are the most common:

1. *Advanced payment.* Payment before treatment is the most desirable, since billing, collection problems, and accounts receivable are eliminated.

2. *Fixed amount.* The total fee is divided by the approximate number of sessions projected for completion of the treatment, and a fixed amount is expected from the patient at each visit, regardless of the actual charge for particular treatment rendered during the visit.

3. *Divided payments.* The total fee is divided into three amounts. The initial payment, usually larger then the other two, is collected when treatment commences. The balance, which is divided in half, is due when treatment is half completed and a visit or two before treatment is completed.

4. *Open account.* The least desirable method of payment is the open account. Patients are sent statements (forms indicating the financial status of their accounts) after treatment is rendered. This method often results in high accounts receivable since most patients are unaware of their obligations until they receive statements, are often unprepared to pay for services rendered, or take a substantial amount of time to complete payment.

Payment methods include cash, checks, money orders, credit cards, and bank plans. Some dentists or dental societies have established loan plans with local banks. These plans enable patients to borrow the needed monies and extend payments to the bank for a year or more, at a minimum interest rate.

Although proper payment arrangements may be made, some patients fail to fulfill their obligations and honor the method of payment to which they have agreed. The business assistant should continuously monitor payment arrangements. As a patient makes the next appointment, the assistant should check to see whether payment is due. If the patient is defaulting and payment is not forthcoming, the assistant should address the issue. Patients should not be given the option of whether to pay, but rather how to pay. If patients offer excuses rather then payments, they should be informed that they may either mail the payment (a stamped, self-addressed envelope should be provided) or bring it in at the next visit.

If a patient continues to default, the assistant should remind the patient that arrangements were agreed upon and determine whether there is a need to renegotiate the contract and ask the patient to select an alternate method of payment. Although many people tend to pay dental obligations last, most will adhere as agreed, after being reminded of their responsibilities.

Statements should be used minimally, as a mechanism for reminding patients of balance to date, when a patient has stopped treatment before completion, or when he or she has finished treatment sooner than expected. They are also used to remind patients of divided payment agreements, noting the dates and amounts of expected payments.

A small percentage of patients complete treatment with an outstanding balance. These patients should be sent several statements at regular intervals (e.g., every 30 days). If the patient does not respond, telephone follow-up should be initiated. If these efforts are unsuccessful, the patient should be informed that if payment is not received on a specified date, the matter will be referred for collection. Most people are concerned with collection referral, since their credit rating is often jeopardized.

F. Third-Party Payments (insurance procedures)

An increased number of people have dental insurance coverage, and it is estimated that this population will be enlarged annually. As a result, insurance claim management is an important duty of the business assistant. Managing insurance coverage in a positive manner often results in practice growth because:

1. Patients accept comprehensive care, since the cost of treatment is defrayed by coverage.
2. People who previously did not seek oral health care are taking advantage of third-party coverage.
3. Accounts receivable are often substantially reduced due to payments received directly from insurance carriers.

Many forms of insurance coverage exist. Most companies reimburse the doctor or the patient for services previously rendered. The amount of reimbursement may be based on usual, customary, or reasonable fees (UCR)—an amount considered standard for the procedure in a given community—or on a fixed amount determined by the carrier for each procedure. Some plans are organized on a prepayment basis where the doctor receives a fixed amount of money for each patient for a specified period of time. Under this system, also known as capitation, the dentist receives the same amount of money regardless of the type and amount of care delivered. Patients covered by this type of insurance seek care only from participating dentists, who constitute a closed panel. The business assistant should be familiar with the organization of different types of coverage and understand how they affect the payments between the dentist and the patient.

For maximum efficiency, a patient's insurance forms should not be located with his or her clinical records. A separate insurance file should be maintained and periodically checked to ensure prompt claim processing.

The insured patient should be aware of individual benefits, and the business assistant can often increase or clarify this understanding. This knowledge encourages acceptance of total treatment plans because the patient understands his or her financial responsibilities and those of the insurer. The doctor's treatment planning may also be affected by this type of coverage. When a patient calls for an appointment, he or she should be told that all forms, benefit booklets, and other relevant information should be brought to the office at the first visit. The business assistant then has the opportunity to initiate the payment process and alleviate or diminish any potential problems.

G. Inventory Systems

For efficiency, every office must maintain a well-organized inventory system. Careful planning and periodic evaluation can result in several advantages:

1. The office does not run out of critically needed material in the midst of patient treatment.
2. Anyone in the office can order supplies simply by referring to the system.
3. Information about the quantity of any given material used in a time period enables the office to take advantage of savings resulting from quantity buying.
4. Awareness of the rise of the price of materials enables the dentist to adjust fees using cost accounting.

An inventory system can be created simply by using index cards or the pages of a loose leaf binder. Each major disposable item used in the office has its own card or page and contains the following information:

1. The name of the item (e.g., anesthetic)
2. The brand name (e.g., Carbocaine 2%)
3. The name of the supplier and the supplier's address and telephone number
4. How the item is sold (e.g., box, case, package)
5. The quantity to order for the most advantageous price
6. The time at which the item should be reordered (e.g., when only three cases of a material are left)

7. Back orders, which are items previously ordered but not shipped by the supplier because of temporary unavailability.

A large pad is kept in the supply area, and when an item is removed it is recorded on the pad. Once a week the pad should be compared with the individual cards or sheets to update all inventory records. When new supplies are ordered the assistant must not change the inventory record until the items are actually delivered in order to keep an accurate accounting of what is on hand and what is backordered.

H. The Office Manual

An office manual is a reference guide that contains detailed descriptions of all office policies and procedures. Information about the following aspects of the practice should be included:

1. The doctor's philosophy of practice (i.e., goals and objectives)
2. Job descriptions for all members of the dental team
3. Employment policies (e.g., working hours, vacation, sick leave, overtime, holidays)
4. Office policies for the staff (e.g., dress code, conduct, staff meetings)
5. Guidelines for appropriate office communication (e.g., telephone technique, reception policies, written correspondence, patient education)
6. Policies for management of office records (e.g., clinical and financial patient records, payment and collection procedures, accounts receivable, accounts payable, insurance coverage, recalls, inventory)
7. Guidelines for clinical procedures (e.g., preparation of tray setups, sterilization techniques, prescriptions, laboratory interaction).

The guidelines set forth in this book summarize office policy, reflect the characteristics of the practice, and enable the office to run smoothly from both a clinical and management perspective. In addition, when a new employee joins the practice, the manual facilitates his or her integration into the practice. The office manual, which should be updated regularly, is an invaluable resource that promotes sound management and allows the office to run more efficiently.

The business assistant clearly performs an integral role in office administration. Tasks may vary as a function of the managerial style of the dentist, but the application of well-organized management techniques results in a successful office that provides fulfillment to the doctor, staff, and patients. It is the business assistant's responsibility to understand the principles of office administration and to employ them daily.

Question Section

Directions: Each of the questions or incomplete statements below is followed by four suggested answers or completions. Select the BEST answer in each case.

1. Cross-training means
   1. auxiliaries are knowledgeable about each other's jobs
   2. dental assistants can perform some of the procedures usually relegated to the hygienists
   3. auxiliaries are trained in a school environment
   4. auxiliaries receive on-the-job training

2. A dental assistant may expose radiographs
   1. if the dentist gives instructions or permission or both
   2. if he or she is a certified dental assistant
   3. if it is permissible in the state in which he or she is employed
   4. if he or she is supervised by the dentist or hygienist or both

3. If a dental office is managed by sound business principles, the business assistant should make every effort to
   1. conserve the doctor's time

2. refrain from making personal telephone calls

3. arrive promptly every morning

4. complete all the bookkeeping promptly

4. When a patient calls and insists on speaking to the doctor, the assistant should
   1. call the doctor to the phone as promptly as possible
   2. explain to the patient that it is the responsibility of the assistant to respond to phone calls
   3. explain that the doctor is treating a patient and that he or she will return the call as soon as possible
   4. tell the patient to call back at a specific hour

5. A case presentation is
   1. a treatment conference with the patient
   2. a case that is sent to the laboratory for construction
   3. a paper or speech presented by the doctor to a dental society
   4. a study model used to diagnose a case

6. On any given day, a business assistant encounters a good deal of pressure, frustration, and interruption. He or she can cope with this if he or she
   1. can delegate tasks to other auxiliaries
   2. takes the phone off the hook during busy periods
   3. remains calm and systematically completes tasks until they are done
   4. takes a personal day off now and then

7. Patients should come in for a recall
   1. whenever they think they need a checkup
   2. whenever they have a toothache
   3. at periodic intervals designated by the dentist
   4. whenever the hygienist can fit them into the schedule

8. "Third party" refers to
   1. children of patients
   2. insurance carriers
   3. a group of general dentists and specialists
   4. patients receiving public assistance

9. Insurance forms should always be
   1. accompanied by x-ray films
   2. accompanied by study models
   3. duplicated for office records
   4. mailed first class

10. The rights of a patient during the treatment phase do not include

1. the right to be informed about his or her condition
2. the right to refuse treatment
3. the right to confidential records
4. the right to dictate the course of treatment

11. The least desirable method of recall is
    1. telephone
    2. mail
    3. advance appointments
    4. telephone and mail

12. A truth-in-lending form is
    1. a contract signed by the patient
    2. a contract signed by the doctor
    3. a government requirement to protect all patients who pay for treatment in advance
    4. a government requirement to protect patients from hidden finance charges in installment payments

13. Accounts receivable are
    1. money owed to the dentist from insurance carriers
    2. all monies owed to the dentist for completed treatment
    3. all monies that the dentist owes to creditors
    4. all monies owed to the dentist for future treatment

14. All insurance carriers use
    1. the same table of benefits
    2. different tables of benefits depending on the type of coverage to which the subscriber is entitled
    3. a percentage of the dentist's usual and customary fees
    4. closed-panel dental care for their subscribers

15. Assignment of benefits means that
    1. the patient is entitled to complete reimbursement for his or her dental care in each given year
    2. the dentist receives direct payment from the insurance carrier in the amount that the patient's insurance plan designates
    3. all members of the immediate family of the insured are entitled to insurance coverage in a given year
    4. if a patient does not utilize his insurance benefits in a given year, he or she can allot these benefits to an immediate family member

16. An office manual is most effective when it is
    1. purchased from a reputable dental supply company

2. organized by a professional management consultant who has evaluated the practice
3. organized by the dentist and the staff in keeping with the office's philosophy, goals, and objectives
4. a collection of directions that the dentist believes is appropriate for his or her mode of dental care delivery

17. A day sheet in each treatment room provides which of the following data?
    1. any serious medical problem that could affect treatment
    2. the patient's occupation
    3. the procedure to be performed and length of the appointment
    4. the number of visits needed to complete treatment

18. If a patient does not keep a scheduled appointment, the business assistant should
    1. wait until the patient contacts the office
    2. contact the patient as soon as possible
    3. send the patient a statement with a charge for the broken appointment
    4. utilize the time for a coffee break

19. An office manual is
    1. a procedural guide for all office activities
    2. detailed information on how the equipment should be serviced
    3. the doctor's instructions for operating equipment most efficiently
    4. the record that the business assistant keeps for the accountant

20. Change in the office procedure involving auxiliary personnel is best planned
    1. by an accountant
    2. by the patient
    3. at a staff meeting
    4. by a consultant

21. Facts that should be obtained when interviewing for a job are
    1. working hours
    2. vacation policy
    3. length of probation period
    4. all of the above

22. An office aid used to train new personnel is
    1. a pegboard system
    2. a balance sheet
    3. an office manual
    4. a magazine on general dentistry

23. How do most new patients come to a private dental office?

1. they see the dentist's sign and walk in
2. they see the dentist's name in the phone book
3. they are referred by other patients
4. they check the dentist's credentials

24. What is a contract?
    1. an analysis of assets against liabilities
    2. an agreement between two or more people
    3. records of work completed
    4. an unexpected action

25. Before proceeding with treatment, the patient should be notified of the
    1. cost
    2. time needed to accomplish the procedure
    3. any risks the treatment may entail
    4. all of the above

26. An appropriate response when answering the phone is
    1. "This is Dr. Smith's office, Ms. Jones speaking, may I help you?"
    2. "Who's calling?"
    3. "With whom would you like to speak?"
    4. "May I help you?"

27. Postoperative telephone calls
    1. remind patients of postoperative care they should be carrying out
    2. remind patients of their appointment for postoperative treatment
    3. show patients special concern
    4. all of the above

28. A patient calls and complains about the treatment given. The receptionist should
    1. justify the dentist's position
    2. engage in a verbal duel
    3. take the patient's side
    4. allow the dentist to handle the situation

29. A telephone caller asks the price of a full mouth rehabilitation. The receptionist should
    1. estimate the price
    2. ask the patient to come in for an examination
    3. put the dentist on the phone to quote prices
    4. refer the person elsewhere

30. During working hours the receptionist should protect the dentist from
    1. door-to-door salespeople
    2. an unidentified telephone caller
    3. a patient who wishes to change an appointment
    4. all of the above

31. Recordkeeping
    A. improves verbal communication
    B. provides production records
    C. provides a history of treatment success or failure
    D. is needed legally to avoid possible malpractice involvement
    E. avoids the need for an accountant
       1. A, B, and E
       2. B, C, and D
       3. B, D, and E
       4. C, D, and E

32. Patient records are
    1. public information
    2. available only to relatives
    3. confidential
    4. released at the assistant's discretion

33. What records are kept in an inactive file?
    1. records of all patients who have completed treatment
    2. records of patients who will return in one year
    3. records of patients no longer seeking treatment at the office
    4. records of patients who receive treatment at a discount

34. Ethics refers to
    1. accreditation by the ADA
    2. professional standards of conduct
    3. jurisprudence
    4. membership in the ADAA

35. What determines which duties the dental auxiliary can perform?
    1. federal law
    2. state law
    3. common law
    4. the dentist

36. Who is responsible for duties delegated to auxiliaries?
    1. the receptionist
    2. the assistant
    3. the dentist
    4. the patient

37. The period of time in which a patient may bring suit against a dentist is known as
    1. libel
    2. a tort
    3. statute of limitations
    4. the end point

38. A treatment plan is a(n)
    1. approach to collections
    2. inventory control system
    3. peer evaluation system

    4. systematic approach to meet the dental needs of the patient

39. The appointment book and day sheet should contain the following information
    A. patient's name
    B. fee for service
    C. length of appointment
    D. patient's occupation
    E. procedure to be performed
    F. a brief medical history
       1. A, C, and E
       2. B, D, and F
       3. C, D, and E
       4. D, E, and F

40. Which person traditionally controls the appointment book?
    1. dentist
    2. chairside assistant
    3. receptionist
    4. hygienist

41. Appointment control will
    A. increase the percentage of money collected
    B. prevent overcrowding
    C. keep hours within desired limits
    D. prevent faulty dentistry
    E. organize the dentist's production time
       1. A, D, and E
       2. B, C, and D
       3. B, C, and E
       4. C, D, and E

42. Which appointments should be scheduled first?
    1. appointments for the elderly
    2. short appointments
    3. those when auxiliaries perform tasks
    4. long appointments

43. An effective method to ensure the patient will keep an appointment made over the telephone is to
    1. overlap appointments
    2. charge the patient for missed appointments
    3. send a written confirmation
    4. repeat the appointment time before hanging up

44. The most efficient way to schedule appointments is to have
    1. many short appointments
    2. long appointments
    3. all appointments a half-hour in length
    4. 20-minute time units

45. A patient requires several appointments,

each a week apart. The best scheduling would be to assign the patient
1. the same time and day each week
2. randomly
3. Monday the first week, Tuesday the second week, Wednesday the next week, and so forth
4. relative to the payment arrangements

46. Which contingencies are most likely to pose scheduling problems?
A. patients arriving early
B. patients arriving late
C. patients behind in payments
D. drop in emergencies
E. unforeseen complications in a planned procedure
    1. A, C, and D
    2. B, C, and D
    3. B, D, and E
    4. C, D, and E

47. A patient did not show up for his appointment. This situation should be dealt with by
1. overlapping the next appointment
2. closing the patient's file
3. taking no action
4. contacting the patient

48. A patient cancels an appointment an hour before he is due. A good course of action is to
1. close the office at the appointment time
2. allow the dentist to resolve the problem
3. call a patient who is available on short notice
4. announce a coffee break to the dentist and rest of the staff

49. If the dentist is delayed, patients who are waiting should be
1. kept busy as a distraction
2. ignored
3. notified of the delay
4. told to leave

50. Overhead is
1. net income
2. the cost necessary to practice dentistry
3. assets of the practice
4. the breakeven production point

51. The money paid to the dental practice is known as its
1. gross income
2. liabilities
3. net income
4. expenses

52. As accounts receivable age, they
1. increase in value
2. remain the same in value
3. decrease in value
4. are placed in an inactive file

53. Third-party precertification (or prior authorization) will inform the
1. dentist and patient of the obligation assumed by the third party
2. dentist of the correct treatment plan
3. dentist that prepayment is available
4. patient of the dentist's skills

54. A patient denies payment responsibilities. The next course of action is
1. to forget about the bill
2. to contact a collection agency
3. harassment
4. to notify the patient's employer

55. A list of equipment and supplies present in the office is known as
1. liabilities
2. specifications
3. an inventory
4. expendables

56. A running inventory is
1. a system of altering the supply list to know which supplies are present in the office
2. moving the inventory from place to place
3. a billing technique
4. an inventory updated once a year

57. The main advantage of purchasing a large quantity of a particular supply at one time is
1. it is easy to store
2. to save money when buying in bulk
3. the billing is easier
4. the dental materials have an indefinite shelf life

58. An invoice is a
1. statement of money collected
2. statement of items shipped
3. cash receipt
4. form of vertical filing

59. A supply company informs the office that an item that has been ordered is not available and will be shipped when it arrives. This is known as
1. a bad order
2. a back order
3. an extra supply
4. deficit spending

60. What is a group practice?

1. a practice of five or more auxiliaries employed by the same dentist
2. a practice which treats a homogeneous group
3. a practice which cares for the total health of the patient
4. a practice in which several dentists work together

61. Maintenance of oral health is aided by
    1. excellent technical skills of the dentist
    2. an effective recall system
    3. a plaque control program
    4. all of the above

62. Distortions in communication with dental patients may be caused by
    A. redundancy
    B. language the patient does not understand
    C. fear
    D. a summary of what was said
    E. noises in the environment (such as a drill)
    F. allowing questions
       1. A, D, and E
       2. B, C, and E
       3. C, D, and F
       4. D, E, and F

63. Nonverbal communication in the dental office includes
    1. hand signals
    2. dress
    3. facial expressions
    4. all of the above

64. A method of building cohesiveness among members of the dental team is to
    1. encourage competition
    2. let the staff know they are dispensable
    3. have rewards contingent upon cooperation
    4. not tolerate individual differences

65. Norms are
    1. informal rules of behavior
    2. state laws
    3. ethics
    4. the expected actions of most individuals in a particular situation

66. An effect of cohesiveness among members of the dental team is
    1. increased tension
    2. decreased personnel turnover
    3. greater formality
    4. decreased attention to job requirements

Directions: Each of the questions or incomplete statements below is followed by four suggested answers or completions. In each case, select the answer or completion that is *incorrect*.

67. The prime responsibilities of the business assistant are
    1. appointment scheduling
    2. answering the telephone properly
    3. recalling patients for checkups
    4. keeping the treatment area updated with supplies

68. Included in patient's clinical records are the
    1. examination (clinical) chart and permanent record card
    2. health questionnaire
    3. radiographs
    4. insurance forms

69. A controlled appointment book should contain
    1. the patient's name
    2. the procedure to be performed
    3. the specific amount of time needed for each patient
    4. the charge for that particular visit

70. A clinical record is a vital record in a dental office because it
    1. provides a patient's past and present dental history
    2. protects against malpractice involvement
    3. provides the dentist with information concerning productivity
    4. keeps the dentist informed of the current patient load

71. When taking telephone messages, the business assistant should
    1. be prepared by having pencil and message pad near all phones
    2. take sufficient time to obtain the information
    3. date the message and indicate the time it was received
    4. transmit the message to the doctor immediately

72. Factors to be considered in appointment scheduling include
    1. the emergency patient
    2. management of prime time
    3. young children or elderly patients
    4. the business assistant's lunch time

73. A call list is for
    1. patients who need an appointment

2. patients who have stopped treatment before completion
3. patients who wish to be called if an earlier appointment becomes available
4. friends and neighbors who have mentioned that they would like to be patients

74. Supplies can be divided into the following basic categories
    1. capital items
    2. expendables
    3. nonexpendables
    4. receivables

75. When recalling patients by telephone, it is wise for the caller to
    1. call early in the morning
    2. insist that they commit themselves to a specific appointment time
    3. speak to each patient privately beyond the hearing distance of patients in the office
    4. have the patient's recall record in front of him or her

76. Since the receptionist is the first person to meet new patients, he or she should
    1. greet them as soon as they enter
    2. always be neat in personal appearance
    3. keep the office orderly and presentable
    4. see to it that the chairside assistant immediately prepares a treatment room

77. The most common payment arrangements in a dental office are
    1. advance payments
    2. fixed amount each visit
    3. divided payments
    4. open accounts

78. The value of double-entry bookkeeping is that it
    1. clearly shows both the debit and credit for every office transaction
    2. provides the necessary components to balance books
    3. assists the dentist in determining fees
    4. provides a record if a patient's payment card is lost or misplaced

79. Statements are sent to patients to remind them
    1. that payment is due for treatment in progress
    2. that there is a balance remaining on treatment rendered
    3. of the total cost of dental care when treatment commences
    4. that payment has not been received for a service previously rendered

Answers and Explanations

1. **1** It is important for every dental assistant to be aware of his or her own job description and be capable of fulfilling those specific tasks in the most efficient manner. A dental assistant who is cross-trained also has a working knowledge about the procedures assigned to other assistants and is capable of performing those tasks should it become necessry in time of absence or during a particularly busy period.

2. **3** The duties that can be legally performed by an assistant are determined by the Dental Practice Act of each state. It is the responsibility of a dental assistant to be aware of legal constraints.

3. **1** While a competent business assistant will arrive promptly, refrain from making personal calls and complete all assigned tasks, his or her prime responsibility is to conserve the doctor's time. Since the income of the office is in direct proportion to how thoughtfully time is managed by the business assistant, time and productivity are synonymous.

4. **3** In an effort to conserve the doctor's time and also permit him or her to provide the appropriate attention to the patient in the chair, the business assistant should make every effort to cope with all telephone calls. In those situations wherein it is necessary for the patient to speak to the doctor, the assistant should explain that the doctor will return the call as soon as possibe. It is then the assistant's responsibility to see that this promise is kept.

5. **1** The case presentation is the treatment conference where the dentist explains to the patient the findings of the examination and discusses what treatment procedures are necessary in order to restore the patient's mouth to optimum oral health.

6. **3** The prime personality trait of a good business assistant is being able to remain calm and to complete all tasks of the day systematically.

7. **3** At the completion of a course of treatment, a patient should be informed of the necessity of returning for a checkup at regular intervals designated by the dentist.

8. **2** In a dental office, third party refers to an insurance carrier. All money paid by a particular insurance company is known as third-party payment.

9. **3** Insurance forms, records, x-ray films, study models, etc., that leave the office for any reason should be duplicated in case of loss.

10. **4** While patients have many rights pertaining to professional care, the right to determine the proper course of treatment belongs to the dentist.

11. **3** Advance appointments are the least desirable form of recall because they fill up the appointment book unrealistically. It is difficult to accurately be assured of one's availability six months in the future. Often situations change in patients' lives which prevent them from honoring long-standing appointments. Additionally, many office situations also change (e.g., dentist goes on vacation, to a convention, a continuing education program).

12. **4** Any office that makes arrangements for patients to pay for their dentistry via installments is required by law to provide the patient with a truth-in-lending form. This form indicates whether or not a finance charge will be added if there is a default on payment.

13. **2** All treatment that has been completed and is unpaid is considered an account receivable.

14. **2** It is important that benefits be determined before treatment begins and that the patient be made aware of how much (or little) he or she might receive from the insurance company.

15. **2** The dental office that accepts assignment of benefits must be sure the patient signs that portion of the insurance form that indicates the money should be sent directly to the dentist. This is done before treatment commences.

16. **3** An office manual that is compiled from the direct input of the dentist and the staff is one that is the most likely to be utilized effectively. This occurs because the entire dental team (doctor and auxiliaries) believe in its contents and are also willing to abide by it.

17. **3** A day sheet provides the dentist and office staff with the day's procedures and the length of each appointment.

18. **2** It must be made very clear to all patients that the time scheduled for appointments is specifically reserved for them and that broken appointments are unacceptable behavior.

19. **1** Every office should have a current manual that details all office tasks, policies, and pro-

cedures, in addition to goals, objectives, and philosophy of practice.

20. **3** Changes in a dental office with multiple auxiliary personnel should occur with input from those individuals the change will affect. An excellent technique is to have a staff meeting to resolve potential problems and permit input into decision-making.

21. **4** The interview is the process by which the potential employee (assistant, in this case) meets the employer (dentist or representative) and obtains information such as job description, the office policy on working hours, vacation policy, and probation period.

22. **3** The office manual is an aid that can be used to train new personnel. Its contents typically describe office duties, tray setups, and common procedures.

23. **3** In most private general practices patients are referred by friends or neighbors. Most patients receiving institutional care in hospitals, dental schools, the armed services, and so on, usually are unable to select the person who will deliver their dental care.

24. **2** A contract is a legal agreement between two or more people. Contracts may be explicit (verbal or written) or implicit (implied, not explicitly expressed). Examples of dental contracts are schedule arrangements, payment arrangements, and job duties.

25. **4** Before proceeding with treatment an explicit contract should be made between the office and the patient. It should include cost, payment arrangements, time schedule, risk of treatment, and prognosis.

26. **1** An excellent response when answering the phone is, "This is Dr. Smith's office, Ms. Jones speaking, may I help you?" The most important part of this communication is the identification of the office.

27. **4** Postoperative calls are usually made at the end of the day to patients who have had difficult procedures performed during the day. The rationale for these calls is to show the patients concern, to remind patients of their postoperative responsibilities (e.g., taking medications, rinsing), and to remind them of their next appointment.

28. **4** The receptionist should allow the dentist to resolve patient problems dealing with the patient's dissatisfaction with treatment. Technical explanations are often required, which are the responsibility of the dentist.

29. **2** Fees have many contingencies that cannot be determined over the telephone; therefore, patients seeking fee quotations should be scheduled for an examination.

30. **4** The production of dental services is the main function of the dentist. To maximize the services produced it is necessary to keep delaying factors to a minimum. Delaying factors include most telephone calls and unexpected salespeople.

31. **2** Important reasons for recordkeeping are that it legally avoids possible malpractice involvement, provides an accurate history of treatment success and failure, provides production records, enables others to carry on treatment, and allows future treatment to be based on past performances, such as anesthesia and payment.

32. **3** Patient records are a confidential written history of financial and treatment experiences. These records should not be released or made public without the permission of the patient.

33. **3** The two patient records that are filed as active or inactive are treatment and financial records. The treatment record is placed in an inactive file if the patient is no longer seeking care at the office. The financial record is placed in an inactive file if the account has been fully paid.

34. **2** Ethics is the moral obligation that dictates the standards of conduct expected by the dental profession. The ADAA has a written code of ethics to which the assistant is expected to adhere.

35. **2** The various State Dental Practice Acts determine which duties the dental auxiliary can perform. These laws, as all laws, are subject to change and many have recently been revised to expand the duties of auxiliaries.

36. **3** The dentist is responsible for duties delegated to auxiliaries on his or her dental team. He or she must supervise the performance of these duties and ensure the quality of the final product.

37. **3** The statute of limitations specifies a period of time in which a patient may bring suit against a dentist. This time varies according to many factors, such as the age of the patient and the reason for the suit.

38. **4** A treatment plan is a systematic approach to accomplishing the dental needs of the patient. This plan is made after evaluating the diagnostic materials gathered from and about the patient (e.g., medical and dental histories, radiographs, study models, clinical examination). Elements of a treatment plan include the procedure, the priority of the procedure, who will perform the task, and the amount of time the procedure requires.

39. **1** The appointment book and day sheet should contain the following information: patient's name, time and length of the appointment, and procedures to be performed.

40. **3** One person should control the appointment book at all times; it is usually the receptionist in an office where several auxiliaries are employed.

41. **3** Appointment control will prevent overcrowding, keep hours within desired limits, organize the dentist's production time, assign tasks to the proper individual, and provide patients with definite appointment information.

42. **4** Schedule longer appointments first because it is easier to fill in unused time units with shorter appointments.

43. **3** To ensure the patient will keep an appointment made over the telephone the receptionist should send a written confirmation.

44. **2** The most efficient way to schedule is to have long appointments rather than numerous short appointments. The rationale is that each change of patient requires five to 10 minutes of chair down time. The fewer the changes (by utilizing longer appointments) the less the total down time. A short appointment might be necessary for an extremely apprehensive patient, for medical reasons, or because of the patient's desire.

45. **1** A patient needing a series of visits should be given appointments at the same time and day each week. This pattern helps the patient remember the appointments.

46. **3** Contingencies that cause scheduling problems are lateness, drop in emergencies, unforeseen complications in planned procedures, cancellations, broken appointments, boisterous patients, and patients with emotional problems.

47. **4** Broken appointments should be handled by contacting the patient to find out the reason for the broken appointment and emphasizing the importance of keeping appointments. Repeated disappointments may necessitate dismissing the patient from the office.

48. **3** A cancellation close to the appointed time can be handled by calling a patient who is available on short notice, by extending the visit of the patient who is present before the cancellation, or by moving a patient to be seen late in the day into the time slot.

49. **3** If the dentist is delayed, patients who are waiting should be notified of the delay. The patient's time must be respected if the dental office expects the same in return. If the delay is extensive, the patients should have the right to reschedule their appointments.

50. **2** Overhead is the cost needed to produce dentistry. It includes rent, supplies, and salary.

51. **1** The money paid to the dental practice is its gross income. The gross income less the overhead results in the net income.

52. **3** As accounts receivable age, they decrease in value and become more difficult to collect; therefore, firm payment arrangements are a necessity for a successful practice.

53. **1** Third-party precertification will inform the dentist and patient of the obligation assumed by the third party. The money allocated by the insurance company is usually partial payment and given to the patient or dentist after treatment is completed.

54. **2** Each office has a policy about payment. If a patient has had dental work completed and then denies payment responsibility the dentist will usually contact a collection agency to begin appropriate legal action.

55. **3** A list of equipment and supplies on hand is known as an inventory. One person in the office should be responsible for maintaining the inventory.

56. **1** A running inventory is a system of altering the supply list to know what is present in the office. This list is updated continuously as the supplies are used. This type of system is especially important with disposable supplies.

57. **2** The advantage of purchasing a large quantity of a particular supply at one time is to save money. The drawbacks are the storage space needed and the shelf life of the material, which might expire before the material is used.

58. **2** An invoice is an itemized bill of supplies sent to the dentist. Before paying this bill the invoice should be checked against the supplies received.

59. **2** A back-ordered item is a supply that is currently unavailable and will be shipped when it is available.

60. **4** A group practice is several dentists working together. It may consist of various types of specialists or generalists in any combination.

61. **4** Oral health is maintained by the placement of excellent dental work, an effective plaque control program, and periodic recall visits.

62. **2** Sources of distortion in communications with dental patients may be caused by language the patient does not understand, fear, noises in the environment, and interfering or misleading cues (such as letting a child have a piece of candy as a reward).

63. **4** Nonverbal communication in the dental office includes hand signals, dress, facial expressions, office structure and decor, and body orientation.

64. **3** Methods of building group cohesiveness are: to have staff recognize that practice goals are dependent on cooperation; to build interdependence among staff; and to decrease situations in which one staff member's gain is another's loss.

65. **1** Norms are informal rules of behavior which are important in group functioning. These rules are usually followed because the group members believe they exist and enforce them.

66. **2** Effects of group cohesiveness are decreased personnel turnover and absenteeism, greater attention to the needs of the patient, decreased tension, and increased productivity.

67. **4** The responsibility for keeping the treatment area updated with supplies is usually assumed by the chairside assistant. In most offices he or she is the one in daily touch with the dental needs.

68. **4** In an effort to maintain current knowledge of patient's insurance coverage, most efficient offices keep insurance forms separate from clinical records. However, as a control measure, there is usually a notation in the clinical records noting the patient's insurance status.

69. **4** The fee (or charge) for treatment is usually recorded in an office's bookkeeping system rather than in the appointment book.

70. **4** Clinical records are vital because they pertain to the doctor-patient relationship in terms of treatment. The appointment book keeps the dentist informed of the current patient load.

71. **4** A competent dental assistant should be able to manage most telephone calls without disturbing the doctor. The doctor may request that certain calls be transmitted immediately (e.g., those from family members or colleagues). All others should be noted and given to the doctor when he or she is free to return calls.

72. **4** While it is necessary for the business assistant to have a lunch break, this is not considered a prime factor in appointment scheduling. The patient always comes first.

73. **4** Call lists are usually not used for solicitation of prospective patients, but rather for those who are current patients of record. The primary use of a call list is for those patients who wish to be contacted when an earlier appointment becomes available.

74. **4** Receivables refer to money outstanding for treatment completed.

75. **1** Unless it is specifically indicated on a patient's recall card that he or she can be reached only by telephoning early in the morning, such calls are disturbing and often irritating. Sometimes a patient will be annoyed to the point of not making any appointment.

76. **4** It is not always possible to prepare a treatment room immediately as soon as a patient arrives. However, it is important for the business assistant to alert the doctor and chairside assistant immediately that the patient has arrived.

77. **4** Open accounts are the most difficult ones to collect, since statements on open accounts are usually sent to patients after treatment has been rendered. This gives patients the option of paying at their convenience, which can increase the office's accounts receivable status.

78. **3** Fees are determined by a careful analysis of expenses, (e.g., office overhead). The purpose of a double-entry bookkeeping system is to record income (both collected and outstanding).

79. **3** If a dentist wishes to reinforce the treatment conference (e.g., the case presentation) before treatment commences, a postconsultation letter is sent.

Bibliography

Cooper, T.M. and Di Biaggo, J.A. *Applied Practice Management,* St. Louis: The C. V. Mosby Co., 1979.

Domer, L.R.; Snyder, T.L.; and Heid, D.W. (eds). *Dental Practice Management,* St. Louis: The C. V. Mosby Co., 1980.

Howard, W.W. *Dental Practice Planning,* St. Louis: The C. V. Mosby Co., 1975.

Ladley, B.A. and Patt, J.C. *Office Procedures for the Dental Team,* St. Louis: The C. V. Mosby Co., 1977.

Schwarzrach, S.P. and Jensen, J.R. *Effective Dental Assisting,* 5th ed. Dubuque, Iowa: William C. Brown Co., 1978.

9

First Aid

Course Synopsis

Introduction

Auxiliaries must be ready to support the dentist in the treatment of dental emergencies. It is easy to be prepared for day-to-day routine procedures because of the repetition of certain tasks. However, it is difficult to be continually prepared for the unexpected emergency that can occur in the office. Being prepared for an emergency requires planning in advance for resources, conveniently located equipment, and a staff capable of carrying out the necessary procedures.

Emergency Prevention

The best way to treat an emergency is to prevent its occurrence. This can be done by collecting information about patients' medical and dental histories, which will inform the office of patients' needs and potential emergency situations. These histories must be continuously updated to provide current information.

Office Preparation for an Emergency

In order to prevent tragic results in an emergency situation, the office must follow certain procedures. All auxiliaries should be trained to participate in emergency situations and to simulate such situations so that each role is clearly understood. Emergency telephone numbers should be available and posted in conspicious locations near telephones.

It is particularly important for all personnel to remain calm and to prevent panic. Procedures should be routine, and materials should be readily available and uncomplicated. An emergency kit should be assembled, and each staff member should be familiar with its use. Basic components of this kit should include emergency equipment, noninjectable drugs, and injectable drugs.

The basic emergency equipment includes an oxygen delivery system, a suction system with tips, syringes, tourniquets, and airways.

Noninjectable drugs should include oxygen, a respiratory stimulant (aromatic ammonia), a vasodilator (nitroglycerin), a bronchodilator (epinephrine), and an antihypoglycemic (sugar).

Injectable drugs that can be used include epinephrine for allergic reactions, diazepam as an anticonvulsant, chlorpheniramine as a antihistamine, hydrocortisone succinate as a corticosteroid, and 50% dextrose glucogen as an antihypoglycemic. However, these injectible drugs are administered only by specially trained medical or dental personnel.

Medical Emergencies

Fear and anxiety about dental treatment can aggravate existing medical conditions for some patients. In addition, accidents can occur that necessitate immediate administration of first aid. The most common categories of medical emergencies follow.

Respiratory Emergencies

In a respiratory emergency, a patient's breathing stops or is reduced to a level at which the body cannot support its oxygen needs. Since nerve tissue can easily be injured from loss of oxygen, an interruption of breathing of 4–6 minutes can easily result in permanent damage.

Respiratory failure can occur from obstruction of the airway, hyperventilation, bronchial asthma, heart failure, or acute pulmonary edema. Dental patients are most likely to experience respiratory difficulties from hyperventilation as a result of anxiety. Symptoms include impaired consciousness (loss of consciousness is very rare), lightheadedness, and a feeling of faintness. Breathing may be prolonged, rapid, or deep. Usual treatment is to discontinue dental treatment, make the patient comfortable, and have him or her breathe into a paper bag to correct respiratory alkalosis by increasing the blood level of CO_2.

Bronchial asthma may also cause respiratory difficulty. These attacks may be precipitated by inhalation of materials that produce an allergic reaction or caused by irritating inhalants, infections or emotional upset. Dental treatment should be stopped and a bronchial dilator or oxygen, or both, may be administered.

Heart failure and acute pulmonary edema also can lead to respiratory problems as a result of the body's inability to transport oxygen adequately. Left-sided heart failure leads to pulmonary congestion, while right-sided failure results in vascular congestion. Patients suffering from these diseases should not be treated in a supine position, and, should a problem occur, they should be placed in an upright position and given oxygen while medical assistance is summoned.

In cases of respiratory difficulty, when the heart has stopped beating, artificial respiration should be instituted. Cardiopulmonary resuscitation requires special training and should be attempted only by individuals possessing these skills. The objective of artifical respiration is to maintain an open airway and mechanically breathe for the victim.

The mouth-to-mouth technique is accepted as the most effective method of artificial respiration. The mouth-to-nose method is used in certain cases. Table I lists the steps involved in both techniques.

Table I

Steps in Administering Artificial Respiration

Mouth-to-Mouth

1. Place victim on his or her back on the ground.

2. Kneel perpendicular to the victim's body and next to his or her head.

3. Wipe any foreign matter from the victim's mouth with two fingers.

4. Open airway.

5. Tip the victim's head back until the chin is pointing upward.

6. Place your left ear very close to the victim's mouth and look at the chest. Look, listen, and feel for breathing.

7. If the victim is not breathing, pinch the nostrils with the fingers of the hand on the forehead and place your mouth over the victim's mouth and deliver four quick, full breaths. Do not allow time for the lungs to deflate between breaths.

8. Add a breath every five seconds until help has arrived, the victim begins to breathe, or exhaustion overtakes you.

Mouth-to-Nose

1. Tip the victim's head as for mouth-to-mouth resuscitation.

2. Using the hand supporting the victim's neck, seal the victim's mouth closed.

3. Blow in the nose.

4. Place left ear close to the victim's mouth and observe the chest. Look, listen, and feel for breathing.

5. Continue with steps seven and eight in mouth-to-mouth respiration, adapting appropriately.

If the victim's stomach bulges during the administration of either method of artificial respiration, it is an indication that air is being forced into the stomach. Turn the victim's head to one side and place the palm of the hand on the upper abdomen between the rib margin and the navel. Press downward and upward to force the air out of the stomach. (This may cause some regurgitation.)

Shock

Shock occurs when the body's vital functions reach a depressed state. It can be caused by trauma, infection, heart attack, smoke, burns, poisoning, lack of oxygen, or obstruction or injury to the air passage. Shock can be exacerbated by abnormal changes in the body's temperture, pain, rough handling, and delay in treatment. In some cases it can be life-threatening.

There are two stages of shock. In the early stage the skin is either pale and cold or the individual is weak and exhibits a rapid pulse. Breathing may be shallow or deep and irregular, and nausea, vomiting, or anxiety may occur. In the late stage symptoms become more acute. The person becomes unresponsive and the eyes appear vacant, with dilated pupils. Blood pressure falls and temperature decreases; loss of consciousness or even death can occur.

Treating shock in a dental office requires that those rendering first aid be skilled in the use of a sphygmomanometer, stethoscope, and oxygen delivery system as well as be knowledgeable about the principles of cardiac and respiratory resuscitation. If it is suspected that a patient is in shock, the following steps should be taken: stop dental treatment; record vital signs; place the patient in supine position; keep the patient comfortable at room temperature; maintain airway; provide oxygen; and immediately summon medical assistance.

Some causes of shock for patients during dental treatment are cardiogenic shock from acute heart failure, hematogenic shock from hemorrhage, neurogenic shock from fear and apprehension, anaphylactic shock from severe allergic reaction to a foreign substance, and insulin shock from hypoglycemia.

Cardiovascular Emergency

Congestive heart failure (CHF) is a broad classification of heart problems that result from an inability of the heart to handle the blood supply. CHF results from several cardiovascular problems; patients suffering from this disability usually have trouble lying in a supine position because of fluid retention in the lungs.

Congestive heart failure is usually the first indication of other heart diseases, most importantly coronary heart disease (CHD), which includes three major categories: arteriosclerotic heart disease (ASHD), myocardial infarction (MI), and angina pectoris.

Arteriosclerotic heart disease is a progressive narrowing of the coronary vessels that develops over a number of years. By depriving the heart muscle of the necessary blood supply, damage occurs.

Myocardial infarction is caused by a sudden deficiency of blood to the heart. When dental treatment is given to patients who have previously suffered an MI, fear and anxiety must be diminished. Steps that can be taken include administering nitrous oxide sedation, decreasing the length of appointments (no more than 60 minutes), and, with permission of the patient's physician, administering nitrous oxide analgesia. In general, systemically released epinephrine which is produced by the body as a reaction to anxiety is more dangerous than a properly given anesthetic with 1:100,000 concentration of epinephrine. Dentists treating a patient who has suffered an MI should consult with the attending physician concerning choice of anesthesia.

Angina pectoris is a painful condition resulting from a transient deficiency of the blood supply to the heart. The pain can be caused by exertion or excitement. Nitroglycerin, a fast-acting vasodilator, is given for relief. Consultation with the patient's physician is suggested prior to dental treatment, and each patient should have emergency medication readily available.

Chest pain that may or may not be caused by a cardiac emergency is managed by stopping dental treatment, shifting the patient to a comfortable position, and administering oxygen if necessary. If the pain does not subside, the patient might be suffering from a serious cardiac disorder; medical assistance should be summoned immediately.

If a patient loses consciousness, basic life support techniques should start. This includes placing the patient in a supine position, maintaining the airway, checking the pulse, and administering artificial respiration or oxygen if necessary. If the pulse disappears, cardiopulmonary resuscitation (CPR) should be begun immediately. CPR is a technique that supplements artificial respiration with manual artificial circulation. Special training is required before an individual attempts CPR, and an individual who lacks the required skills may actually cause damage to the patient.

Cerebrovascular Accident

A cerebrovascular accident (CVA or stroke) is a neurological disorder in the brain caused by a vascular insufficiency resulting from hemorrhage or formation of blood clots that interfere with or stop blood flow. Transischemic attacks (TIA) are minor strokes that last for minutes or hours and may include symptoms of headache, confusion, difficulty in speech, dizziness, ringing in the ears, weakness in arms and legs, and personality changes. TIAs may be warnings for major CVAs.

If a patient undergoing dental treatment suffers a TIA, the procedure should be stopped and medical attention should be suggested to the patient. Signs and symptoms of major strokes may include unconsciousness, paralysis or weakness of upper or lower extremities, difficulty in breathing, and a problem with speech. If a patient suffers a major stroke, signs and symptoms should be managed and medical assistance should be summoned immediately. It might be necessary to supply life support, including CPR.

Diabetes Mellitus

Diabetes mellitus is a chronic disease associated with carbohydrate, fat, and protein metabolism. The diabetic patient in the dental office can present several types of emergencies, including those related to the vascular consequences of the disease (MI, angina, and stroke); however, most emergencies will be caused by insulin therapy, resulting in a blood sugar level that is either too high or too low.

Hypoglycemia, a condition resulting from below-normal levels of blood sugar, is characterized by disorientation, cool and moist skin, and excessive hunger. Treatment includes administration of oral carbohydrates such as orange juice or chocolate.

If a patient suffers from hyperglycemia as a result of above-normal levels of blood sugar, he or she may suffer abdominal pain, nausea or vomiting, and intense thirst. The individual's breath might have an acetone odor, and the skin might appear dry and flushed. Medical assistance should be summoned immediately.

Avoidance of an emergency associated with diabetes mellitus can be enhanced by following general rules. Diabetic patients should be treated in the morning and questioned to determine whether diet and insulin therapy is properly coordinated.

Hyperthyroidism

Hyperthyroidism is a disease caused by excessive production of thyroid hormones. In general, patients with this problem have an increased basal metabolic rate that might be manifested in rapid heart rate, sweating, headache, increased blood pressure, and anxiety. In addition, there might be an increase in the possibility of cardiac problems. If these symptoms appear, dental treatment should be stopped, and a medical consultation should be suggested. Additionally, local anesthesia containing epinephrine should never knowingly be given to such patients, since it may intensify the condition.

Epilepsy

Epilepsy is a chronic disease characterized by convulsion-like seizures. These episodes may be mild (petit mal) and symptomized by twitching muscles and momentary disorientation or more severe (grand mal), including symptoms of muscle spasms, thrashing, foaming or drooling at the mouth, rolling eyes, and a loss of consciousness. Management of grand mal seizures includes placing the patient in a supine position, loosening tight clothing, maintaining an open airway, if possible placing a soft object between the teeth, and removing objects that might injure a thrashing patient. Medical assistance might be necessary. It should be remembered that the patient might feel very embarrassed by the incident, and the oral health care delivery team should be supportive of the patient's emotional needs.

Other Emergencies That Can Arise During Dental Treatment

Postural hypotension, also known as orthostatic hypotension, is a common cause of transient unconsciousness in the dental office. This difficulty occurs when the body's nervous system is unable to compensate for changes in blood pressure resulting from changes in the body position. This is most likely to occur when the patient's position is changed too quickly. Factors that contribute to its occurrence are antihypertensive, narcotic, and antiparkinsonian medications; prolonged confinement to a bed; and poor postural reflexes. Treatment includes placing the patient in a supine position, maintaining the airway, administering oxygen if necessary, and slowly changing the patient's position before dismissal.

Fainting is a transient loss of consciousness that can occur during any phase of dental treatment. It is usually a harmless situation, but all loss of consciousness must be regarded as potentially life-threatening. Contributing factors include anxiety, fear, emotional stress, exhaustion, and poor physical condition. The patient should be placed in a supine position with the feet slightly elevated. The airway should be established, and tight clothing should be loosened. Spirits of ammonia and oxygen may also be administered.

Simple bleeding can occur as a result of certain dental procedures. Careful medical histories should be elicited so the doctor can be aware of any conditions that might predispose a patient to prolonged bleeding. There are three sources of bleeding: arterial bleeding, when the blood is bright red and spurting; venous bleeding, when the blood is darker and flows continuously; and capillary bleeding, when the blood is bright red and flows slowly and steadily. Most bleeding can be controlled by isolating the area and applying pressure as directly as possible. The patient should be watched carefully for signs of shock. If bleeding does not subside with pressure, the area should be anesthetized in preparation for further treatment. If the bleeding is of capillary origin, sponges impregnated with epinephrine hydrochloride (1:1000) or absorbable gelatin sponges can be packed in the bleeding site. Closing the wound tightly with sutures can also stop the bleeding.

Complications may also arise from local anesthesia. Allergic reactions have decreased dramatically with the introduction of amide anesthesia. (The traditional anesthesia is of the ester type.) Some reactions do occur, however, and may range from a simple dermatitis to fatal anaphylactic shock. Often these reactions occur in response to preservatives or other ingredients in the anesthestic solution. The most common reaction from local anesthesia is tachycardia caused by an exogenous release of epinephrine. Dental treatment should be stopped, and the patient should be made comfortable in a supine position until symptoms subside.

An overdose of anesthesia can cause convulsive reactions or even death. Factors that can affect the dosage are age (younger and older patients are more sensitive), low body weight, impaired liver and kidney function, or a metabolic disorder. Since an overdose of anesthesia is preventable, it is incumbent upon the dentist to evaluate each patient for correct dosage. If the patient has a reaction to the anesthestic, dental treatment should be stopped, basic life support steps should be undertaken, and medical assistance should be summoned if needed.

Eye injuries can also occur during dental treatment. The dentist and auxiliaries are especially susceptible to these injuries and should wear safety glasses to prevent damage from flying objects. If an eye injury should occur, the area should not be rubbed. Additionally, no one should attempt to remove an object by inserting an instrument, but skilled medical assistance should be obtained.

Choking, while not common during dental treatment, may occur from aspirated filling or impression materials or dental prostheses. The patient should be placed in a comfortable position and encouraged to cough in order to remove the obstruction. If the patient is in severe distress, four sharp blows should be delivered between the victim's shoulder blades and followed by four upward abdominal thrusts. If the choking is not relieved by these measures, medical assistance should be sought immediately. If breathing stops, basic life support measures must be started.

Burns from open flames or hot materials can also occur in the dental office either to the patient or to a member of the dental team. Cold water or cold compresses should be applied. If a dressing is necessary, only dry sterile cloth should be used; ointments or salves should not be applied.

Medications are named by one of two broad classes: (1) brand names given by a manufacturer and protected by a trademark and (2) generic names, which reflect the product's chemical composition.

A prescription is a written order to a pharmacist directing him or her to dispense a certain drug with specific instructions to a patient. The dentist is the only member of the oral health care delivery team who is legally allowed to prescribe drugs. Commonly used drugs in dentistry include antibiotics, analgesics, and hyponotics.

Antibiotics are organic substances that destroy or inhibit the growth of bacteria. These drugs are used to prevent or alleviate bacterial infections and prophylactically prevent them. Common antibiotics used in dentistry include penicillin, tetracycline, and sulfonamides. For example, they are given to patients in whom cellulitis or an abscess develops. In addition, antibiotics are prophylactically prescribed for patients who have certain chronic diseases in order to prevent postoperative complications.

Analgesics are administered to relieve pain. Mild analgesics include aspirin and acetaminophen. More potent analgesics are available only by prescription and include codeine, opiate, and synthetic opiate compounds. These drugs are sometimes prescribed for patients who have experienced painful procedures such as extraction.

Hypnotic and antianxiety drugs are used to control anxiety. Low doses of hypnotic drugs are considered sedatives. These drugs, rarely prescribed in dentistry, act to depress the central nervous system, facilitating the reduction of anxiety.

The interaction of one drug with another might result in a deleterious effect on the patient. It is particularly important for an auxiliary who has taken a medical history to alert the doctor if the patient is currently taking medication in order to prevent future problems with additionally prescribed medications. For example, aspirin should not be prescribed for a patient taking an anticoagulant drug, because these two drugs enhance each other's effect, and the patient could develop difficulties controlling bleeding as a result.

Question Section

Directions: Each of the questions or incomplete statements below is followed by four suggested answers or completions. Select the BEST answer in each case.

1. Knowledge of the patient's medical and dental history might affect
   1. the treatment plan
   2. the drugs prescribed
   3. the frequency of appointments
   4. all of the above

2. When treating a patient with a history of rheumatic fever, the patient should
   1. be prophylactically given antibiotics
   2. be treated with the operator wearing gloves
   3. be treated without any special precautions
   4. never be placed in a supine position

3. The definition of first aid is
   1. the immediate and temporary care given the victims of an accident until the services of a physician can be obtained
   2. the temporary care given the victim of an accident or sudden illness
   3. the immediate care given to a person who has been injured or has been suddenly taken ill
   4. the care and treatment given to a victim of an accident or sudden illness

4. Symptoms of inflammation are
   A. swelling
   B. pain
   C. hypoventilation
   D. redness
   E. heat
   F. hyperventilation
      1. A, C, D, and E
      2. A, B, D, and E
      3. B, D, E, and F
      4. C, D, E, and F

5. Acute symptoms are
   1. severe, with quick onset
   2. dull and steady
   3. of long duration
   4. somniferous

6. Chronic symptoms are
   1. of short duration
   2. sharp and quick
   3. of long duration
   4. extremely painful

7. Chronic respiratory problems affect the
   1. type of prosthesis a patient can wear
   2. prognosis of root canal therapy
   3. positioning of the patient
   4. design of cavity preparation

8. Breathing air containing insufficient oxygen, carbon monoxide, or other toxic gases may cause

1. acute asthma
2. asphyxia
3. circulatory collapse
4. inhalation collapse

9. If you are a lone rescuer with a victim with no pulse and no breathing, which of the following would you use in CPR techniques?
   1. one breath for 10 compressions; 40 compressions per minute
   2. two breaths for 15 compressions; 50 compressions per minute
   3. one breath for 5 compressions; 60 compressions per minute
   4. two breaths for 15 compressions; 80 compressions per minute

10. Proper preparation of a victim for artificial respiration is
    1. wipe foreign matter from mouth and tilt head backward with chin pointing upward
    2. wipe foreign matter from mouth and tilt head backward with chin pointing upward. Put one hand under victim's neck and lift; place heel of other hand on forehead and rotate backward. Pinch nostrils shut and seal your mouth tightly around the victim's mouth
    3. tilt head backward with chin pointing upward, put one hand under victim's neck, and lift. Place heel of other hand on forehead and rotate backward. Pinch nostrils shut and seal your mouth tightly around the victim's mouth.
    4. wipe foreign matter from mouth and tilt head forward with chin pointing downward. Put one hand under victim's neck and lift. Place heel of other hand on forehead and rotate backward. Pinch nostrils shut and seal your mouth tightly around victim's mouth.

11. Insulin shock is due to
    1. too much blood sugar
    2. too much insulin in the blood
    3. too little insulin in the blood
    4. all of the above

12. A method used for removing swallowed objects on which a victim is choking is the
    1. Silvester method
    2. Herman method
    3. Albin method
    4. Heimlich maneuver

13. A patient taking anticoagulation medication could pose a problem related to
    1. the length of the appointment

2. control of hemorrhage
3. stress and anxiety of the dental situation
4. all of the above

14. An administration of an excess amount of a drug is known as
    1. an overdose
    2. an overkill
    3. hyperactivation
    4. hypokinesis

15. When treating for shock, the body position is
    1. head lower than the rest of the body
    2. based on the injury
    3. head and shoulders raised 8–12 inches
    4. flat with head turned to the side

16. A reason for first aid training is to
    1. prevent accidents
    2. eliminate the need for a physician in emergency situations
    3. avoid contagious diseases
    4. increase the patient's dental IQ

17. The depressed state of many body functions is called
    1. shock
    2. depression
    3. psychosis
    4. mental retardation

18. The condition of the skin when a patient is in shock is
    A. pale
    B. red
    C. warm
    D. cold
    E. moist
       1. A, C, and E
       2. A, D, and E
       3. B, C, and E
       4. B and D

19. The first aid measures for a person in shock in the dental office are
    A. administer stimulants
    B. maintain a comfortable temperature
    C. keep the patient lying down
    D. be encouraging to the patient
    E. keep the patient moving
       1. A, B, and C
       2. A, C, and D
       3. B, C, and D
       4. B, D, and E

20. Sharp cuts bleeding freely are
    1. abrasions
    2. incisions
    3. lacerations
    4. punctures

21. Wounds that are jagged, irregular, and associated with considerable tissue damage are
    1. abrasions
    2. incisions
    3. lacerations
    4. punctures

22. The first aid measure for a deep incision in a finger is to
    1. allow the finger to bleed freely
    2. place the finger in warm water
    3. place ice over the gash
    4. apply direct pressure over the incision

23. The proper sequence in an emergency is
    1. treat for shock, control severe bleeding, restore breathing
    2. restore breathing, treat for shock, control severe bleeding
    3. restore breathing, control severe bleeding, treat for shock
    4. control severe bleeding, restore breathing, treat for shock

24. To prevent foreign objects, such as amalgam, from flying in the eyes, the dentist and assistant should
    1. blink frequently
    2. turn away from foreign objects when working on them
    3. wear safety glasses
    4. work under water

25. If a foreign object is embedded in a person's eye
    1. rub the eye with the back of the hand
    2. attempt to remove the object with a tweezer
    3. irrigate the eye with tap water
    4. seek medical attention

26. To avoid injuries to teeth while playing contact sports, athletes should
    1. keep their mouths closed
    2. chew gum
    3. have fluoride treatments before each game
    4. wear mouth guards

27. If a permanent central incisor is accidently evulsed, what is the treatment?
    1. throw the tooth away
    2. prompt reinsertion of the tooth
    3. extract the tooth adjacent
    4. render no treatment

28. Syncope refers to
    1. a sudden state of excitement
    2. a lack of blood to the brain
    3. dizziness after an injection
    4. high blood pressure

29. Some causes of syncope in the dental office are
    A. fear
    B. hyperglycemia
    C. seeing blood
    D. smoking
       1. A, B, and D
       2. A and C
       3. B, D, and E
       4. D and E

30. If a patient faints, the assistant should
    1. seat the patient upright
    2. place the patient's head lower than the rest of the body
    3. hold the patient's head in his or her lap
    4. slap the patient's face sharply

31. Inhalation of spirits of ammonia is used in
    1. insulin shock
    2. respiratory collapse
    3. circulatory collapse
    4. syncope

32. If circulatory collapse occurs, the patient should be
    1. given a drink of warm water
    2. left alone
    3. given external cardiac massage
    4. seated upright

33. An antidote
    1. counteracts the effects of a poison
    2. is a form of artificial respiration
    3. is a central nervous system stimulant
    4. all of the above

34. Some symptoms of an allergic reaction are
    A. numbness of extremities
    B. itching
    C. excessive salivation
    D. rash
    E. swelling
       1. A, B, and C
       2. B, C, and D
       3. B, D, and E
       4. A, C, and E

35. Anaphylactic shock is
    1. preceded by hysterical laughter
    2. the result of aspirating a foreign object
    3. a sudden violent allergic reaction
    4. a reaction to mental depression

36. The drug that best counteracts anaphylactic shock is
    1. Novocaine
    2. Xylocaine
    3. epinephrine
    4. a barbiturate

37. Angina pectoris is
    1. an embolism in the brain
    2. a painful condition of the heart
    3. cancer of the heart
    4. a spasm of a chest muscle

38. The drug given to alleviate an attack of angina pectoris is
    1. epinephrine
    2. Lidocaine
    3. nitroglycerin
    4. alcohol

39. To reduce the possibility of injury during an epileptic seizure, the operator or assistant should
    1. hold the patient's tongue between the thumb and forefinger
    2. place padded tongue depressors between the patient's teeth
    3. attempt to hold the patient absolutely still
    4. seat the patient in a straight-back chair

40. If a patient begins to have convulsions in the waiting room, the operator or assistant should
    1. place his or her hand on the patient's mouth
    2. tie the patient's hands together
    3. administer stimulants orally
    4. protect the patient from injury by moving objects out of reach

41. A patient walking to the operatory suddenly keels over; there is no pulse or breathing. What should be done?
    1. cover the patient
    2. do not treat until help arrives
    3. keep the patient's head below his or her feet
    4. summon help and begin artificial respiration and external cardiac massage

42. A partial denture becomes lodged in a patient's throat. The proper first aid measure is to
    1. give the patient a glass of milk
    2. allow the patient to cough out the object
    3. attempt to quiet the patient
    4. ask the patient to jump up and down

43. Hot compound drips on the operator's finger. What is the first aid treatment?
    1. wash the area with soap and warm water
    2. place the finger in cold water
    3. ignore the injury
    4. gently peel away the injured skin

44. Etching acid accidently contacts the assistant's hand. What is the first aid treatment?
    1. wave the hand in the air
    2. blow air on the area
    3. wash the area thoroughly
    4. hold the hand high in the air

Answers and Explanations

1. **4** A patient's medical and dental history can affect all phases of a patient's treatment, including appointments and prescriptions.

2. **1** Patients who have a history of rheumatic fever must be protected against bacterial infections which could lead to further heart complications by prophylactically prescribed antibiotics.

3. **3** First aid is the immediate care given to a person who has been injured or has been suddenly taken ill.

4. **2** The symptoms of inflammation are pain, swelling, redness, and heat.

5. **1** Acute symptoms are those that are severe and occur with a quick onset.

6. **3** Chronic symptoms are characterized by their long duration.

7. **3** Patients with chronic respiratory problems must be positioned in such a manner that may facilitate the breathing process and comfort. In many cases, these patients cannot be placed in a supine position.

8. **2** Asphyxia, or suffication, may occur when the air does not contain sufficient oxygen to support the respiratory process.

9. **2** A lone rescuer should give two breaths for each 15 compressions at the rate of approximately 50 compressions per minute.

10. **2** Clearing foreign matter from the mouth; tilting the head backward with chin pointing up; putting one hand behind the victim's neck to lift it and rotating the forehead backward maintains an open airway. Pinching the nostrils shut and sealing the victims's mouth maximizes the air supply.

11. **2** Insulin shock results from excess insulin in the blood and can be counteracted by eating a high-sugar-content food.

12. **4** The Heimlich maneuver includes placing the victim in a forward-bending position, standing behind him or her, and placing arms around the victim's waist. A fist is made and placed one hand's length above the patient's navel. The rescuer makes quick inward and upward thrusts, forcing air through the trachea to dislodge trapped particles.

13. **2** Patients taking anticoagulation medication must be watched for bleeding problems, because this medication diminishes the ability of the blood to clot.

14. **1** An overdose is the term used to identify administeration of an excess amount of a drug.

15. **1** When treating a patient for shock, the victim's feet should be raised 8–12 inches above the rest of the body to increase blood circulation in the head.

16. **1** Some reasons for first aid training are to promote prevention of accidents, provide emergency care, and prevent additional injury due to improper care.

17. **1** The depressed state of many body functions is called shock. The severity of shock depends on the cause. Some forms of shock are neurogenic, insulin, and anaphylactic.

18. **2** The condition of the skin when a patient is in shock is pale, cold, and moist.

19. **3** First aid measures for a person in shock in a dental office are to maintain a comfortable temperature, keep the patient lying down, be encouraging to the patient, loosen any tight clothing, and call the patient's physician.

20. **2** Incised wounds are caused by sharp objects. The amount of bleeding depends on their depths and the tissues that are cut.

21. **3** Lacerated wounds are jagged and irregular. They are associated with considerable tissue damage and with free bleeding if blood vessels are severed.

22. **4** The first aid measures for a deep incision in a finger are to apply direct pressure over the incision, elevate the arm, and apply pressure to the brachial artery if bleeding does not stop.

23. **4** The proper sequence in an emergency situation is to control bleeding, restore breathing, and treat for shock.

24. **3** To prevent foreign objects from flying into a person's eye, the best precaution is to wear safety glasses.

25. **4** If a foreign object is embedded in a person's eye, an eye patch should be placed over both eyes and medical attention sought. Attempting to remove an embedded foreign body may result in further irritation and damage.

26. **4** To avoid injuries to teeth while participating in contact sports, athletes should wear mouth guards. Mouth guards are usually made of flexible materials that will absorb some of the impact of a traumatic blow.

27. **2** The treatment for an accidently evulsed central incisor is to rinse the tooth in lukewarm water, reinsert it as soon as possible, and stabilize the reinserted tooth.

28. **2** Syncope refers to the lack of blood to the brain for a short period. This is caused by dilation of blood vessels in the body and results in loss of consciousness.

29. **2** Some causes of syncope in the dental office are fear, visual disturbances (such as seeing blood or a needle), pain, and the injection of local anesthesia directly into a blood vessel.

30. **2** The treatment for syncope is to place the head lower than the rest of the body, administer aromatic ammonia inhalant, loosen tight clothing, administer oxygen, and give reassurance.

31. **4** Inhalation of spirits of ammonia is used as a reflex stimulant which causes a patient to regain consciousness after fainting. It is stored in individual vials that are broken at the time of use.

32. **3** If circulatory collapse occurs, the patient should be given external cardiac massage. This procedure artificially continues the circulation until the patient's heartbeat has been restored or until medical help arrives.

33. **1** An antidote counteracts the effect of a toxic drug.

34. **3** Some symptoms of an allergic reaction are itching, rash, swelling, hives, and breathing difficulties.

35. **3** Anaphylactic shock is a sudden violent allergic reaction. Two drugs used in dentistry that may cause this reaction are local anesthesia and penicillin. A detailed accurate medical history of past adverse drug reactions could indicate whether a drug could cause this reaction.

36. **3** The drug that best counteracts anaphylactic shock is epinephrine. 0.5 ml of 1:1000 epinephrine is injected subcutaneously for this purpose.

37. **2** Angina pectoris is a painful condition of the heart caused by a lack of blood to the heart muscles. Patients who have this condition should be treated with techniques that decrease anxiety, pain, and other stressful situations that may promote an attack.

38. **3** The drug of choice when treating patients suffering from angina pectoris is nitroglycerin. The method of administration is placing a tablet under the patient's tongue (sublingual). The drug acts as a vasodilator, allowing increased blood supply to the cardiac tissue.

39. **2** The first aid measures that should be rendered to a patient during an epileptic seizure are moving objects away from the patient, placing padded tongue depressors between the patient's teeth, loosening the patient's clothing, supporting the patient's breathing if necessary, allowing the patient to rest, and reassuring the patient.

40. **4** If a patient begins to have convulsions in the waiting room, the operator or assistant should protect the patient from injury by moving objects out of his or her reach.

41. **4** If a patient suddenly keels over with no pulse or breathing, summon help immediately, support respiration by mouth-to-mouth resuscitation, and support circulation with external cardiac massage.

42. **2** If a foreign object, such as a denture, becomes lodged in a patient's throat, allow the patient to cough the object out first. If this is not successful, use the Heimlich maneuver and begin artificial respiration. If there is complete obstruction, attempt to remove the object physically. If the patient loses consciousness and cannot breath, a tracheotomy is the last resort.

43. **2** Hot compound contacting a finger causes a first-degree burn. The treatment is to immerse the finger in cold water and dress the wound, if necessary.

44. **3** Chemicals used to etch the enamel of teeth are strong acids. If they contact the skin they will cause a chemical burn. The treatment is to wash the area thoroughly for several minutes and to dress the wound.

Bibliography

American Red Cross. *Advanced First Aid and Emergency Care,* 2nd ed. New York: Doubleday and Co., Inc., 1980.

American Red Cross. *Standard First Aid and Personal Safety,* 2nd ed. New York: Doubleday and Co., Inc., 1979.

Malamed, S.F. *Handbook of Medical Emergencies in the Dental Office,* 2nd ed. St. Louis: The C. V. Mosby Co., 1982.

McCarthy, F.M. *Emergencies in Dental Practice; Prevention and Treatment,* 3rd ed. Philadelphia: W. B. Saunders Co., 1979.

Soltero, D.J. and Whitacre, R.J. *Vital Signs,* Seattle: Instructional Services, 1978.